D1348502

TREATMENT OF THE HOSPITALIZED CYSTIC FIBROSIS PATIENT

LUNG BIOLOGY IN HEALTH AND DISEASE

Executive Editor

Claude Lenfant
Director, National Heart, Lung and Blood Institute
National Institutes of Health
Bethesda, Maryland

ADDITIONAL VOLUMES IN PREPARATION

Asthma and Immunological Diseases in Pregnancy and Early Infancy, *edited by Michael Schatz, Robert S. Zeiger, and Henry Claman*

Dyspnea, *edited by Donald A. Mahler*

Inflammatory Mechanisms in Asthma, *edited by Stephen T. Holgate and William W. Busse*

Self-Management of Asthma, *edited by Harry Kotses and Andrew Harver*

Physiological Basis of Ventilatory Support, *edited by John J. Marini and Arthur S. Slutsky*

Proinflammatory and Antiinflammatory Peptides, *edited by Sami L. Said*

Biology of Lung Cancer, *edited by Madeleine A. Kane and Paul Bunn, Jr.*

Eicosanoids, Aspirin, and Asthma, *edited by Andrew Szczeklik, Ryszard Gryglewski, and John R. Vane*

Pulmonary Edema, *edited by Michael A. Matthay and David H. Ingbar*

The opinions expressed in these volumes do not necessarily represent the views of the National Institutes of Health.

TREATMENT OF THE HOSPITALIZED CYSTIC FIBROSIS PATIENT

Edited by

David M. Orenstein

*University of Pittsburgh School of Medicine
and Children's Hospital of Pittsburgh
Pittsburgh, Pennsylvania*

Robert C. Stern

*Case Western Reserve University School of Medicine
and Rainbow Babies and Children's Hospital
Cleveland, Ohio*

MARCEL DEKKER, INC.   NEW YORK · BASEL · HONG KONG

ISBN: 0-8247-9500-8

The publisher offers discounts on this book when ordered in bulk quantities. For more information, write to Special Sales/Professional Marketing at the address below.

This book is printed on acid-free paper.

Marcel Dekker, Inc.
270 Madison Avenue, New York, New York 10016

Currrent printing (last digit):
10 9 8 7 6 5 4 3 2 1

PRINTED IN THE UNITED STATES OF AMERICA

INTRODUCTION

Cystic fibrosis is one of the diseases that point to the wonders of molecular genetics and its application. The discovery of the cystic fibrosis gene in the mid-1980s and the ensuing attempt to apply gene replacement or gene therapy in cystic fibrosis patients sent a wave of hope through the scientific community and among the patients and their families. However, this hope has now been tempered by the realization that although the potential of genetic approaches remains enormous, their application is still distant as more basic research work remains to be done. Unquestionably, our enthusiasm for gene therapy of cystic fibrosis must be as high as the caution with which we should approach it and promulgate it among the patients.

And so, the question today is "Where does this leave the patient's hope for a better and longer life?" Much progress has been made during the last decade as a result of the convergence of several factors: a better understanding of the pathogenesis of this disease, the enthusiasm of the scientific and clinical community for further and continued investigation, and, not least, a public expression of support for research. As a result, patients who would have died in their teens or shortly thereafter are now living a good life for several decades.

Nevertheless, many of these cystic fibrosis patients see their normal life interrupted frequently by hospitalization, which often requires highly specialized and intensive care. That is the subject of this book.

Volume 64 of this series was titled *Cystic Fibrosis*. Its editor, Dr. Pamela B. Davis, ended her Preface to the book with the following sentence: "It is devoutly to be hoped that cystic fibrosis can soon be relegated to an item of historical interest in the annals of the advances of medicine. Such a day cannot come soon enough for the patients and their families." That day is on the horizon, and this new contribution to the Lung Biology in Health and Disease series is one vehicle that moves us closer to it.

Practitioners, patients, and their families will be the beneficiaries of this scholarly volume which addresses such an important subject, treatment of the hospitalized cystic fibrosis patient. As the executive editor, I am grateful to the editors and authors for this contribution and for the opportunity to include it in this series.

Claude Lenfant, M.D.
Bethesda, Maryland

PREFACE

Cystic fibrosis is a generalized exocrinopathy, affecting most organs with epithelial surfaces, especially the tracheobronchial tree, pancreas, intestines, liver, and reproductive tract. It is the most common life-shortening disease of whites (incidence 1 in 2500 live births). The CF gene, termed the cystic fibrosis transmembrane regulator (CFTR), is located on chromosome 7. The CFTR protein normally plays a key role in the regulation and transport of chloride and sodium. In CF, the abnormal protein results in impaired chloride transport at the lumenal surface and increased sodium transport in the opposite direction. Although alternative, calcium-dependent chloride channels exist, they are not used under most conditions. The abnormality in sodium and chloride transport accounts for the abnormal transepithelial bioelectric potential difference and the long-recognized dehydration of lumenal secretions. Although these abnormalities allow a reasonably acceptable pathophysiological explanation of gastrointestinal, pancreatic, hepatic, and reproductive manifestations of the disease, a complete understanding of the respiratory problems (e.g., the high incidence of infection with *Pseudomonas aeruginosa*) is not yet available. Definitive medical treatment, if it is possible, awaits further elucidation of pathophysiology.

The estimated 30,000 cystic fibrosis patients in the United States account for many hospital days. Thirty percent of them are hospitalized 1–3 times and

4% are hospitalized 4–20 times in a given year; the mean duration of these hospitalizations is 11 days. Clinicians have gradually developed relatively successful treatment approaches to many of the serious complications of the disease, and this no doubt contributed to the improved prognosis for these patients. However, the dissemination of this information has been largely by rumor.

With the help of many experienced clinician contributors, we have gathered information on indications for hospitalization, continued hospital stay, general principles that apply to inpatient treatment of these patients, and optimal treatment for specific problems. Whenever possible, we have cited objective data for these recommendations, but when no such data exist, we have not shied away from making recommendations anyway. Of necessity, there is some overlap between inpatient and outpatient care; we have tried to include all aspects of care needed for inpatient management.

The care of these patients is complex and may involve input from many consultants. However, we think it is especially important that each patient have a primary CF physician who is overseeing all aspects of care. This primary CF physician gains the trust and understanding of the patient and family over many years and is most likely to see the forest of an overall plan through the individual trees of specific components of its treatment.

This book is intended primarily to help physicians who take care of hospitalized CF patients, but we hope it will also be useful to medical students, physicians in postgraduate training programs, nurses, respiratory therapists, and other health professionals.

Robert C. Stern, M.D.
David M. Orenstein, M.D.

CONTRIBUTORS

Thomas F. Boat, M.D. Department of Pediatrics, University of Cincinnati College of Medicine, and Director, Research Foundation, Children's Hospital Medical Center, Cincinnati, Ohio

Drucy Borowitz, M.D. Associate Professor of Clinical Pediatrics, Department of Pediatrics, State University of New York at Buffalo, and Acting Chief, Pediatric Pulmonology, The Children's Hospital of Buffalo, Buffalo, New York

Christine Coburn-Miller, M.S.R.D. Registered Dietician, Cystic Fibrosis Center, The Children's Hospital of Buffalo, Buffalo, New York

Pamela B. Davis, M.D., Ph.D. Professor of Pediatrics, Department of Pediatrics, and Chief, Pediatric Pulmonology, Case Western Reserve University School of Medicine, Rainbow Babies and Childrens Hospital, Cleveland, Ohio

Thomas M. Egan, M.D., M.Sc. Associate Professor of Surgery and Associate Division Chief for General Thoracic Surgery, Department of Surgery, University of North Carolina School of Medicine, Chapel Hill, North Carolina

Howard Eigen, M.D. Professor of Pediatrics, Asssociate Chairman for Clinical Affairs, Director, Section of Pulmonary and Intensive Care, Department of

Pediatrics, Indiana University School of Medicine, and James Whitcomb Riley Hospital for Children, Indianapolis, Indiana

Bartley P. Griffith, M.D.   Henry T. Bahnson Professor of Surgery, and Chief, Division of Cardiothoracic Surgery, Department of Surgery, University of Pittsburgh School of Medicine, University of Pittsburgh Medical Center, and Presbyterian University Hospital, Pittsburgh, Pennsylvania

Geoffrey Kurland, M.D.   Associate Professor of Pediatrics, Department of Pediatrics, University of Pittsburgh School of Medicine, and Children's Hospital of Pittsburgh, Pittsburgh, Pennsylvania

Blakeslee E. Noyes, M.D.   Assistant Professor of Pediatrics, Department of Pediatrics, St. Louis University School of Medicine, and Director, Pulmonary Medicine, Cardinal Glennon Children's Hospital, St. Louis, Missouri

David M. Orenstein, M.D.   Professor of Pediatrics, Department of Pediatrics, University of Pittsburgh School of Medicine, and Director, Cystic Fibrosis Center and Pulmonary Division, Children's Hospital of Pittsburgh, Pittsburgh, Pennsylvania

Michael D. Reed, Pharm.D., F.C.C.P., F.C.P.   Professor of Pediatrics, Case Western Reserve University School of Medicine, and Director, Pediatric Clinical Pharmacology/Toxicology, Rainbow Babies and Childrens Hospital, Cleveland, Ohio

Frederick J. Rescorla, M.D.   Associate Professor of Surgery, Department of Pediatric Surgery, Indiana University School of Medicine, and James Whitcomb Riley Hospital for Children, Indianapolis, Indiana

Beryl J. Rosenstein, M.D.   Professor of Pediatrics, Director, Johns Hopkins University School of Medicine, and Director, Cystic Fibrosis Center, Johns Hopkins Hospital, Baltimore, Maryland

Robert J. Rothbaum, M.D.   Associate Professor of Pediatrics, Division of Pediatric Gastroenterology and Nutrition, Department of Pediatrics, Washington University School of Medicine, and St. Louis Children's Hospital, St. Louis, Missouri

Michael Spino, Pharm.D.   Apotex, Inc., Weston, Ontario, Canada, and Professor, Faculty of Pharmacy, University of Toronto, and Hospital for Sick Children, Toronto, Ontario, Canada

Robert C. Stern, M.D.   Professor of Pediatrics, Department of Pediatrics, Case Western Reserve University School of Medicine, Cleveland, Ohio

John C. Stevens, M.D.   Clinical Associate Professor of Pediatrics, Pulmonology Section, Department of Pediatrics, Indiana University School of

Medicine, and James Whitcomb Riley Hospital for Children, Indianapolis, Indiana

William B. Zipf, M.D. Professor and Director of Pediatric Endocrinology, Department of Pediatrics, The Ohio State University, and Children's Hospital, Columbus, Ohio

CONTENTS

1

Making and Confirming the Diagnosis

BERYL J. ROSENSTEIN

Johns Hopkins University School of Medicine
and Johns Hopkins Hospital
Baltimore, Maryland

I. Introduction

The incidence of cystic fibrosis (CF) in the United States is 1 in 2750 live births. Although it occurs most frequently in whites, the diagnosis needs to be considered in patients of diverse racial and ethnic backgrounds; 3.1% of patients in the United States Cystic Fibrosis Foundation Data Registry are black (1). There are certain population groups and geographic areas in which there is an unusually high frequency of CF, probably related to random genetic drift and founder effect. These include Northern Ireland (1:1700), parts of Brittany (1:377), American Amish (1:640 to 1:1200), and southwest Africa (1:1192) (2).

Although CF is a well-characterized genetic disorder, it remains a clinical diagnosis based on the phenotypic (clinical) features of the patient with confirmation by demonstration of an elevated concentration of electrolytes in the sweat. The disease is marked by great variability in the frequency and severity of clinical manifestations and complications. CF should never be "ruled out" because a patient with suspicious clinical findings appears "too healthy." In most cases, the diagnosis should be established before age 1 year, usually within the first several months of life (Fig. 1). Approximately 10% of CF patients have relatively intact exocrine pancreatic function, however, and this subset of

1

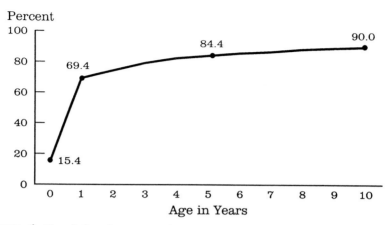

Figure 1 Cumulative frequency of age-at-diagnosis among newly diagnosed CF patients, 1993; 15.4% of patients were diagnosed prenatally, or in the newborn period, and 69.4% by age 1 year. (Courtesy of the Cystic Fibrosis Foundation, Bethesda, MD.)

patients is characterized by milder clinical course, better nutritional status, better pulmonary function, and, consequently, a distinctly later age at diagnosis compared with patients with pancreatic insufficiency (3,4). Although genotype is predictive of pancreatic function status (4,5), for most CF alleles, no such correlation has been established for pulmonary outcome (6,7).

The frequency of common presenting manifestations among patients reported to the United States Cystic Fibrosis Foundation Data Registry is listed in Table 1. In most cases, the family history is negative for CF.

II. Clinical Presentations by Age Group

A. Prenatal

High-Risk Pregnancies

The prenatal diagnosis of CF is usually established in pregnancies that are known to be at increased risk based on the CF carrier status of the parents (8). When the genotype status of the parents is known, or when the parents are "informative" for restriction fragment length polymorphisms (RFLPs) known to be associated with the CF gene, the diagnosis of CF can be confirmed or excluded with a very high degree of sensitivity and specificity by direct muta- tion analysis (9) or DNA linkage analysis (10) performed on fetal cells obtained by chorionic villus sampling (10 weeks' gestation) or cultured amniotic fluid cells (15 to 18 weeks' gestation). In pregnancies at increased risk but in which the genotype status of one or both parents is unknown, or when the parents are

Table 1 Characteristics at Diagnosis in Newly Diagnosed Patients

CF Diagnosis Suggested by:	Percent
Acute/persistent respiratory symptoms	45.1
Failure to thrive/malnutrition	35.9
Steatorrhea/malabsorption	26.7
Meconium ileus/intestinal obstruction	17.7
Family history of CF	16.9
Electrolyte imbalance	6.2
Neonatal screening	4.5
Genotype	3.4
Rectal prolapse	2.9
Nasal polyps/sinus disease	2.9
Prenatal diagnosis (CVS, amnio)	1.8
Liver problems	0.7

Source: Courtesy of the Cystic Fibrosis Foundation, Bethesda, Maryland.

not informative for RFLPs, analysis of amniotic fluid (16 to 18 weeks' gestation) for concentrations of microvillar intestinal enzymes (11,12), and linkage disequilibrium analysis (13) can be helpful. If the fetus is affected by CF, there is a reduced concentration of leucine aminopeptidase, alkaline phosphatase, gamma-glutamyl transpeptidase, and disaccharidases in the amniotic fluid, presumably secondary to in utero intestinal blockage secondary to viscous meconium. The accuracy of these assays is in the range of 95%–98% (false-positive rate 1%–4%; false-negative rate 6%–8%) when performed on a pregnancy with a 1 in 4 risk of CF. Analysis of microvillar enzymes is not recommended for the detection of CF in routine pregnancies. Several polymorphic markers on the centromeric and telomeric sides of the CF locus show strong linkage disequilibrium with the CF gene. In the North American white population, 86% of CF chromosomes occur with a particular RFLP haplotype that is present on only 14% of normal chromosomes. Linkage disequilibrium can be used to refine the risk of heterozygosity in a person who has no family history of CF (9,10). Prenatal testing should always be carried out in conjunction with an experienced geneticist or genetic counselor. It is mandatory to carry out postnatal sweat testing in all cases in which the diagnosis of CF has been made or excluded on the basis of prenatal genotyping or intestinal enzyme assays.

Fetal Intestinal Obstruction

In pregnancies not known to be at increased risk for CF, the diagnosis is sometimes suggested by the finding on prenatal ultrasonography of persistently increased echogenicity of the fetal bowel pattern suggestive of meconium ileus

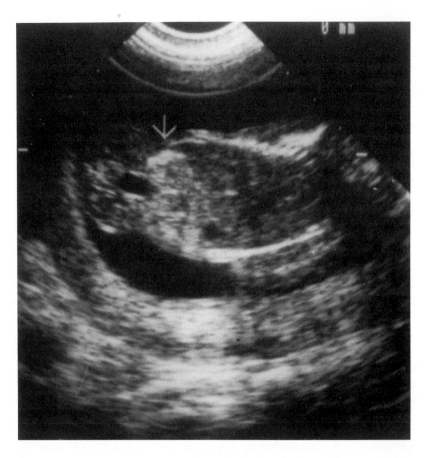

Figure 2 Sagittal scan at 22 weeks' gestation demonstrating a hyperechoic bowel pattern (arrow). Parental testing revealed that both parents were carriers of ΔF508 deletion; subsequent amniocentesis confirmed the intrauterine diagnosis of CF. (From Ref. 15.)

(14,15) (Fig. 2). In approximately 13% of such cases, the diagnosis of CF is confirmed (15). Hyperechoic bowel occurring as a benign variant is distinguished by spontaneous resolution, usually before the third trimester of pregnancy. In pregnancies in which there is a fetal hyperechoic bowel, carrier testing for CF gene mutations can be carried out in the parents. If both parents are carriers of a CF mutation, the diagnosis of CF in the fetus is highly likely and can be confirmed by direct mutation analysis of amniotic fluid cells.

Meconium peritonitis secondary to small bowel perforation in utero can also be detected by prenatal ultrasonography. However, only 7% of such cases are associated with CF (16). The presence of abdominal calcifications is significantly associated with causes of meconium peritonitis other than CF. Conversely, the absence of calcifications favors the diagnosis of CF (16). Parental CF carrier testing with fetal mutation analysis in at-risk couples could be useful in such cases.

B. Neonatal

Meconium Ileus

Approximately 15% of patients with CF present with intestinal obstruction in the immediate postnatal period secondary to inspissation of tenacious meconium in the ileum. Clinically, there is progressive abdominal distention, bilious vomiting, poor feeding, and failure to pass meconium (17,18). Impacted intraluminal meconium may be palpable as a doughy, rubbery substance on the right side of the abdomen. Abdominal radiography shows dilated loops of bowel, usually without air–fluid levels, and a granular ground-glass appearance in the area of the terminal ileum, indicating the mixture of air bubbles with meconium ("soap-bubble" sign). Contrast enema shows a small-caliber, unused microcolon (Fig. 3). Approximately 50% of cases are complicated by peritonitis, volvulus, atresia, necrosis, perforation, or pseudocyst formation (17,18). Among full-term neonates with meconium ileus, CF is confirmed in approximately 98% of cases.

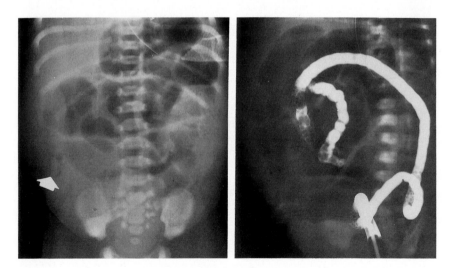

Figure 3 Newborn with intestinal obstruction. Abdomen film (left) shows distended bowel loops with "bubbly" pattern of inspissated meconium in terminal ileum (arrow). Contrast enema (right) shows an unused miscrocolon.

Patients should be presumptively treated for this diagnosis and parents appropriately counseled, pending the results of confirmatory sweat testing or mutation analysis.

Meconium Plug Syndrome

Meconium plug syndrome, in which there is transient distal colonic obstruction relieved by the passage of a meconium plug, may also be the presenting mani-

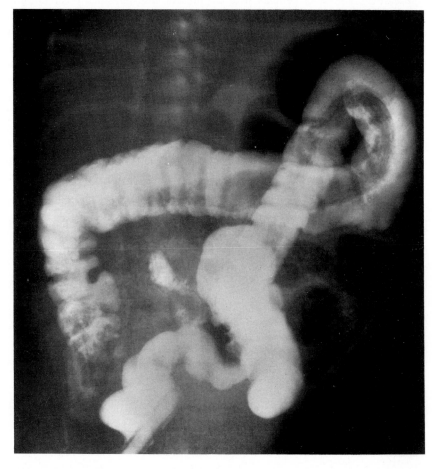

Figure 4 Contrast enema at 72 hours of age in an infant with intestinal obstruction. There is a long continuous filling defect in the transverse and proximal descending colon consistent with a meconium plug.

festation of CF in the neonatal period (19,20) (Fig. 4). The meconium plug syndrome may also occur in association with prematurity, hypotonia, hyper-magnesemia, sepsis, and hypothyroidism, and as the earliest manifestation of Hirschsprung's disease, but its presence should always be an alert to the possibility of CF. The presence of calcified scrotal masses in male infants secondary to in utero meconium peritonitis may also be a presenting manifestation of CF in the neonatal period (21). A sweat test should be performed in every neonate with a meconium abnormality.

It is important to distinguish meconium ileus and the meconium plug syndrome from meconium disease or inspissated meconium syndrome seen in infants of very low birth weight (22). This entity is characterized by the development of obstructive symptoms at several days of age after the initial passage of meconium. Meconium plugs are found in the distal ileum and proximal colon. The inspissated meconium syndrome often occurs in association with respiratory distress syndrome and is not associated with CF.

Liver Disease

Neonates with CF may have prolonged obstructive jaundice (23,24), presumably secondary to obstruction of extrahepatic bile ducts by thick bile along with intrahepatic bile stasis (25). There may be associated hepatomegaly. Approximately 50% of cases occur in association with meconium ileus (24). Massive hepatomegaly with steatosis (fatty replacement) may occur (26), probably related to protein–calorie malnutrition or essential fatty acid deficiency.

Pulmonary Manifestations

Respiratory symptoms may begin during the first month of life. Manifestations include cough, wheezing, retractions, and tachypnea. Symptomatic infants always have radiographic evidence of hyperinflation. Segmental or lobar atelectasis, particularly involving the right upper lobe (Fig. 5), is highly suggestive of CF. Other infants may have severe respiratory distress associated with a bronchiolitic-like syndrome (27).

Growth Failure

Failure to regain birth weight within the appropriate time or inadequate weight gain at 4 to 6 weeks of age is a common finding in neonates with CF. Growth failure often occurs despite a normal or even increased caloric intake. Many of these infants cry after feedings, appear irritable, and are mistakenly diagnosed as having colic or milk allergy.

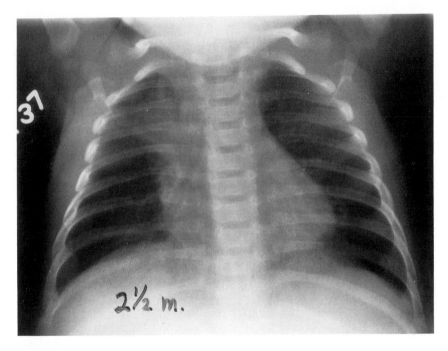

Figure 5 Chest radiograph of a 2-month-old infant with tachypnea and respiratory distress. There is atelectasis in the area of the right upper lobe.

C. Infancy and Childhood

In infants and young children, the diagnosis of CF is usually suggested by respiratory tract symptoms or steatorrhea, often in association with some degree of failure to thrive.

Upper Respiratory Tract

The upper respiratory tract is usually involved secondary to abnormal mucous gland secretions and hypertrophy and edema of the mucous membranes. Nasal polyps occur frequently and may be present at a very early age (28,29) (Fig. 6). The presence of a nasal polyp in a child is always an indication for a sweat test. Sweat testing should also be considered in a child with recurrent or chronic sinusitis refractory to antimicrobial therapy (30). Rarely, a patient with CF is seen with unilateral proptosis secondary to a mucocele of the underlying sinus (31,32) (Fig. 7). Radiographic evidence of opacification of the paranasal sinuses is present in almost all CF patients and may be a helpful diagnostic finding (33).

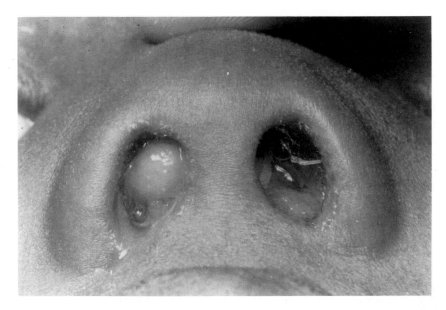

Figure 6 Nasal polyps of recent onset in 9-year-old-boy with CF. He had been followed up in allergy clinics since age 2 years because of recurrent episodes of mild wheezing.

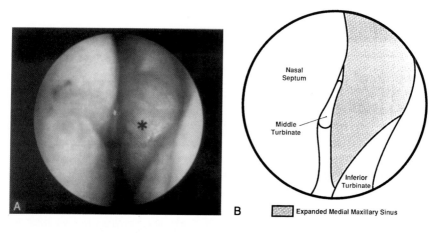

Figure 7 A 13-month-old girl seen for evaluation of chronic nasal congestion and rhinorrhea. Endoscopic view of the left nasal cavity shows a bulging area of lateral nasal wall (*) from maxillary mucocele expansion anterior to middle turbinate. (From Ref. 32.)

Lower Respiratory Tract

In approximately 45% of CF patients, the diagnosis is first considered because of pulmonary symptoms (1). Although the lower respiratory tract is almost invariably involved, manifestations may not appear until months or even years after birth. Cystic fibrosis should be considered in every patient with chronic or recurrent lower respiratory tract findings such as prolonged or recurrent pneumonia, bronchiolitis, bronchitis, bronchiectasis, atelectasis, refractory asthma, and empyema. The most consistent feature of pulmonary involvement is chronic cough. Often, cough is initiated by an upper respiratory infection, after which, it persists for weeks and may never resolve. At first, the cough may be dry and hacking, but, with progression, it becomes paroxysmal and may be associated with gagging, choking, and vomiting. Older patients may expectorate mucopurulent sputum, particularly in association with pulmonary exacerbations.

There may be crackles, rhonchi, wheezes, retractions, and tachypnea. Progressive airway obstruction leads to air trapping with an increase in the anterior–posterior diameter of the chest. Digital clubbing is almost universal in symptomatic patients older than 4 years of age.

Chest radiograph findings are not diagnostic of CF but may be helpful in suggesting the diagnosis. Air trapping and bronchial wall thickening are the earliest radiographic findings (Fig. 8). Persistent air trapping, mucoid impaction of the bronchi (34), and atelectasis of the right upper lobe are highly suggestive of CF.

Isolation of a mucoid variant of *Pseudomonas aeruginosa* from a respiratory tract culture is almost uniquely associated with CF and is always an indication for a sweat test (35).

Gastrointestinal Tract

In infants and young children, steatorrhea is strongly suggestive of CF. Other presentations include abdominal protuberance, crampy abdominal pain, flatulence, frequent bulky, oily, malodorous stools, and poor weight gain. There may be associated rectal prolapse (36). Although prolapse may occur as a complication of severe constipation, when seen in the context of loose or bulky stools in industrialized countries, it is highly suggestive of CF (37). In underdeveloped countries, rectal prolapse most often represents parasitic disease.

Apparent steatorrhea can be investigated by formal fat absorption studies. The only direct quantitative assessment of exocrine pancreatic function involves duodenal intubation and measurement of pancreatic enzyme and bicarbonate concentration in duodenal fluid at baseline and following stimulation with intravenous secretin and cholecystokinin (38). This is an invasive, expensive, and time-consuming procedure, which is rarely performed except for research purposes. There are also a number of indirect and noninvasive measurements of

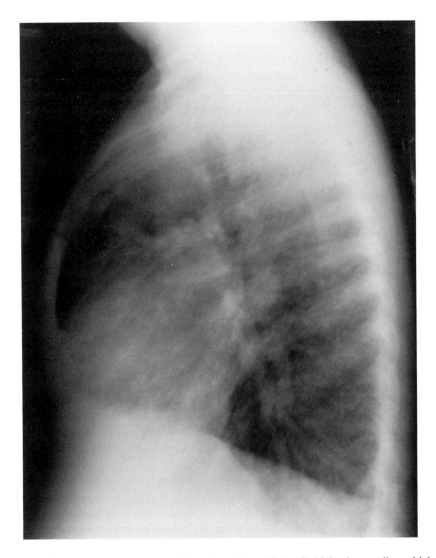

Figure 8 Chest radiograph lateral view shows bronchial wall thickening, peribronchial infiltrates, and marked air trapping.

exocrine pancreatic status that may be useful. These include stool trypsin and chymotrypsin levels (39), microscopic examination of a random stool sample for fat globules, oral administration of measurable tracers [fluorescein dilaurate, (40), *N*-benzoyl-L-tyrosyl-*p*-aminobenzoic acid (41)] bound to a peptide that is specifically cleaved by one of the pancreatic enzymes, measurement of serum

levels of immunoreactive pancreatic lipase (42), cationic trypsin (ogen) (42), pancreatic amylase and amylase isoenzymes (43,44), "pancreatitis-associated protein" (45), and measurement of 72-hour fecal fat output (46). Although cumbersome to perform, this last procedure is probably the most useful of all of the tests to document the presence and degree of steatorrhea. Normally, stool fat output is less than 7% of fat intake (coefficient of absorption > 93%).

Assessment of exocrine pancreatic status is indicated at diagnosis. During infancy, approximately 35% of patients have substantial preservation of pancreatic function (47). However, some of these patients will develop progressive decline of pancreatic function during the first few years of life (47,48). Mutation analysis is helpful in predicting the pancreatic course of such patients (4,49). Patients who have one or two "mild" mutations can be expected to remain pancreatic sufficient, whereas patients who have two "severe" mutations can be predicted to progress to pancreatic insufficiency. Mutations are characterized as "mild" or "severe" only in relation to pancreatic function. These classifications do not relate to pulmonary status.

Other gastrointestinal manifestations of CF in infancy and childhood include recurrent episodes of intussusception (50), pancreatitis (51), gastroesophageal reflux (52), and mucoid impaction (asymptomatic right lower quadrant mass) of the appendix (53). In some patients, the diagnosis of CF has been suggested by the histologic appearance of an appendix removed from a patient with acute or recurrent/chronic abdominal pain (54,55) (Fig. 9). There is an increase in the number of goblet cells and they are often markedly distended with mucus secretions. The crypts are dilated secondary to distention of the lumen by accumulated secretions, and eosinophilic casts of the crypts may extrude into the lumen. These findings are pathognomonic of CF.

Miscellaneous

A variety of clinical presentations related to deficiency of protein, vitamins, minerals, or fat are suggestive of CF.

Infants with CF may present with edema and hypoproteinemia, usually in association with breast milk or soy protein feedings (56,57). Associated findings include anemia, hepatomegaly, elevated concentration of liver enzymes, and rash, called (acrodermatitis enteropathica (58,59) (Fig. 10). The sweat test may initially be negative in such cases (60).

An increased concentration of electrolytes in the sweat may result in a salty taste to the skin, salt crystal formation on the skin, hyponatremic–hypochloremic dehydration secondary to salt depletion, or hypokalemic metabolic alkalosis secondary to chronic salt loss (61–63). This latter presentation is particularly common in hot climates (62). Cystic fibrosis should always be considered in an infant with profound hypoelectrolytemia not accounted for by gastrointestinal losses.

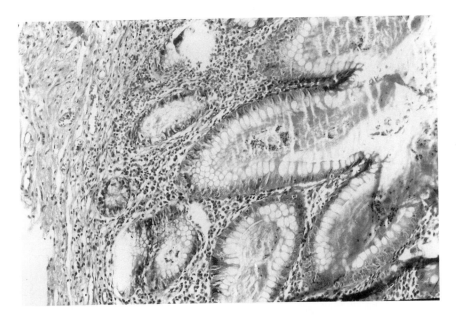

Figure 9 Typical histological appearance of the appendix in CF. There is an increased number of goblet cells distended with mucus. Casts of the crypts extrude into the lumen of the appendix.

Deficiency of fat-soluble vitamins may result in a bulging fontanel (vitamin A) (64), hemolytic anemia (vitamin E) (65,66), and hemorrhagic complications (vitamin K) 67. A sweat test is indicated in all such cases.

The incidental finding of absence of the vas deferens at the time of an orchiopexy or herniorrhaphy may be the initial clue to the diagnosis of CF (68).

D. Adolescents and Adults

In approximately 5%–10% of patients with CF, the diagnosis is first made during adolescence and adulthood (69). Many of these cases have a history of typical, although somewhat mild, respiratory tract and gastrointestinal features of CF with onset in childhood, often associated with a poor growth pattern. In some patients, however, pulmonary symptoms may first become manifest after the age of 13 years (70). Chronic cough, sputum production, recurrent pneumonia, and chest radiograph abnormalities are common presenting features. The diagnosis of CF should also be considered in patients with allergic bronchopulmonary aspergillosis and in those from whom *P. aeruginosa* is recovered from the respiratory tract (71). All adolescents and adults with unexplained chronic lung disease, malabsorption, or both, deserve a sweat test as part of their diagnostic evaluation.

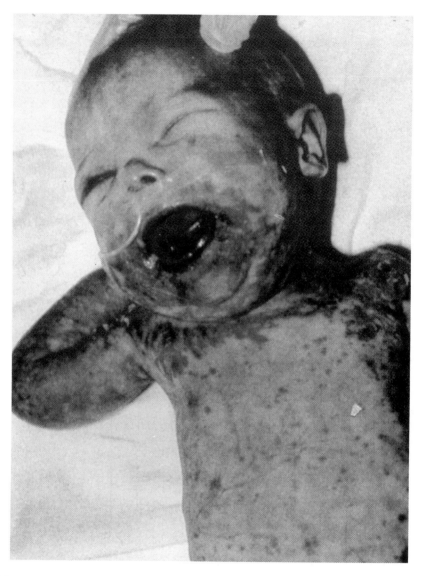

Figure 10 Widespread papulosquamous, desquamating eruption with periorificial accentuation in a 4-month-old infant referred for evaluation of rash, extremity edema, and failure to thrive. (From Ref. 58.)

Table 2 Clinical Manifestations Suggestive of Cystic Fibrosis

Respiratory	Gastrointestinal	Metabolic and other
Atelectasis (lobar or segmental, especially right upper lobe)	Appendix impacted with mucous secretions	Acrodermatitis enteropathica
Bronchiectasis	Cirrhosis and portal hypertension	Alkalosis, metabolic (with hypochloremia and hyponatremia)
Chronic cough	Cholelithiasis	Azoospermia
Digital clubbing	Intestinal obstruction (late)	Edema and hypoproteinemia
Hemoptysis	Intussusception, at atypical age	Failure to thrive
Nasal polyps	Jaundice, prolonged in neonate	Family history of CF
Pansinusitis	Meconium ileus	Salt crystals
Pneumonia, chronic or recurrent, or caused by *Staphylococcus*	Meconium plug syndrome	Salt depletion syndrome
Pseudomonas colonization, especially with mucoid strain	Pancreatitis	Salty taste to skin
Retractions[a]		Scrotal calcification, prenatal or newborn
Tachypnea[a]		Vas deferens, absent
Wheezing and hyperinflation[a]		Vitamin A deficiency (bulging fontanel, night blindness)
		Vitamin E deficiency (hemolytic anemia)
		Vitamin K deficiency (bleeding)

[a]If persistent or refractory to usual therapy.

Older patients may present with cirrhosis in the absence of pulmonary symptoms (70); CF should be considered in the evaluation of any patient with obscure liver disease. Other unusual presentations in older patients include pancreatitis (72), intussusception (50), night blindness (73), and intestinal obstruction (74).

Among adult males who present with infertility (azoospermia) secondary to bilateral absence of the vas deferens, there is a high frequency of identifiable CF mutations. Among such cases, 50% are heterozygous for a known CF mutation and 10%–15% are compound heterozygotes (75,76). Such individuals warrant careful clinical evaluation, sweat testing, and mutation analysis. In the absence of other CF-related symptoms or an elevated sweat electrolyte concentration, however, it is probably best not to label such individuals as having CF. Exceptions are ΔF508/R117H compound heterozygotes, most of whom have a mild form of CF manifested by elevated sweat electrolyte concentrations, pancreatic sufficiency, and variable degrees of pulmonary involvement (6). The relatives of individuals with absence of the vas deferens are at increased risk of being CF carriers and should receive appropriate genetic counseling.

The clinical manifestations suggestive of CF are summarized in Table 2.

III. Diagnostic Testing

A. Sweat Test

The sweat test remains the "gold standard" for the confirmation or exclusion of the diagnosis of CF (77). During the first 24 hours after birth, sweat electrolyte values may be transiently elevated in normal infants (78). After the first 2 days of life, there is a rapid decline in sweat electrolyte concentrations and an elevated value can then be used to confirm the diagnosis of CF. Therefore, sweat test results obtained in the first 48 hours of life should be confirmed by repeat testing. It may be difficult to obtain an adequate sweat sample during the first 4 weeks after birth. This may be a particular problem among preterm infants.

Ideally, sweat testing should be carried out at a time when the patient is clinically stable, well hydrated, free of acute illness, and not receiving mineralocorticoids.

Methodology

Sweat testing should be carried out in accordance with the guidelines of the National Committee for Clinical Laboratory Standards (document 34-A, 1994). It is crucial that testing be carried out by experienced personnel using standardized methodologies in facilities in which adequate numbers of tests are performed to maintain laboratory proficiency and quality control. The only acceptable test for confirmation or exclusion of CF is the quantitative pilocarpine iontophoresis sweat test (79). When a physician orders a sweat test, he or she must know the methodology being used.

Sample Collection

The methods of sample collection approved by the United States Cystic Fibrosis Foundation are the Gibson-Cooke procedure (79) and the Macroduct Sweat Collection System (Wescor, Inc., Logan, UT) (80). In both systems, localized sweating is stimulated by the iontophoresis of pilocarpine into the skin of the flexor surface of the forearm, calf, or thigh, using an electrical charge of approximately 5 mV for 5–10 min. Sweat is then collected on filter paper or gauze (Gibson-Cooke) (Fig. 11) or in microbore tubing (Macroduct) (Fig. 12), the amount of sweat quantitated, and the sample analyzed for chloride concentration, sodium concentration, or both. The minimum acceptable amount for the Gibson-Cooke procedure is 75 mg and for the Macroduct system 15 µL.

If an adequate sweat sample is not obtained, repeat testing may be carried out as soon as practical because the rate of sweating may vary from day to day. Thermal stimulation over the iontophoresis site, use of a warmer for an infant (with careful monitoring of the infant's temperature), or feeding or nursing an infant during the collection period may increase sweat production. When an adequate sweat sample cannot be obtained from one site, collection can be repeated at another site, but inadequate samples from several sites must never be pooled for analysis.

Sweat should not be stimulated or collected from the head (including forehead), trunk, or any area of diffuse inflammation or serous or bloody discharge. Sweat can be collected from a site receiving intravenous fluids as long as good contact between the skin and electrode is possible and the collection technique does not interfere with venous flow.

Sample Analysis

Electrolytes. Sodium concentration in sweat can be determined by flame photometry and chloride concentration with a chloridometer. Even though either electrolyte can be measured, chloride provides better discrimination between CF patients and unaffected individuals (81–83) and is usually the analyte of choice. Among adults, there may be overlap in sweat sodium concentration between CF patients and unaffected individuals, leading to diagnostic confusion 84 (Fig. 13). When there is a borderline sweat sodium concentration, the percentage of suppression of sweat sodium concentration after administrative of a mineralocorticoid has been used to improve diagnostic accuracy, because the concentration of sodium in the sweat of CF patients does not decrease, whereas it does in unaffected individuals. However, there is too much overlap between CF and unaffected patients for this to be useful (84). As a quality control measure, it may be helpful to measure the concentration of both

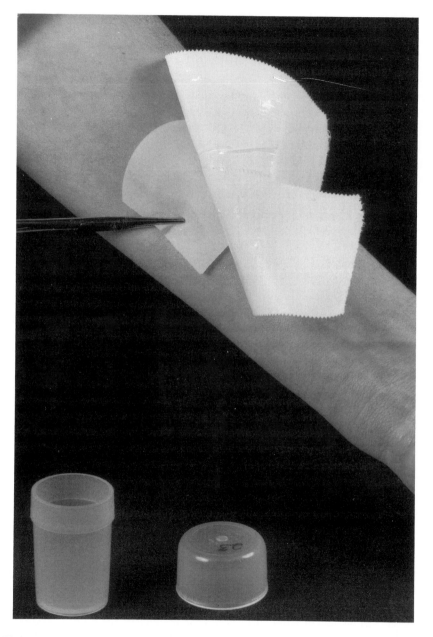

Figure 11 Quantitative pilocarpine iontophoresis sweat test (Gibson-Cooke). Localized sweating is stimulated by the iontophoresis of pilocarpine; sweat is then collected on filter paper or gauze.

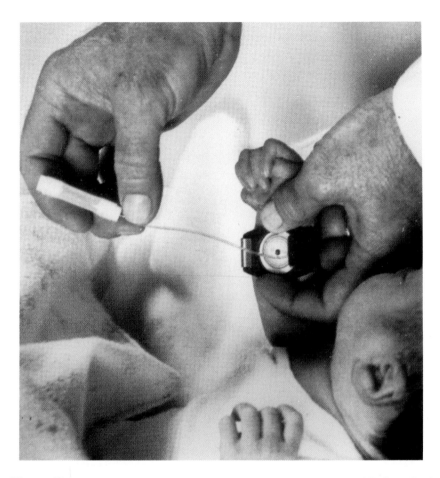

Figure 12 Macroduct sweat collection system (Wescor, Inc., Logan, UT). Localized sweating is stimulated by the iontophoresis of pilocarpine; sweat is then collected in microbore tubing.

sodium and chloride (85,86). Both analytes should be proportionately increased or decreased. Discordant values can indicate problems with collection or analysis. Furthermore, the ratio of sodium to chloride concentrations can help to discriminate between patients with CF and unaffected individuals: in those with CF, the sweat $[NA^+]/[Cl^-]$ ratio is nearly always less than 1.0 (86). One exception may be those with uncommon CF mutations associated with pancreatic sufficiency: one study showed 96% of patients with ΔF508, W1282X, G542X, N1303K, or 1717-1G $\rightarrow$ A (all associated with pancreatic insufficiency) had chloride values higher than sodium, whereas only 40% of those

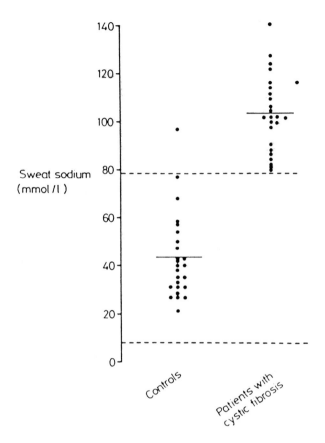

Figure 13 Sweat sodium concentrations in control subjects and adults with cystic fibrosis. Solid horizontal lines indicate means; broken horizontal lines indicate 2 standard deviations for controls subjects. (From Ref. 84.)

with 3849 + 10kb C → T (associated with pancreatic sufficiency) had sweat chloride concentrations higher than sweat sodium (87). Sweat chloride or sodium concentrations greater than 160 mmol/L are not physiologically possible. Procedural errors should be sought and the patient should be retested.

Conductivity. Conductivity represents a nonselective measurement of ions. Sweat conductivity is increased in patients with CF and its measurement has been proposed as a diagnostic test (88). A conductivity analyzer (Wescor Sweat-Chek), designed specifically for use with the Wescor Macroduct sweat collector, has been approved by the Cystic Fibrosis Foundation as a screening method. There is excellent correlation between the results of sweat sodium and chloride concentrations and sweat conductivity (89) (Fig. 14). Any sweat

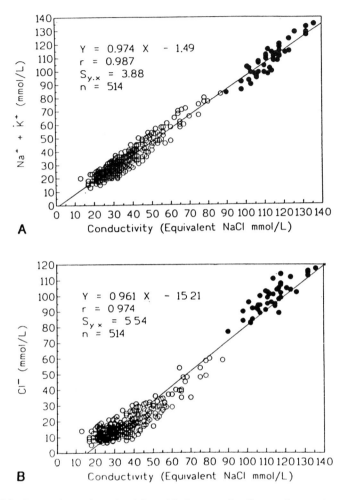

Figure 14 Comparison of conductivity with the sum of sodium and potassium concentrations (A) and with the chloride concentration (B) performed on the same sweat samples taken from patients with CF (dark circles) and without CF (clear circles). r, regression coefficient; $S_{y \cdot x}$, standard error of the estimate. (From Ref. 89.)

conductivity result equal to or greater than 50 mmol/L (equivalent NaCl) is considered positive and should be followed up by a quantitative sweat test.

Osmolality. *Osmolality* of sweat reflects the total solute concentration in mmol per kilogram of sweat. It is necessary to use an osmometer capable of measuring undiluted microsamples of sweat (80,90,91). The reference interval for sweat osmolality in children is approximately 50–150 mmol/kg. Children with CF have sweat osmolality values of more than 200 mmol/kg; values between 150 and 200 mmol/kg are equivocal. Positive or equivocal results should always be followed up by a quantitative sweat test.

Alternative Sweat Methodology

Conductivity. Direct reading in situ tests using ion-selective electrodes or older electrical conductivity measurements are not acceptable as diagnostic tests (92). With direct reading procedures, the amount of sweat collected is not measured and an adequate sample cannot be assured. Unheated cup collectors are unsatisfactory because of condensation.

Paper-Patch Test. The sweat patch test or cystic fibrosis indicator system (CFIS, ScandiPharm) (93,94) is a semiquantitative test in which localized sweating is stimulated by pilocarpine iontophoresis and sweat is then collected on a paper patch, which is designed to complex chloride and give a "positive" color change result when the chloride concentration is greater than 45 mmol/L. This is only a screening procedure and should never be used as the basis of a definitive CF diagnosis. The equipment is easily portable, requires no chemistry equipment, and may be useful as a screening test in areas where access to quantitative sweat testing is limited.

Results Reporting

Reference Values. The results of quantitative analysis of sweat chloride in patients with CF, unaffected siblings, and controls are shown in Fig 15. A chloride or sodium concentration of more than 60 mmol/L is consistent with the diagnosis of CF (95). The test results should be interpreted with regard to the patient's age because some unaffected adults can have values of more than 60 mmol/L. Nevertheless, the sweat test remains the gold standard confirmatory test in adults (96,97) (Fig. 16). Borderline sweat chloride concentrations in the range of 40 to 60 mmol/L occur in approximately 4%–5% of all sweat tests. In such cases, repeat sweat testing may yield results that clearly fall within the normal or abnormal range. Analysis of the ratio of sodium to chloride also may be helpful. In patients with CF, the chloride concentration is usually higher than the sodium; whereas, in normal subjects, the reverse usually occurs (86).

Diagnostic Criteria. Results from the measurement of chloride and sodium concentrations in sweat should be interpreted in relation to the patient's clinical picture by a physician knowledgeable about CF. The test results need to be consistent with the clinical picture; no single laboratory result is sufficient to establish or rule out the diagnosis of CF. The diagnosis should be made only if there is an elevated sweat chloride or sodium concentration, or both, on two separate occasions (or one elevated sweat test result plus identification of two CF mutations) in a patient with clinically significant findings such as chronic lung disease, exocrine pancreatic insufficiency, meconium ileus, or a family history of CF. In 0.1%–1.0% of cases, the diagnosis of CF is established (nasal

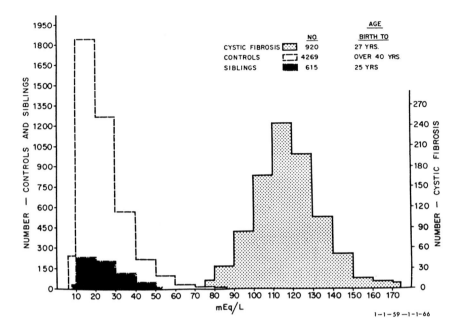

Figure 15 Chloride concentrations in patients with CF, healthy persons, and healthy siblings of patients with CF. (From Ref. 95.)

potential difference measurement, histopathology, mutation analysis) in patients with borderline or normal electrolyte concentrations (98,99). As more information becomes available concerning the phenotypic expressions of the CF genotype, this number may increase.

Sources of Error. The incidence of erroneous sweat test results is probably in the range of 10%–15%. Although most errors represent false-positive results, false-negative results are also a serious problem (100). Sweat electrolyte values may vary depending on the method of sweat stimulation, weight of the sweat sample, sweat secretory rate, salt intake, and nutritional and hydration status. However, it is rare for these factors to interfere with the diagnostic validity of the test results. Most errors are caused by the use of unreliable methodology, inadequate sweat collection, technical errors, and misinterpretation of results (101,102). Problems are also attributable to inexperienced laboratory personnel and lack of appropriate quality assurance.

Technical problems associated with sweat testing include failure to obtain an adequate sweat sample; skin contamination by salt-containing materials; failure to dry the patient's skin before sweat collection; evaporation of the sweat sample during collection, transfer, and transport; failure to include condensate

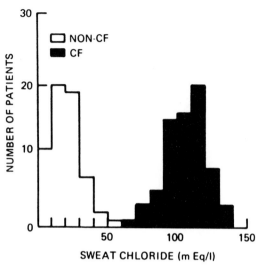

Figure 16 Distribution of sweat chloride values in 75 adults with CF and 60 unaffected adults. (From Ref. 97.)

in the sweat sample when using gauze or filter paper; and errors in sample weighing, dilution, elution, electrolyte analysis, and result computation.

Duplicate sweat collection and analysis may be useful for purposes of quality assurance. These is generally a good correlation between the amount of sweat collected at different sites and the electrolyte concentrations (85). Chloride values from two different collection sites usually agree within 10 mmol/L for values less than or equal to 60 mmol/L and within 15 mmol/L for values greater than 60 mmol/L.

Errors in interpretation include establishment of a diagnosis of CF on the basis of a single positive test, failure to repeat a test giving borderline results, and failure to repeat a test in a patient with a negative result but a clinical picture highly suggestive of CF. Transiently negative sweat electrolyte results have been reported in CF patients in the presence of edema and hypoproteinemia (60). In such cases, the test must be repeated after resolution of the edema.

Other Diseases Associated with Elevated Sweat Electrolyte Concentrations

A variety of diseases other than CF may be associated with moderately elevated concentrations of sodium and chloride in sweat (103) (Table 3). However, with few exceptions these conditions do not represent a problem in differential diagnosis.

There is evidence that there may be physiological variability of sweat electrolyte concentrations over time, and that there may be transient elevation of sweat electrolyte values in unaffected persons (104). Transient elevations in

Table 3 Conditions Other than Cystic Fibrosis Associated with an Elevated Sweat Electrolyte Concentration

Adrenal insufficiency (untreated)[a]	Hypoparathyroidism, familial[a]
Anorexia nervosa[a]	Hypothyroidism (untreated)[a]
Atopic dermatitis[a]	Klinefelter's syndrome
Autonomic dysfunction	Mauriac's syndrome
Celiac disease	Mucopolysaccharidosis Type I
Ectodermal dysplasia	Malnutrition[a]
Environmental deprivation	Nephrogenic diabetes insipidus[a]
Exercise, especially in the heat[a]	Nephrosis[a]
Familial cholestasis (Byler's disease)	Prostaglandin E_1 infusion, long-term[a]
Fucosidosis	Protein-calorie malnutrition[a]
Glucose-6-phosphate dehydrogenase deficiency	Pseudohypoaldosteronism[a]
Glycogen storage disease Type 1	Psychosocial failure to thrive[a]
Hypogammaglobulinemia	

[a]Sweat test reverts to normal with resolution of underlying condition.

electrolyte concentrations have also been reported in infants and young children with environmental deprivation (nonorganic failure to thrive) (105) and in adolescents with anorexia nervosa (106). Repeat testing after medical stabilization is indicated in such cases.

When an elevated sweat electrolyte concentration is not consistent with the patient's clinical picture, there is marked variability in electrolyte concentrations on repeat testing, the sweat electrolyte concentration is higher than a "physiologically possible" level, or there is a discrepancy among the medical history, examination, laboratory results, and response to treatment, it is important to consider the possibility of Munchausen syndrome by proxy (107).

Indications for Repeat Sweat Testing

(1) All positive sweat tests must be repeated; the diagnosis of CF should never be based on a single positive test. (2) All borderline sweat test results (chloride concentration 40–60 mmol/L) should be repeated; if results remain in an indeterminate range, additional ancillary tests may be helpful (Fig. 17). (3) Sweat testing should be repeated in patients thought to have CF who do not follow an expected clinical course (108). As patients are followed up, the clinical, laboratory, and chest radiograph findings should be consistent with the diagnosis of CF. It is especially important to reevaluate those patients in whom the diagnosis was suggested primarily on the basis of failure to thrive or a positive family history, the clinical features prompting the initial sweat test disappear, the patient's course is consistent with asthma without evidence of suppurative lung disease, or there is a normal growth pattern without evidence

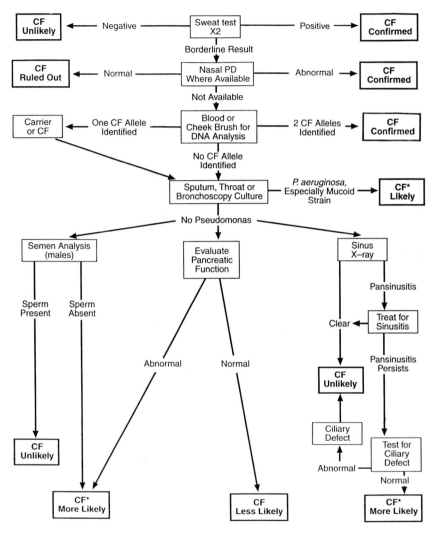

* Treat as though has CF until definitive diagnosis possible.

Figure 17 Algorithm of approach to the patient with clinical features consistent with CF and with no family history of CF.

of digital clubbing, *Pseudomonas* colonization, or typical chest radiograph findings.

Repeat testing can be carried out at any time after the initial testing, but preferably at a time when the patient is clinically stable, well hydrated, free of acute intercurrent illness, and not receiving mineralocorticoids.

Indeterminate Sweat Test Results

Patients who have persistent borderline sweat chloride or sodium concentrations present a difficult diagnostic challenge. In such cases, it is important to assess exocrine pancreatic function quantitatively. Ancillary findings such as azoospermia in postpubertal males, isolation of a mucoid strain of *P. aeruginosa* from the respiratory tract, and radiographic evidence of pansinusitis may be helpful (see Fig. 17).

B. Mutation Detection

Worldwide, among patients reported to the Cystic Fibrosis Genetic Analysis Consortium, 13 mutations occur at a frequency greater than 1% and account for 87.3% of CF alleles (109) (Table 4). However, there can be wide variation from one population to another. The most common mutation, ΔF508, is present on approximately 70% of CF alleles in the United States, but the frequency increases to as high as 80% in Denmark. In discrete populations, however, the frequency of non-ΔF508 mutations is significantly higher. Among Ashkenazi Jews, W1282X (60%), ΔF508 (22%), and 3849 + 10kb C $\rightarrow$ T (15%) account for almost all CFTR mutations (109). Among African-Americans, ΔF508 accounts for 43% of CF alleles, a subset of common mutations for 24% and private mutations for 22% (110). Familiarity with these population differences can be very helpful in selecting diagnostic testing and carrier screening programs.

There is also considerable interest in genotype-phenotype correlations. Genotype is known to be highly predictive of pancreatic status (4,5,49). There

Table 4 CFTR Gene Mutations Reported to the Cystic Fibrosis Genetic Analysis Consortium with Relative Frequency of $\geq 1\%$

Mutation	Relative frequency
Delta F508	67.2
G542X	3.4
G551D	2.4
W1282X	2.1
3905insT	2.1
N1303K	1.8
3849 + 10kb C $\rightarrow$ T	1.4
R553X	1.3
621 + G $\rightarrow$ T	1.3
1717 − 1G $\rightarrow$ A	1.1
1078delT	1.1
2789 + 5G $\rightarrow$ A	1.1
3849 + 4A $\rightarrow$ G	1.0

Source: Ref. 109.

are a number of "mild" mutations, i.e., R117H, R334W, R347P, A455E, P574H, G551S, T338I, and 3849 + 10kb C → T, which are almost always associated with pancreatic sufficiency (5,49,111). The T338I mutation has been identified in patients with isolated hypotonic dehydration in the absence of pancreatic or pulmonary disease (112). In general, genotype does not correlate with pulmonary or overall clinical severity (6,7,113), but several mutations (R117H, 3849 + 10kb C → T, and G551S) are more likely to be associated with a mild pulmonary phenotype, often with normal or borderline sweat chloride concentrations (99,109,111). Genotype is not predictive of liver disease (114), diabetes (115), or meconium ileus except that, with rare exception, these complications are seen only in patients with two "severe" mutations, e.g., ΔF508 and evidence of pancreatic insufficiency.

The ability to detect mutations in the CF gene may be helpful in ambiguous clinical situations. In a patient with clinical features consistent with CF, the identification of two CF mutations confirms the diagnosis; the identification of a CF mutation on one allele does not confirm the diagnosis but it does increase the likelihood that the patient has a variant form of CF and it can provide information for genetic counseling. From a practical standpoint, however, mutation analysis is often not helpful in patients with atypical clinical features or borderline sweat test results, because such patients often do not carry the mutations present in diagnostic screening panels. Alternatively, in a patient with two CF mutations but without a consistent clinical picture, a CF diagnosis is not warranted. CF is a clinical rather than a genetic diagnosis. The sensitivity and utility of mutation analysis will undoubtedly improve as we increase our knowledge of the distribution of CF mutations in discrete populations and subsets of patients with atypical clinical features.

C. Potential Difference Measurement

In patients with CF, increased sodium absorption and decreased chloride permeability results in a significantly higher maximal transepithelial voltage, or potential difference (PD), across the respiratory and intestinal tract epithelia (116-117) (Fig. 18). Also, superfusion of the luminal surface with the sodium transport inhibitor amiloride results in a greater reduction in voltage in CF patients compared with that in unaffected control subjects (116,117) (Fig. 19), and there is absence of a voltage response to beta-adrenergic agonists (e.g., isoproterenol) in CF patients. The in vivo measurement of voltage across the nasal epithelium coupled with the response to amiloride and isoproterenol can be used to differentiate CF patients (including those with borderline or even normal sweat test results) from patients with other disorders (117–119) (Fig. 20). Although PD measurement has been primarily a research tool, the proce-

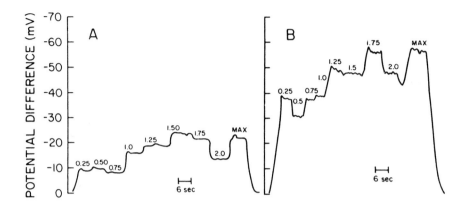

Figure 18 Recording of nasal potential difference as measured under inferior turbinate in a healthy control subject (A) and a patient with CF (B). Numbers above the tracing represent distance (in centimeters) from the anterior tip of the inferior turbinate. (From Ref. 117.)

dure is relatively noninvasive and it can be used as a useful diagnostic adjunct in patients of all ages, including neonates (117). Although this procedure is currently available only at a limited number of centers, its diagnostic utility has been widely confirmed, and it should now be considered a useful procedure in ambiguous clinical situations.

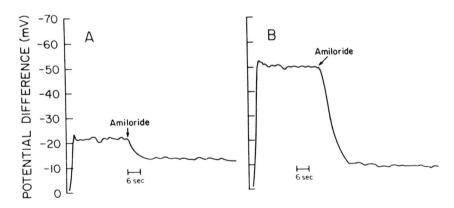

Figure 19 Recordings of nasal potential difference before and during superfusion with amiloride in a healthy control subject (A) and a patient with CF (B). (From Ref. 117.)

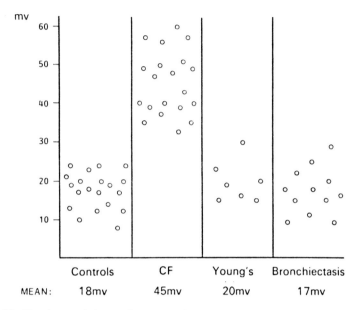

Figure 20 Nasal potential recordings (in mV, lumen negative) in control subjects and in patients with cystic fibrosis, Young's syndrome, and bronchiectasis. (From Ref. 119.)

IV. Caveats

The most commonly encountered errors regarding the diagnosis of CF are as follows:

1. Failure to consider the diagnosis because the patient is not white, the patient looks "too healthy," or pancreatic function is normal.
2. Use of unacceptable sweat test methodology.
3. Misinterpretation of sweat test result because of inadequate sweat sample; confusing values for sweat weight, osmolality, and electrolyte concentration; failure to repeat positive and borderline results; and failure to repeat negative sweat test in a patient with a highly suggestive clinical picture.
4. Failure to reconsider the diagnosis in a patient who does not follow the "usual" or "expected" clinical course.

V. Carrier Screening

Mutation detection enables us to carry out CF carrier (heterozygote) screening in the general population. However, there is agreement that such screening should not be undertaken until approximately 95% of mutations can be detected (120). At this detection rate, 90% of couples at risk of having a child with CF would be identified. This is currently possible in only a few ethnically and geographically discrete populations throughout the world (Ashkenazi Jewish; Saguenay-Las St. Jean) in which CF is probably the result of founder effect (121). As more mutations are identified and detection strategies evolve, screening may become feasible even in the ethnically diverse population of North America. Successful implementation of population-based screening also will require an extensive commitment to public education and genetic counseling. In the interim, carrier screening is not recommended for individuals who do not have a family history of CF (120).

VI. Neonatal Screening

Because of well-documented delays in diagnosis, there has been considerable interest in establishing a satisfactory method for the neonatal detection of CF (122). The goals of newborn screening include the presymptomatic identification and early treatment of patients with CF and the identification and counseling of at-risk families.

A. Meconium Screening

Initially, CF neonatal screening programs were based on the detection of an elevated albumin concentration in meconium, either by a semiqualitative test strip (123) or by quantitative immunochemical methods (124). Although meconium screening is simple, noninvasive, and relatively inexpensive, it has been associated with major disadvantages including a high incidence of false-positive and false-negative test results (125). Sample collection was a problem. The test did not lend itself to automation, and variables of storage and transfer affected test results. Because of these problems, meconium screening was never widely implemented in the United States.

B. Immunoreactive Trypsin Screening

Current screening programs are based on the observation that newborns with CF have persistently elevated concentrations of immunoreactive cationic trypsin(ogen) (IRT), a pancreatic enzyme precursor, in their blood secondary to pancreatic ductular blockage and leakage of enzyme into the circulation (126) (Fig. 21). A number of studies throughout the world have documented that screening for IRT in dried blood spots can identify affected newborns, including those without steatorrhea, and that population-based screening programs are feasible (127–131). Timely access to reliable quantitative pilocarpine iontophoresis sweat testing is a crucial component of any CF screening program.

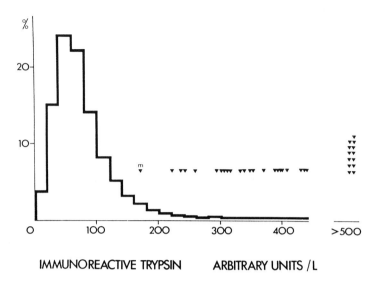

Figure 21 Distribution of IRT values in dried blood samples from 10,244 neonates. Values in samples are from neonates with CF detected by screening 75,000 babies. *m*, CF missed by screening. (From Ref. 127.)

In the most common screening strategy, IRT is measured on the blood spot routinely collected for metabolic screening on postnatal day 1 to 4 followed by a repeat test (generally on about day 28) in those infants whose IRT value is above a predetermined "cutoff" point, followed by a sweat test on those with a persistently elevated IRT value. Because of an age-related decline in blood IRT values, both in CF patients and unaffected newborns (132), the sensitivity of screening is increased by using a lower cutoff value for the repeat test.

With this strategy, the recall rate, specificity (false-positive results), and sensitivity (false-negative results) vary according to the cutoff value selected. In the largest U. S. experience (in Colorado), the recall rate was 3.2 per 1000 (131). The false-positive rate was 92% for initial testing and 25.8%–67.7% (depending on the cutoff value) for repeat testing. The false-negative rate (excluding infants with meconium ileus) was 4.9%. In a number of other screening programs throughout the world, sensitivity has ranged from 91% to 98%. Most groups have found it necessary to do between eight and 20 second blood tests and two or three sweat tests per case detected to achieve a final sensitivity of 90%–95% (133). Given the current technology, 100% sensitivity is unattainable in CF neonatal screening and missed cases are unavoidable.

An alternative strategy proposed for neonatal screening involves an initial blood IRT assay followed by direct CF mutation (ΔF508) analysis when the IRT value is higher than the predetermined cutoff value (122,133). This procedure identifies babies homozygous for ΔF508 who will have CF, babies heterozygous for the deletion, some of whom will have an unknown second mutation and a positive sweat test, and babies without ΔF508, most of whom are normal but a small proportion of whom will be homozygous or compound heterozygotes for unknown CF mutations and will be missed. The specificity of this strategy should be 100%. The sensitivity varies according to the frequency of ΔF508 in the population being screened; at a ΔF508 frequency of 70%, sensitivity would be 85%–95%. Testing for a panel of common mutations, especially in ethnically discrete populations, would significantly increase the sensitivity of this screening strategy. This type of screening program is being used in several countries.

The IRT–mutation detection screening strategy should be undertaken with caution, because it will lead to the detection of CF heterozygotes (122,134). Even though this information might be of potential value to families in regard to genetic counseling, it offers no benefit to the carrier children until they reach reproductive age. Also, disclosure of this information may be confusing and anxiety-producing for parents and may place the child at risk of stigmatization and discrimination.

C. Risks and Benefits

The role of population-based neonatal screening in the United States remains controversial (122). Potential benefits include fewer hospitalizations in the first years of life (135), diagnosis and treatment of unsuspected protein malnutrition and vitamin deficiencies (136) (Table 5), earlier genetic counseling, and a reduction in the anxiety associated with delayed diagnosis. Conversely, there are a number of potential risks of screening. Laboratory errors, misdiagnoses, confusion, psychosocial stress, and stigmatization may occur, even in carefully managed programs (122). The possibility exists that early diagnosis of mildly affected patients may lead to inappropriate and expensive therapy that might have untoward consequences (122). Finally, there are psychosocial risks in the families of infants both with false-positive and false-negative results.

Pending demonstration of an overall benefit of early diagnosis, population-based neonatal screening has not been recommended in the United States. In other parts of the world, however, where most cases of CF are diagnosed late or not at all, neonatal screening can be used as an efficient case-finding strategy. Also, the introduction of new therapies (antiinflammatory agents, gene transfer), which are most effective if started before the appearance of significant lung injury, may favor the implementation of newborn screening in the United States.

Table 5 Nutritional Deficits Before 2 Months of Age in 20 Infants with
Cystic Fibrosis Identified by Newborn Screening

Deficit	Percentage of patients tested
Weight percentile	45
Triceps skinfold	88
Serum albumin or total protein	29
Serum prealbumin	81
Serum cholesterol	33

Source: Ref. 136.

D. Immunoreactive Trypsin Testing as an Ancillary Diagnostic Tool

Because sweat testing is often not feasible (inadequate sweat collection) until after 4 weeks of age, IRT testing can be used as a diagnostic screening procedure in infants at increased risk of CF based on a positive family history. In such instances, IRT testing may provide the family with a result within 7 days. However, regardless of the IRT result, a quantitative sweat test is always indicated in such cases. Approximately 25%–40% of newborns with meconium ileus have a negative IRT screen (122,131). In infants with meconium ileus, other forms of intestinal obstruction, or other clinical features suggestive of CF, a quantitative sweat test or mutation analysis should be performed without an initial IRT measurement.

Measurement of IRT is only a screening procedure and should never be used as laboratory confirmation of a CF diagnosis.

Also physicians need to remain alert to the possibility of CF in infants and children with suggestive symptoms and a history of a negative newborn screening test.

VII. Postmortem Diagnosis

A patient may die before the diagnosis of CF can be confirmed or ruled out. Making the diagnosis remains important for family knowledge and family planning. Postmortem diagnosis can sometimes be strongly suggested by the typical histological pattern of the pancreas and intestines (137), particularly the appendix and ileum (138) with hypereosinophilic secretions overfilling mucous glands.

A 1-g section of fresh tissue from any organ, but particularly the liver, can be used for DNA analysis (139,140). The tissue is best obtained within hours of death, but may suffice even within 72 hours. If the tissue is cut, wrapped in foil, and put in dry ice, it should be usable. DNA analysis can, on occasion, be carried out on paraffin-embedded biopsy or autopsy tissue from years before (141), even—in extenuating circumstances—from autopsy slides. The limitations previously discussed for DNA diagnosis also apply. Finding two CF alleles makes the diagnosis likely; finding one or none may modify the estimated likelihood of CF, but does not rule it out.

References

1. FitzSimmons S. The changing epidemiology of cystic fibrosis. J Pediatr 1993; 122:1–9.
2. Boat TF, Welsh MJ, Beaudet AL. Cystic fibrosis. In: Scriver CF, Beaudet AL, Sly WS, Valle D, eds. The Metabolic Basis of Inherited Disease. New York: McGraw-Hill, 1989:2649–2680.
3. Gaskin K, Gurwitz D, Durie P, Corey M, Levison H, Forstner G. Improved respiratory prognosis in patients with cystic fibrosis with normal fat absorption. J Pediatr 1982; 100:857–862.
4. Kerem E, Corey M, Kerem B-S, et al. The relation between genotype and phenotype in cystic fibrosis—analysis of the most common mutation (ΔF508). N Engl J Med 1990; 323:1517–1522.
5. Kristidis P, Bozon D, Corey, et al. Genetic determination of exocrine pancreatic function in cystic fibrosis. Am J Hum Genet 1992; 50:1178–1184.
6. Hamosh A, Corey M, for The Cystic Fibrosis Genotype–Phenotype Consortium. Correlation between genotype and phenotype in patients with cystic fibrosis. N Engl J Med 1993; 329:1308–1313.
7. Lester LA, Kraut J, Lloyd-Still J, et al. ΔF508 Genotype does not predict disease severity in an ethnically diverse cystic fibrosis population. Pediatrics 1994; 93:114–118.
8. Christian CL. Prenatal diagnosis of cystic fibrosis. Clin Perinatol 1990; 17:779–791.
9. Lemna WK, Feldman GL, Kerem B-S, et al. Mutation analysis for heterozygote detection and the prenatal diagnosis of cystic fibrosis. N Engl J Med 1990; 322:291–296.
10. Johnson JP. Genetic counseling using linked DNA probes: cystic fibrosis as a prototype. J Pediatr 1988; 113:957–963.
11. Mulivor RA, Cook D, Muller F, et al. Analysis of fetal intestinal enzymes in amniotic fluid for the prenatal diagnosis of cystic fibrosis. Am J Hum Genet 1987; 40:131–146.
12. Szabo M, Munnich A, Teichmann F, Huszka M, Veress L, Papp Z. Discriminant analysis for assessing the value of amniotic fluid microvillar enzymes in the prenatal diagnosis of cystic fibrosis. Prenatal Diagnosis 1990; 10:761–769.
13. Beaudet AL, Feldman GL, Fernback SD, et al. Linkage disequilibrium in cystic fibrosis and genetic counseling. Am J Hum Genet 1989; 44:319–326.
14. Hogge WA, Hogge JS, Boehm CD, Sanders RC. Increased echogenicity in the fetal abdomen: use of DNA analysis to establish a diagnosis of cystic fibrosis. J Ultrasound Med 1993; 12:451–454.
15. Dicke JM, Crane JP. Sonographically detected hyperechoic fetal bowel: significance and implications for pregnancy management. Obstet Gynecol 1992; 80:778–782.

16. Foster MA, Nyberg DA, Mahony BS, Mack LA, Marks WM, Raabe RD. Meconium peritonitis: prenatal sonographic findings and their clinical significance. Radiology 1987; 165:661–665.
17. Rescorla FJ, Grosfeld JL, West KJ, Vane DW. Changing patterns of treatment and survival in neonates with meconium ileus. Arch Surg 1989; 142:837–840.
18. Holsclaw DS, Eckstein HB, Chir M, Nixon HH. Meconium ileus: a 20-year review of 109 cases. Am J Dis Child 1965; 109:101–113.
19. Rosenstein BJ. Cystic fibrosis presenting with the meconium plug syndrome. Am J Dis Child 1978; 132:167–169.
20. Olsen MM, Luck SR, Lloyd-Still J, Raffensperger JG. The spectrum of meconium disease in infancy. J Pediatr Surg 1982; 17:479–481.
21. Berdon WE, Baker DH, Becker J, De Sanctis P. Scrotal masses in healed meconium peritonitis. N Engl J Med 1967; 277:585–587.
22. Vinograd I, Mogle P, Peleg O, Alphan G, Lernua OZ. Meconium disease in premature infants with very low birth weight. J Pediatr 1983; 103:963–966.
23. Taylor WF, Qaqundah BY. Neonatal jaundice associated with cystic fibrosis. Am J Dis Child 1972; 123:161–162.
24. Valman HB, Wallis PG. Prolonged neonatal jaundice in cystic fibrosis. Arch Dis Child 1971; 46:805–809.
25. Oppenheimer EH, Esterly JR. Hepatic changes in young infants with cystic fibrosis: possible relation to focal biliary cirrhosis. J Pediatr 1975; 86:683–689.
26. Wilroy RS, Crawford SE, Johnson WW. Cystic fibrosis with extensive fat replacement of the liver. J Pediatr 1966; 68:67–73.
27. Lloyd-Still JD, Khaw K-T, Shwachman H. Severe respiratory disease in infants with cystic fibrosis. Pediatrics 1974; 53:678–682.
28. Stern RC, Boat TF, Wood RE, Matthews LW, Doershuk CF. Treatment and prognosis of nasal polyps in cystic fibrosis. Am J Dis Child 1982; 136:1067–1070.
29. Shwachman H, Kulczycki LL, Mueller HL, Flake CG. Nasal polyposis in patients with cystic fibrosis. Pediatrics 1962; 30:389–401.
30. Wiatrak BJ, Myer CM, Cotton RT. Cystic fibrosis presenting with sinus disease in children. Am J Dis Child 1993; 147:258–260.
31. Strauss RG, West PJ, Silverman FN. Unilateral proptosis in cystic fibrosis. Pediatrics 1969; 43:297–300.
32. Tunkel DE, Naclerio RM, Baroody FM, Rosenstein BJ. Bilateral maxillary sinus mucoceles in an infant with cystic fibrosis. Otolaryngol Head Neck Surg 1994; 111:116–120.
33. Ledesma-Medine J, Osman MS, Girdany BR. Abnormal paranasal sinuses in patients with cystic fibrosis of the pancreas. Pediatr Radiol 1980; 9:61–64.
34. Waring W, Brunt CH, Hilman BC. Mucoid impaction of the bronchi in cystic fibrosis. Pediatrics 1967; 39:166–175.
35. Kulczycki LL, Murphy TM, Bellanti JA. *Pseudomonas* colonization in cystic fibrosis. JAMA 1978; 240:30–34.
36. Kulczycki LL, Shwachman H. Studies in cystic fibrosis of the pancreas: occurrence of rectal prolapse. N Engl J Med 1958; 259:409–412.
37. Zempsky WT, Rosenstein BJ. The cause of rectal prolapse in children. Am J Dis Child 1988; 142:338–339.

38. Hadorn B, Zoppi G, Shmerling DH, Prader A, McIntyre I, Anderson CM. Quantitative assessment of exocrine pancreatic function in infants and children. J Pediatr 1968; 73:39–50.

39. Barbero GJ, Sibinga MS, Marion JM, Seibel R. Stool trypsin and chymotrypsin. Am J Dis Child 1966; 112:536–540.

40. Dalzell AM, Heaf DP. Fluorescein dilaurate test of exocrine pancreatic function in cystic fibrosis. Arch Dis Child 1990; 65:788–789.

41. Nousia-Arvanitakis S, Arvanitakis C, Greenberger NJ. Diagnosis of exocrine pancreatic insufficiency in cystic fibrosis by the synthetic peptide N-benzoyl-L-tyrosyl-p-aminobenzoic acid. J Pediatr 1978; 92:734–737.

42. Cleghorn G, Benjamin L, Corey M, Forstner G, Dati F, Durie P. Serum immunoreactive pancreatic lipase and cationic trypsinogen for the assessment of exocrine pancreatic function in older patients with cystic fibrosis. Pediatrics 1968; 77:301–306.

43. Wolf RO, Taussig LM, Ross ME, Wood RE. Quantitative evaluation of serum pancreatic isoamylases in cystic fibrosis. J Lab Clin Med 1976; 87:164–168.

44. Taussig LM, Wolf RO, Woods RE, Deckelbaum RJ. Use of serum amylase isoenzymes in evaluation of pancreatic function. Pediatrics 1974; 54:229–235.

45. Iovanna JL, Ferec C, Sarles J, Dagorn JC. The pancreatitis-associated protein (PAP). A new candidate for neonatal screening of cystic fibrosis. Comptes Rendus de l Academie des Sciences—Serie Iii, Sciences de la Vie 1994; 317 (6):561–564.

46. Durie PR, Gaskin KJ, Corey M, Kopelman H, Weizman Z, Forstner GG. Pancreatic function testing in cystic fibrosis. J Pediatr Gastroenterol Nutr 1984; 3 (suppl 1):S89–98.

47. Waters DL, Dorney SFA, Gaskin KJ, Gruca MA, O'Halloran M, Wilcken B. Pancreatic function in infants identified as having cystic fibrosis in a neonatal screening program. N Engl J Med 1990; 322:303–308.

48. Couper TRL, Corey M, Moore DJ, Fisher LJ, Forstner GG, Durie PR. Decline of exocrine pancreatic function in cystic fibrosis patients with pancreatic sufficiency. Pediatr Res 1992; 32:179–182.

49. Durie PR. Pathophysiology of the pancreas in cystic fibrosis. Neth J Med 1992; 41:97–100.

50. Holsclaw DS, Rocmans C, Shwachman H. Intussusception in patients with cystic fibrosis. Pediatrics 1971; 48:51–58.

51. Atlas AB, Orenstein SR, Orenstein DM. Pancreatitis in young children with cystic fibrosis. J Pediatr 1992; 120:756–759.

52. Thomas D, Rothberg RM, Lester LA. Cystic fibrosis and gastroesophageal reflux in infancy. Am J Dis Child 1985; 139:66–67.

53. Dolan TF, Meyers A. Mild cystic fibrosis presenting as an asymptomatic distended appendiceal mass: a case report. Clin Pediatr 1975; 14:862–863.

54. Shwachman H, Holsclaw D. Examination of the appendix at laparotomy as a diagnostic clue in cystic fibrosis. N Engl J Med 1972; 286:1300–1301.

55. Oestreich AE, Adelstein EH. Appendicitis as the presenting complaint in cystic fibrosis. J Pediatr Surg 1982; 17:191–194.

56. Gunn T, Belmonte MM, Colle E, Dupont C. Edema as the presenting symptom of cystic fibrosis: difficulties in diagnosis. Am J Dis Child 1978; 132:317–138.

57. Lee PA, Roloff DW, Howatt WF. Hypoproteinemia and anemia in infants with cystic fibrosis. JAMA 1974; 228:585–588.

58. Darmstadt GL, Schmidt CP, Wechsler DS, Tunnessen WW, Rosenstein BJ. Dermatitis as a presenting sign of cystic fibrosis. Arch Dermatol 1992; 128:1358–1364.

59. Hansen RC, Lemen R, Revsin B. Cystic fibrosis manifesting with acrodermatitis enteropathica-like eruption. Arch Dermatol 1983; 119:51–55.

60. Goldman AS, Travis LB, Dodge WF, Daeschner CW. Falsely negative sweat tests in children with cystic fibrosis complicated by hypoproteinemic edema. J Pediatr 1961; 59:301.

61. Ruddy R, Anolik R, Scanlin TF. Hypoelectrolytemia as a presentation and complication of cystic fibrosis. Clin Pediatr 1982; 21:367–396.

62. Beckerman RC, Taussig LM. Hypoelectrolytemia and metabolic alkalosis in infants with cystic fibrosis. Pediatrics 1979; 63:580–583.

63. Kennedy JD, Dinwiddie R, Daman-Willems C, Dillon MJ, Matthew DJ. Pseudo-Bartter's syndrome in cystic fibrosis. Arch Dis Child 1990; 65:786–787.

64. Abernathy RS. Bulging fontanelle as a presenting sign in cystic fibrosis, vitamin A metabolism and effect on CSF pressure. Am J Dis Child 1976; 130:1360–1362.

65. Wilfond BS, Farrell PM, Laxova AN, Mischler E. Severe hemolytic anemia associated with vitamin E deficiency in infants with cystic fibrosis. Clin Pediatr 1994; 33:2–7.

66. Dolan TF Jr. Hemolytic anemia and edema as the initial sign in infants with cystic fibrosis. Clin Pediatr 1976; 15:597–600.

67. Tortenson OL, Humphrey CG, Edson JR. Cystic fibrosis presenting with severe hemorrhage due to vitamin K malabsorption: A report of three cases. Pediatrics 1970; 45:857–860.

68. Goshen R, Kerem E, Shoshani T, et al. Cystic fibrosis manifested as undescended testis and absence of vas deferens. Pediatrics 1992; 90:982–984.

69. Fitzpatrick SB, Rosenstein BJ, Langbaum TS. Diagnosis of cystic fibrosis during adolescence. J Adolesc Health Care 1987; 7:38–43.

70. Stern RC, Boat TF, Doershuk CF, Tucker AS, Miller RB, Matthews LW. Cystic fibrosis diagnosed after age 13. Ann Intern Med 1977; 87:188–191.

71. Reynolds HY, di Sant' Agnese PA, Zierdt CH. Mucoid *Pseudomonas aeruginosa*: a sign of cystic fibrosis in young adults with chronic pulmonary disease? JAMA 1976; 236:2190–2192.

72. Shwachman H, Lebenthal E, Khaw K-T. Recurrent acute pancreatitis in patients with cystic fibrosis with normal pancreatic enzymes. Pediatrics 1975; 55:86–95.

73. Petersen RA, Petersen VS, Robb RM. Vitamin A deficiency with xerophthalmia and night blindness in cystic fibrosis. Am J Dis Child 1968; 116:662–665.

74. Holsclaw DD, Rocmans C, Shwachman H. Abdominal complaints and appendiceal changes leading to the diagnosis of cystic fibrosis. J Pediatr Surg 1974; 9:867–873.

75. Patrizio P, Asch RH, Handelin B, Silber SJ. Aetiology of congenital absence of vas deferens: genetic study of three generations. Hum Reprod 1993; 8:215–220.

76. Anguiano A, Oates RD, Amos JA, et al. Congenital bilateral absence of the vas deferens: a primarily genital form of cystic fibrosis. JAMA 1992; 267:1794–1797.

77. di Sant' Agnese PA, Darling RC, Perera GA, Shea E. Abnormal electrolyte composition of sweat in cystic fibrosis of the pancreas. Pediatrics 1953; 12:549–562.

78. Hardy JD, Davison SHH, Higgins Mu, Polycarpou PN. Sweat tests in the newborn period. Arch Dis Child 1973; 48:316–318.
79. Gibson LE, Cooke RE. A test for concentration of electrolytes in sweat in cystic fibrosis of the pancreas utilizing pilocarpine by iontophoresis. Pediatrics 1959; 23:545–549.
80. Webster HL, Barlow WK. New approach to cystic fibrosis diagnosis by use of an improved sweat induction/collection systems and osmometry. Clin Chem 1981; 27:385–387.
81. Gleeson M, Henry RL. Sweat sodium or chloride? Clin Chem 1991; 37:112.
82. Hall SK, Stableforth DE, Green A. Sweat sodium and chloride concentrations— essential criteria for the diagnosis of cystic fibrosis in adults. Ann Clin Biochem 1990; 27:318–320.
83. Kirk JM, Keston M, McIntosh I, Al Essa S. Variation of sweat sodium and chloride with age in cystic fibrosis and normal populations: further investigations in equivocal cases. Ann Clin Biochem 1992; 29:145–152.
84. Hodson ME, Beldon I, Power R, Duncan FR, Bamber M, Batten JC. Sweat tests to diagnose cystic fibrosis in adults. BMJ 1983; 286:1381–1383.
85. Shwachman H, Mahmoodian A, Neff R. The sweat test: sodium and chloride values. J Pediatr 1981; 98:576–578.
86. Green A, Dodds P, Pennock C. A study of sweat sodium and chloride; criteria for the diagnosis of cystic fibrosis. Ann Clin Biochem 1985; 22:171–176.
87. Augarten A, Hacham S, Kerem E, Kerem BS, Szeinberg A, Laufer J, Doolman R, Altshuler R, Blau H, Bentur L, Gazit E, Katznelson D, Yahav Y. The significance of sweat Cl/Na ratio in patients with borderline sweat test. Pediatr Pulmonol 1995; 20:369–371.
88. Shwachman H, Mahmoodian A, Kopito L, Khaw KT. A standard procedure for measuring conductivity of sweat as a diagnostic test for cystic fibrosis. J Pediatr 1965; 66:432–434.
89. Hammond KB, Turcios NL, Gibson LE. Clinical evaluation of the macroduct sweat collection system and conductivity analyzer in the diagnosis of cystic fibrosis. J Pediatr 1994; 124:255–260.
90. Schoni MH, Kraemer R, Bahler P, Rossi E. Early diagnosis of cystic fibrosis by means of sweat microosmometry. J Pediatr 1984; 104:691–694.
91. Barnes GL, Vaelioja L, McShane S. Sweat testing by capillary collection and osmometry: suitability of the Wescor Macroduct system for screening suspected cystic fibrosis patients. Aust Paediatr J 1988; 24:191–193.
92. Denning CR, Huang NN, Cuasay, et al. Cooperative study comparing three methods of performing sweat tests to diagnose cystic fibrosis. Pediatrics 1980; 66:752–757.
93. Yeung WM, Palmer J, Schidlow D, Bye MR, Huang NN. Evaluation of a paper-patch test for sweat chloride determination. Clin Pediatr 1984; 23:603–607.
94. Warwick WJ, Hansen LG, Werness ME. Quantification of chloride in sweat with the cystic fibrosis indicator system. Clin Chem 1990; 36:96–98.
95. Shwachman H, Mahmoodian A. Pilocarpine iontophoresis sweat testing: results of seven years' experience. In: Rose E, Stoll E, eds. Modern Problems in Pediatrics. New York: 1967:158–182.
96. Davis PB, Del Rio S, Muntz JA, Dieckman L. Sweat chloride concentration in adults with pulmonary diseases. Am Rev Respir Dis 1983; 128:34–37.

97. di Sant' Agnese PA, Davis PA. Cystic fibrosis in adults: 75 cases and a review of 232 cases in the literature. Am J Med 1979; 66:121–32.

98. Davis PB, Hubbard VS, di Sant' Agnese PA. Low sweat electrolytes in a patient with cystic fibrosis. Am J Med 1980; 69:643–646.

99. Strong TV, Smit LS, Turpin SV, et al. Cystic fibrosis gene mutation in two sisters with mild disease and normal sweat electrolyte levels. N Engl J Med 1991; 325:1630–1634.

100. LeGrys VA, Wood RE. Incidence and implications of false-negative sweat test reports in patients with cystic fibrosis. Pediatr Pulmonol 1988; 4:169–172.

101. Rosenstein BJ, Langbaum TS, Gordes E, Brusilow SW. Cystic fibrosis: problems encountered with sweat testing. JAMA 1978; 240:1987–1988.

102. Shwachman H, Mahmoodian A. Quality of sweat test performance in the diagnosis of cystic fibrosis. Clin Chem 1979; 25:158–161.

103. Birkrant DJ, Stern RC. Sweat testing in the 90's. American Journal of Asthma and Allergy for Pediatricians. 1991; 4:194–198.

104. Palmer J, Huang NN, Schidlow D, Bye M. What is the true incidence and significance of false-positive and false-negative sweat tests in cystic fibrosis? 12 years experience with almost 6,000 tests. Cystic Fibrosis Club Abstracts 1984; 25:43

105. Christoffel KS, Lloyd-Still JD, Brown G, Shwachman H. Environmental deprivation and transient elevation of sweat electrolytes. J Pediatr 1985; 107:231–234.

106. Beck R, Goldberg E, Durie PR, Levison H. Elevated sweat chloride levels in anorexia nervosa. J Pediatr 1986; 108:260–262.

107. Orenstein DM, Wasserman AL. Munchausen syndrome by proxy simulating cystic fibrosis. Pediatrics 1986; 78:621–624.

108. Rosenstein BJ, Langbaum TS. Misdiagnosis of cystic fibrosis. Clin Pediatr 1987; 26:78–82.

109. Tsui L-C. The cystic fibrosis transmembrane conductance regulator gene. Am J Respir Crit Care Med 1995; 151S47–S53.

110. Macek M Jr, FitzSimmons S, Mackova A, et al. Distribution of CF mutations in African-Americans reflects admixture and the presence of native alleles. Pediatr Pulmonol 1995; S12:210.

111. Augarten A, Kerem B-S, Yahav Y, et al. Mild cystic fibrosis and normal or borderline sweat test in patients with 3849 + 10kb C → T mutation. Lancet 1993; 342:25–26.

112. Leoni G, Pitzalis S, Podda R, et al. A specific cystic fibrosis mutation (T3381) associated with the phenotype of isolated hypotonic dehydration. J Pediatr 1995; 127:281–283.

113. Burke W, Aitken ML, Chen S-H, Scott CR. Variable severity of pulmonary disease in adults with identical cystic fibrosis mutations. Chest 1992; 102:506–509.

114. DeArce M, O'Brien S, Hegarty J, et al. Deletion delta F508 and clinical expression of cystic fibrosis–related liver disease. Clin Genet 1992; 42:271–272.

115. Rosencker J, Eichler I, Kuhn L, et al. Genetic determination of diabetes in patients with cystic fibrosis. J Pediatr 1995; 127:441–443.

116. Knowles M, Gatzy J, Boucher R. Increased bioelectric potential difference across respiratory epithelia in cystic fibrosis. N Engl J Med 1981; 305:1489–1495.

117. Gowen CW, Lawson EE, Gingras-Leatherman J, Gatzy JT, Boucher RC, Knowles MR. Increased nasal potential difference and amiloride sensitivity in neonates with cystic fibrosis. J Pediatr 1986; 108:517–521.

118. Alton EWFW, Currie D, Logan-Sinclair R, Warner JO, Hodson ME, Geddes DM. Nasal potential difference: a clinical diagnostic test for cystic fibrosis. Eur Respir J 1990; 3:922–926.

119. Alton EWFW, Hay JG, Munro C, Geddes DM. Measurement of nasal potential difference in adult cystic fibrosis, Young's syndrome, and bronchiectasis. Thorax 1987; 42:815–817.

120. NIH statement. Statement from the National Institutes of Health Workshop on population screening for the cystic fibrosis gene. N Engl J Med 1990; 323:70–71.

121. Cutting GR, Curristin SM, Nash E, et al. Analysis of four diverse population groups indicates that a subset of cystic fibrosis mutations occur in common among Caucasians. Am J Hum Genet 1992; 50:1185–1194.

122. Farrell PM, Mischler EH. Newborn screening for cystic fibrosis. Adv Pediatr 1992; 39:35–70.

123. Stephan U, Busch EW, Kollberg H, Hellsing K. Cystic fibrosis detection by means of a test-strip. Pediatrics 1975; 55:35–38.

124. Ryley HC, Neale LM, Brogan TD, Bray PT. Screening for cystic fibrosis in the newborn by meconium analysis. Arch Dis Child 1979; 54:92–97.

125. Bruns WT, Connell TR, Lacey JA, Whilser KE. Test strip meconium screening for cystic fibrosis. Am J Dis Child 1977; 131:71–73.

126. Crossley JR, Elliott RB, Smith PA. Dried-blood spot screening for cystic fibrosis in the newborn. Lancet 1979; 1:472–474.

127. Wilcken B, Brown ARD, Ruwin, Brown DA. Cystic fibrosis screening by dried blood spot trypsin assay: results in 75,000 newborn infants. J Pediatr 1983; 102:383–387.

128. Cassio A, Bernardi F, Piazzi S, et al. Neonatal screening for cystic fibrosis by dried blood spot trypsin assay. Acta Paediatr Scand 1984; 73:554–558.

129. Ryley HC, Deam SM, Williams J, et al. Neonatal screening for cystic fibrosis in Wales and the West Midlands: evaluation of immunoreactive trypsin test. J Clin Pathol 1988; 41:726–729.

130. Heeley AF, Bangert SK. The neonatal detection of cystic fibrosis by measurement of immunoreactive trypsin in blood. Ann Clin Biochem 1992; 29:361–376.

131. Hammond KB, Abman SH, Sokol RJ, Accurso FJ. Efficacy of statewide neonatal screening for cystic fibrosis by assay of trypsinogen concentrations. N Engl J Med 1991; 325:769–774.

132. Rock MJ, Mischler EH, Farrell PM, et al. Newborn screening for cystic fibrosis is complicated by age-related decline in immunoreactive trypsinogen levels. Pediatrics 1990; 85:1001–1007.

133. Bowling FG, McGill JJ, Shepherd RW, Danks DM. Screening for cystic fibrosis: use of ΔF508 mutation. Lancet 1990; 335:925–926.

134. Wilfond BS, Fost N. The cystic fibrosis gene: medical and social implications for heterozygote detection. JAMA 1990; 263:2777–2783.

135. Wilcken B, Chalmers G. Reduced morbidity in patients with cystic fibrosis detected by neonatal screening. Lancet 1985; 2:1319–1321.

136. Reardon MC, Hammond KB, Accurso FJ. Nutritional deficits exist before 2 months of age in some infants with cystic fibrosis identified by screening test. J Pediatr 1984; 105:271–274.

137. Rosenstein BJ, Langbaum TS, Winn K. Unexpected diagnosis of cystic fibrosis at autopsy. South Med J 1984; 77:1383–1385.

138. Tomashefski JF Jr., Abramowski CR, Dahms BB. The pathology of cystic fibrosis. In: Davis PB, ed. *Cystic Fibrosis*. New York: Marcel Dekker, 1993:467.

139. Ozguc M, Tekin A, Erdem H, Yilmaz E, Ayter S, Coskun T, Can A, Gogus S, Caglar M, Kale G, Akcoren Z. Analysis of delta F508 mutation in cystic fibrosis pathology specimens. Pediatr Pathol 1994; 14 (3):491–496.

140. Salcedo M, Chavez M, Ridaura C, Moreno M, Lezena JL, Orozco L. Detection of the cystic fibrosis delta-F508 mutation at autopsy by site-directed mutagenesis. Am J Med Genet 1993; 46(3):268–270.

141. Palacios J, Ezquieta B, Gamallo C, Limeres MA, Benito N, Rodriguez JI, Molano J. Detection of delta F508 cystic fibrosis mutation by polymerase chain reaction from old paraffin-embedded tissues: a retrospective autopsy study. Mod Pathol 1994; 7(3):392–395.

2

The Newly Diagnosed Patient

DAVID M. ORENSTEIN

University of Pittsburgh School of Medicine
and Children's Hospital of Pittsburgh
Pittsburgh, Pennsylvania

Making the diagnosis of cystic fibrosis is the first step in initiating a treatment program that can extend a patient's life—and improve its quality—many fold. Because of the huge prognostic difference that aggressive treatment can make, and because of the complexity of that treatment, hospital admission is almost always indicated for institution of the treatment program. If the patient is sick at diagnosis, hospitalization for intensive treatment may be essential; it is usually indicated in the asymptomatic patient as well. So many devastating misconceptions abound about CF, many of them "confirmed" by a relative's decades-old nursing textbook or encyclopedia, that the diagnosis of CF constitutes a psychological and educational emergency, even when the patient is relatively well. In addition, hospitalization at diagnosis has the effect of emphasizing that this is a serious disease.

Educating the family of a newly diagnosed infant and educating the patient and family when the diagnosis is made later should be carried out largely by, and entirely under the direction of, the patient's attending CF physician. Teaching should begin with a detailed discussion of the disease, including pathophysiology, rationale of treatment, genetics, and prognosis for morbidity and survival. The origin of the name ("cystic fibrosis of the pancreas") must be included in this discussion. Many physicians and counselors find it helpful to present a historical overview as part of their initial discussion: an average survival of 30 years is not a satisfactory situation in and of itself; however, this median prognosis has increased by approximately 27 years since the introduction of comprehensive treatment programs in the late 1950s, providing hope for even more progress during the patient's lifetime. It can also be helpful to point out that our understanding of the cellular and molecular bases of CF has increased tremendously since seminal physiological advances and the isolation of the gene in the 1980s. This information can be expected to lead to even better treatment.

It may be useful to ask the family what they know or have heard about CF. This provides the opportunity to correct misconceptions and address particular concerns. Different families are disturbed by different aspects of CF. It is not unusual, for example, for parents to sit impassively during the discussion of lung destruction and their infant's potentially dramatically shortened life, only to decompensate when they hear about the 98% likelihood of male infertility.

Education can be facilitated by visual aids, and these may be particularly vivid if they are drawn for the family by the physician-educator. The education concerning treatment must include in-person demonstrations, followed by supervised trials by the family as they explain the procedures to their teachers. This approach is important for virtually all aspects of CF treatment and is essential for some such as chest physical therapy and postural drainage, enzyme administration for infants, and introduction of the "flutter" valve device (see Chapter 4.)

There are several useful teaching aids for families, including an excellent video tape and accompanying pamphlet available from McNeil Pharmaceuticals (1000 Route 202, Raritan, NJ 08869-0602; telephone 908-218-6000), a book, *Cystic Fibrosis: A Guide for Patient and Family* by David M. Orenstein, published by Lippincott-Raven Press, and a series of pamphlets available from Genentech, Inc. (460 Point San Bruno Blvd, South San Francisco, CA 94080-4990; telephone 415-225-1000). None of these aids can substitute for the active involvement of the primary CF physician. One approach that many physicians have found useful is to have an initial education session, after which the family can be given the video. The video sensibly suggests taking several breaks during the tape. Then, after an hour or so, the physician, perhaps with various members of the CF care team, can return to field questions. This approach gives the family some time alone, which can be important at this difficult time.

During this initial education and treatment hospitalization, it is important to establish several principles that will serve as the foundation for the rest of the patient's life: (1) the availability of the primary CF physician and the care team, (2) the team's willingness to answer questions and provide education about CF, and (3) the optimism underlying (and justified by) the *aggressive* therapeutic program and worldwide research effort.

If the newly diagnosed patient has a productive cough and pulmonary overinflation, immediate aggressive in-hospital treatment with bronchodilator aerosols, airway clearance techniques, and intravenous antibiotics is usually warranted. Choice of antibiotics is covered in more detail in Chapter 4. These antibiotics should cover *Staphylococcus aureus* and common CF gram-negative pathogens, at least until throat, sputum, or bronchoscopy specimens are available to guide therapy. A typical and effective combination of antibiotics for intravenous administration for the newly diagnosed infant, child, or adolescent is an aminoglycoside and ceftazidime or an aminoglycoside and Timentin.

In addition to intravenous antibiotics, initial hospital treatment usually includes aerosolized bronchodilator (e.g., albuterol), at least in older patients in whom a positive response to bronchodilator is demonstrated on pulmonary function testing. This treatment can be undertaken as a therapeutic trial, with careful monitoring of, for example, oxyhemoglobin saturation, respiratory effort and rate, and auscultatory findings, before and after the treatment. If there is clear benefit, the treatment should continue; if there is clear worsening, it should be stopped. With an equivocal or unclear response, the decision to continue is more difficult. Some experts recommend continuing these treatments because of benefits that are mainly theoretical, or at least more difficult to measure in the acute clinical setting: improved mucociliary transport rates have been reported with beta-agonist bronchodilators in patients with CF (1), and these agents and theophylline may also augment ventilatory muscle strength and endurance in adults with chronic obstructive pulmonary disease (2,3), although this has not been confirmed in CF patients. Many centers continue this treatment despite lack of clear-cut immediate benefit because of the variability of the bronchodilator response in CF: a patient's response at one time is not predictive of the response later, and most have a measurable positive response at some time (4,5). Few patients with mild or moderate disease have a negative response, so benefit at some time is likely and harm is unlikely. The physician should be alert to the possibility that bronchodilators may worsen gastroesophageal reflux, and, therefore, contribute indirectly to worsening of pulmonary status. In a preliminary study (6), CF patients given aerosolized albuterol seem to have maintained better pulmonary function tests than similar CF patients on placebo. Oral beta-agonist agents are usually not very helpful.

Chest physical therapy (PT) and other methods of airway clearance should be instituted at diagnosis. The initial hospitalization is the ideal time for parents to be taught how to administer these treatments. The parents can watch treatments and then be supervised by experienced therapists as they administer the treatments themselves. The opportunity for repeated visits by the instructor (usually a respiratory therapist) and repeated demonstrations by the family makes the inpatient setting ideal for this teaching. Patients may seem to learn the technique in one session, only to discover that they have not fully mastered it. The mucus-clearing procedures should be performed immediately after or during bronchodilator aerosols (allowing the greatest bronchial caliber for maximum clearance). If antibiotic aerosols are to be administered, they should follow chest PT because removing the mucus first provides better access of the inhaled antibiotic to organisms deep in the tracheobronchial tree.

The initial hospitalization gives a convenient setting for assessing pancreatic function. It was long believed that 85%–90% of patients with CF were pancreatic insufficient (7) and thus required enzyme supplementation for optimal growth and nutrition. With the advent and broad application of newborn screening programs, it became clear that, at birth, the incidence of pancreatic insufficiency is considerably lower than originally believed (8). In some infants, the history and physical examination (especially if there happens to be a full diaper) may be suggestive enough to justify the institution of enzyme supplementation. In others, especially in breast-fed infants, however, the stool history may be similar to that of healthy infants, and growth may be good. In these infants, it is reasonable to assess pancreatic exocrine function before instituting pancreatic enzyme therapy. Stool collection and quantification is more likely to be done accurately in the hospital.

If pancreatic insufficiency is obvious clinically or is confirmed by laboratory analysis, either with a formal 72-hour stool fat collection and quantitative analysis or with a qualitative fat stain of a "spot" stool sample or other test, enzyme supplementation can begin. Experienced nurses and nutritionists can help parents learn "tricks" of administering enzymes to newly diagnosed patients (infants, toddlers, or older patients), thus avoiding the frequent frustration that parents of newly diagnosed patients feel in not knowing whether they are giving the enzymes correctly. Hospital personnel can demonstrate the most successful methods of administering the enteric-coated beads.

The confidence that can be instilled in parents in learning, under close supervision, the foundations of the many parts of the complex treatment plan that will be carried out for the rest of the patient's life—influencing the length of that life—is probably not attainable outside the hospital.

References

1.   Wood R, Wanner A, Hirsch J, Farrell P. Tracheal mucociliary transport in patients with cystic fibrosis and its stimulation by terbutaline. Am Rev Respir Dis 1975; 111:733–738.

2. Nava S, Crotti P, Gurrieri G, Fracchia C, Rasmpulla C. Effect of a β_2-agonist (broxaterol) on respiratory muscle strength and endurance in patients with COPD with irreversible airway obstruction. Chest 1992; 101(1):133–140.

3. Murciano D, Auclair M-H, Pariente R, Aubeir M. A randomized, controlled trial of theophylline in patients with severe chronic obstructive pulmonary disease. N Engl J Med 1989; 320(23):1521–1525.

4. Hordvik N, Koenig P, Morris D, Kreutz C, Barbero G. A longitudinal study of bronchodilator responsiveness in cystic fibrosis. Am Rev Respir Dis 1985; 131:889–893.

5. Pattishall E. Longitudinal response of pulmonary function to bronchodilators in cystic fibrosis. Pediatr Pulmonol 1990; 9:80–85.

6. Konig P, Gayer D, Barbero G, Shaffer J. Short-term and long-term effects of albuterol aerosol therapy in cystic fibrosis: a preliminary report. Pediatr Pulmonol 1995; 20:205–214.

7. Wood R, Boat T, Doershuk C. State of the art: cystic fibrosis. Am Rev Respir Dis 1976; 113:833–878.

8. Gaskin K, Waters, D, Dorney S, Gruca M, O'Halloran M, Wilcken B. Assessment of pancreatic function in screened infants with cystic fibrosis. Pediatr Pulmonol 1991; (suppl 7):69–71.

3

General Care of the Hospitalized Cystic Fibrosis Patient

ROBERT C. STERN

Case Western Reserve University School of Medicine
Cleveland, Ohio

I. Introduction

Optimal care of the cystic fibrosis (CF) patient requires attention to the same general principles that apply to any other hospitalized patient. Only more so. When otherwise normal people are hospitalized briefly for an acute illness or surgical procedure, they may be irked by hospital routine, but their long-term health is rarely affected adversely. They live to joke about hospital life. These "healthy" patients with self-limited or curable illnesses may even sustain mild physical injury or unnecessary mental stress due to seemingly incompetent personnel or inane hospital rules, but they generally recover and then often forget the incident altogether.

Editors' note: This chapter differs from the others in that it presents a personal approach of one physician to the hospitalized patient. No one will agree with all of this chapter. However, a chapter such as this one is clearly needed, and this chapter will give many of us food for thought, will provide the next generation of CF caregivers with the opportunity to see hospitalized CF patients through the eyes of an experienced CF physician, and will allow the non-CF world some insight into the problems that physicians encounter when these complex patients are hospitalized. Much of what is covered applies to patients with other chronic illnesses as well.

Cystic fibrosis patients are different. The background level of anxiety is often higher for them and their families. They have a health-threatening (and often a life-threatening) disease. They are destined to be hospitalized many times, perhaps for prolonged periods, and, when they perceive themselves to be victims of hospital incompetence or indifference, or to be at risk for actual physical injury from errors, their attitudes toward physicians and medical care are often profoundly affected. With repeat hospitalizations, CF patients begin to view these episodes as unnecessary and preventable. Some patients may perceive them as almost intentional. Minor physical inconveniences (e.g., "blown veins," "lab errors," delayed initiation of treatment, missed meals, medication errors, inaccurate information) may have only minimal direct impact on physical health but can have indirect (attitudinal) effects that compromise treatment by undermining the patient's and family's faith in the entire medical establishment.

It should be the CF center physician's responsibility to diminish or prevent these minor traumas. To do so, the *physician* must (1) be "on record" as insisting that all hospital personnel be sympathetic to patients' reasonable requests and be responsive to their legitimate complaints, (2) insist on being informed of incidents that threaten patient care, comfort, or confidence in the hospital, and (3) when adverse incidents do occur, reassure the patient and family that the general situation that led to the incident is being addressed. There is seemingly no limit to the variety of ways that hospital routine is stressful. I address some examples in detail, touch on a few more, and list the rest. It will not be difficult for you to think of other examples.

This chapter also discusses some general medical issues, especially those with psychosocial overtones that transcend individual organ system involvement, including addressing non-CF medical problems, performing painful procedures, and advising and recruiting patients for research studies.

II. Psychosocial Issues

A. Continuity of Care

Ideally, from the viewpoint of patient care, the same center physician should see the patient at all outpatient visits and continue to follow up the patient during all inpatient stays. There may be logistic reasons that make this goal difficult to accomplish. However, I doubt that many senior CF center physicians really believe that discontinuous care is intrinsically better than continuous care. How many CF center physicians accept rotating physicians for their own chronic illness care? How many would accept hospital care for a life-threatening illness from a physician whom they have never seen after having been followed by an equally capable specialist as an outpatient for several years? How many would accept specialty care from a physician whom he or she does not like?

There may be reasons that continuous care is difficult to provide, and some compromises may be necessary. However, the need for compromise is not a valid reason for developing a theory of treatment that makes discontinuity of care seem like a platonic ideal. The concept of a "team approach" should be an adjunct to physician continuity, not an excuse to abandon or deemphasize it.

If there is only one CF physician at the center, that physician cannot be expected to be continuously available to every patient around-the-clock every day of the year. However, that does not mean that the physician cannot resume care of the patient as soon as possible. Patient care by a fellow is intrinsically limited to a maximum of 3 years (i.e., the length of the fellowship). That does not preclude the fellow's care being supervised by the same senior attending physician who then takes over continuity care when the fellow moves on. "Protected time for young faculty" has become essential to faculty recruitment. This protection does not have to be "absolute"; perhaps CF patients could be an exception. How many CF patients does a junior faculty member have? How much time is really involved? Some discontinuity may be inevitable, but it should not be worshiped as a major advance in the theory of patient care.

Furthermore, "continuity of care" means true continuity. It extends to both inpatient and outpatient care. What is the point of outpatient continuity if, after several years of seeing the same physician (during relatively good health), a serious complication develops that requires the patient to be hospitalized, and then the patient has to deal with a new supervising physician (or, worse yet, the vagaries of "the service"), just when he or she is sickest and feels most vulnerable?

The First Hospitalization

When a patient is about to be admitted to the center hospital for the first time (or the first time a child is admitted after age 3 years), the physician or CF nurse should give some overview of hospitalization—what to expect, what to demand, what is not worth fussing about. This discussion might include the following:

1. *Hospital personnel:* Residents and interns, medical students, nurses, respiratory therapists, and dieticians, among others, provide direct patient care. Clergy, social workers, child life personnel, music therapists, and others provide ancillary services. The overall responsibility of the senior CF physician should be clearly understood by the patient and the physician—it is the physician who is ultimately responsible for overseeing the patient's total care, including everything from medical treatment to the availability of Froot-Loops for breakfast. The physician may choose to assign the minute-to-minute management of some of these areas to other personnel, but the doctor is responsible for them nonetheless.

2. *Hospital routines:* Topics include the importance of "vital signs" versus the unimportance and nuisance of obtaining excess vital signs, the importance of following the patient's weight versus the insanity of weighing the patient too often, the usefulness of following intake and output versus the lack of need for detailed intake and output measurements in all patients, the pros and cons of calorie counts, the need for and anticipated frequency of follow-up blood tests versus a strategy for minimizing the number of venipunctures, and the "reasons" that sleeping patients are disturbed by nurses at night, seemingly for no rational purpose.

3. *Insurance worries:* Topics include utilization review and retrospective denials, uncovered services, lifetime caps and logical ways to reduce hospital bills, and hospital and insurance policy concerning leaves of absence from the hospital.

4. *Medical risks of hospitalization:* Topics include contagion, medication errors, psychological trauma, sleep deprivation, refusal to eat, acquisition of bad self-care habits after talking with other patients, depression, and psychological regression. Older patients should be told that they have the right to refuse any treatment if they think that it will harm them or is inconsistent with the center physician's plan (e.g., a teenager should not be afraid to refuse a newly ordered drug if he or she remembers having had a serious reaction to it previously.

5. *Other risks of hospitalization:* Topics include falling behind in school work, theft (children should not keep valuables such as money, jewelry, expensive watches, or easily portable, expensive electronic equipment), and kidnapping and random violence (explain safeguards used at the hospital, but acknowledge that the risk can never be reduced to zero).

6. *Parents' decisions and responsibilities:* Discuss whether parents should stay with the child (see below) and the need to "keep the child's life going," for example, to obtain school work and inform physicians of when immunizations are due. Allow (and encourage) the child to interact directly with physicians and other personnel.

7. *Positive features of hospitalization:* Topics include exposure to a "different slice of life" (i.e., interacting with a wide variety of people), learning to cope and interact with medical personnel, learning to survive without a parent present, learning about non-CF medical care and learning about hospitals.

8. *The basics of intravenous treatment* (see also Section III.B, Painful Procedures): The following points should be discussed:
   a. Some drugs cannot be given orally because of inactivation by the gastrointestinal tract or inadequate absorption. Often these drugs

must be given intravenously. Other drugs can be given orally under other circumstances, but the higher doses needed can only be achieved by intravenous (IV) administration.

b. The ease of venous access varies from patient to patient. Congenitally "bad veins" are not correlated with any other aspect of health. (Also, the ability to insert IVs is not necessarily correlated with how well a physician performs in other patient-care arenas; however, physician indifference to the importance of the mechanical aspects of IV therapy to the patient is not a good sign.)

c. The three major (most common) concerns of patients with regard to IV therapy are not warranted:

  (i)   There is no reason to stay awake all night worrying about air bubbles. Patients and parents may spend hours watching a bubble that is adherent to the plastic tube, worried about its breaking free, entering the vein, and causing death. Bubbles of air are frequently infused accidentally. For all practical purposes, this is not dangerous. Television plots that rely on a murder by "a bubble of air" have no basis in fact. It would take approximately 15 full-length IV tubings of air (approximately 100 mL) to threaten the life of an adult man. Theoretically, a bubble of air could traverse an open foramen ovale, gain access to the systemic circulation, enter a carotid artery, and cause a stroke, but has anyone ever actually heard of such a case?

  (ii) What if the IV bottle runs dry? Patients and families may be worried that if the fluid in their IV bottle is used up, air will enter the vein. When the skin is violated (e.g., by a scrape or cut), blood comes out, air does not enter. The same is true of gravity-based IV drips. Infusion pumps have air bubble detectors; they stop infusing and sound an alarm when air is encountered in the tubing.

  (iii) Other patients have the "opposite" worry, that is, that if all the IV fluid in the bottle or bag is used up, a large amount of their blood could back up in the tubing. Even though some blood may enter the tubing, air pressure keeps it to a minimum.

B. Achieving Independence

When fundamentally normal babies, toddlers, and young school-aged children are hospitalized for an acute illness or surgery, around-the-clock presence by a parent or other close family member is widely advocated. This approach is certainly reasonable. It is unrealistic to expect acutely ill or postoperative children to be able to cope with an unfamiliar and frightening environment. In addition, healthy children are rarely hospitalized for very long and are unlikely to have repeated hospital stays. These patients have no need to develop the complex coping skills needed for prolonged life in the hospital.

Cystic fibrosis inpatients may face a much different future. Even if dramatically improved treatment is theoretically attainable, it is possible that it will not be available in time for many of today's patients. Center physicians must act on the assumption that their patients will need the psychological skills to deal with the disease for many years.

Cystic fibrosis is one of only a few chronic diseases that extend from infancy to (potentially late) adulthood. Children with the disease must develop the psychological tools to become the primary decision makers (sometime during teenage years) and to allow their parents to play a less prominent role. Self-sufficiency as hospital inpatients is an essential skill for CF patients. Learning to deal with hospital routine and the diverse personalities of their hospital caretakers takes time.

Appropriate planning early in the patient's "hospital career" can pay important dividends later. Consider suggesting the following to parents: (1) When nurses and doctors ask questions that are directed at or clearly revolve around present symptoms, parents should refrain from immediately giving the answer. Parents should expect the child to answer and give the child a chance to do so. (2) As the child becomes more adapted to the hospital environment, parents should leave the child alone for short periods (e.g., to "go eat," to "make a phone call," to meet someone in the lobby) and gradually lengthen the time they are away from the ward. At first, these absences can be timed to coincide with the presence of a child life worker, but eventually can be extended to other times as well. When the time seems right, the parent should leave the child for the night. This first night alone should be coordinated with the nurse and physician to help ensure that no invasive procedures are done that night, and that the child's only task is to sleep alone. (3) The medical staff should do their best to give the child some feeling of mastery over the hospital environment by accommodating requests that originate with and are presented to them by the child. (4) For somewhat older children, contact with carefully chosen patients ("hospital veterans") can be helpful.

C. Drug-Seeking Behavior and Recreational Use of Drugs

Narcotic addiction and chemical dependency is a complex issue. The diagnosis of drug-seeking behavior is important, however, and CF center physicians should be alert to its possibility in their patients. The patient's socioeconomic background should not be used to "rule out" the possibility of drug abuse and chemical dependency. The diagnosis should be considered in CF patients with one or more of the following findings: (1) sudden request for oral narcotics, particularly for a specific drug and especially for drugs containing hydrocodone or oxycodone (e.g., Histussin, Percodan, Percocet), (2) very frequent requests for refill of any codeine-containing cough syrup, (3) sudden onset of an apparently new problem (e.g., symptoms of nephrolithiasis), which causes severe pain (and requires narcotic analgesia) on the first day of a hospitalization for another indication, (4) failure (refusal) to convert from narcotic to nonnarcotic analgesia after surgery, (5) persistent pain that superficially could be CF-related, but seems to be lasting too long, such as pancreatitis after amylase levels are normal or pleurisy for longer than 1 week, (6) suspicion that the patient is getting narcotic prescriptions from more than one physician or has asked that prescriptions be telephoned in to more than one pharmacy, (7) previous claims of "lost prescription" for narcotic, (8) no evidence of pain (e.g., grimacing or guarding site of alleged pain) during sleep before awakening to ask for the next narcotic dose.

These patients should be told that their use of narcotics is worrisome and that the "pain service" or the "chemical dependency service" will be consulted for help. The only acceptable goal is for the patient to be drug free ("clean and serene") long enough to have a negative urine toxicology screen. If the physician wants to take every possible precaution, he or she could insist that a nurse be present when the urine specimen is obtained.

Drug-seeking behavior can consume virtually all of the patient's energy, thus compromising ability to perform self-care. In extreme cases, it can lead to unnecessary surgery and prolonged hospitalizations. Dealing with these patients can also be stressful for center physicians and nurses. It is best to confront the issue as soon as it is suspected. Similarly, the first time a patient unexpectedly asks for narcotic treatment, it may be worthwhile to insist on a urine sample before the first dose (either to demonstrate that it is free of narcotic metabolites or to freeze and save it, in case such a demonstration might be clinically helpful later.)

Recreational use of drugs is common among CF patients. In addition to their use of the common drugs (e.g., marijuana and cocaine) by the usual routes, many patients have indwelling central venous catheters that they can use for IV injection of virtually any drug. Patients can empty the contents of oral capsules (e.g., antihistamines, antiemetics), mix them with water, and inject the slurry intravenously. If the physician is suspicious, the central access device can be removed and examined for inert powder (the filler of the capsule). Occasionally, this method of drug abuse can be definitively proved by seeing talc in or near pulmonary blood vessels after lobectomy or at autopsy.

D. Child Abuse and Neglect, Munchausen's Syndrome and Munchausen's Syndrome by Proxy, School Phobia, and Malingering

Patients with serious chronic illnesses are not immune to the major psychosocial problems that afflict otherwise healthy persons. When the patient's symptoms and course are atypical, then factitious or fraudulent illness must be considered. Drug-seeking behavior, as discussed, is one of many possible explanations.

Sometimes the patient or family is consciously trying to outwit the physician and "the system." For example, nonmedical issues, unknown to members of the CF team (or forgotten by them), may make prolongation of hospitalization seem advantageous. The patient may be planning to use prolonged hospitalization as legal "ammunition" for a disability claim (or some other insurance purpose). Patients in legal difficulties, particularly if they are facing jail terms, may hope that prolonged hospitalization or the confirmed presence of a complex, severe, or life-threatening medical problem will be seen as a possible extenuating circumstance in their sentencing. Children and teenagers may simply want to delay facing up to undone homework or lack of preparation for an examination. The patient may have made an agreement with a roommate or another patient to stay in the hospital "as long as you do!" Despite the transient nuisance of invasive procedures, patients from poor psychosocial environments (from any socioeconomic group) may find hospital life (with its playroom and child life workers, its comparatively good food and regular mealtimes, its safety from the chaos of their neighborhood and school, or its shelter from drunk or abusive parents) superior to their existence at home.

More serious family psychopathology, such as Munchausen's syndrome or Munchausen's syndrome by proxy and other forms of child abuse should also be considered. Even the diagnosis of CF may have to be reconsidered if there is circumstantial evidence that a parent might be falsifying laboratory data, and the CF team must be alert for these problems.

Serious child neglect for which legal action may be considered (e.g., overt neglect of serious symptoms or illness; failure to supply food, water or shelter; not arriving to take the child home when hospital treatment is no longer needed) is usually easy to detect, and, fortunately, is not very common. However, less obvious child neglect (perhaps "indifference" or "callousness" are better terms), usually not necessitating legal intervention, can be less obvious, but equally important. The most common such problem is (temporary) "abandonment," that is, a parent or other family member "drops" the patient at the hospital, fulfills the admission process, including the admission interview by the nurse and physician, but then never visits until it is time to pick the child up at discharge. When the child's roommates are frequently visited by parents, siblings, pets, and school friends, and receive showers of get-well cards and presents and seemingly continuous phone calls, the comparison may be devastating.

Furthermore, the child with CF may stay long enough to see several sets of roommates come and go. Abandonment is not always detected by hospital personnel who work in shifts and can miss the significance of an "unvisited patient" during their 8-hour duty time. Lonely appearing children should be asked about their last contact from home; those who appear "abandoned" should receive appropriate empathy and extra attention from a child life worker. For some, all that is needed is a medical request that parents visit, call, or write. Alternatively, the child may need help (and, in some hospitals, money) to call home.

School phobias (actually a fear of leaving home) are not uncommon. A young child with a school phobia usually responds well to "treatment" (usually enforced school attendance is all that is needed). When a child who normally does well in school (receives grades of As and Bs) is hospitalized for a puzzling problem for a long period of time, school phobia should be strongly considered, especially if the patient is not overtly worried about missing schoolwork. These children may be difficult to differentiate from those who find that hospital life (e.g., receiving good food and adult attention) is so much better than their home life that prolongation of hospitalization is worth its drawbacks.

Physicians and nurses who are normally astute at detecting these behaviors in healthy children may be confused by the fact that the patient is known to have a potentially life-threatening chronic illness, particularly one like CF, which has many unusual complications, and thus can produce a great variety of symptoms.

E. Group Meetings

Almost all large CF centers have experimented with group meetings. Outpatient group meetings (patients, families, or both), educational meetings for anyone, and panel discussions are not discussed in this chapter. However, there is also a temptation to organize inpatient group meetings (either of patients alone or of patients and families).

The key questions regarding the desirability of group meetings are (1) Whether the sessions help enough people and help them enough to justify having the meeting, and (2) with what frequency would the psychosocial status of the patients or family actually worsen as a result of these meetings.

Most CF team members have formed strong opinions about this issue. The benefit of these sessions probably varies considerably. It is probably not essential to offer group meetings to inpatients. If they are offered, however, some guidelines should be followed: (1) Meetings should not be instituted unless the "leader" or "facilitator" is a stable member of the CF team, one who is likely to be around for several years. (2) Patients must be told that attendance is strictly optional and that persons can leave any meeting at any time if they are not interested in or are not ready to confront the subject being discussed. (3) When a meeting is about to start, a general announcement should be made. (4) No one should be individually "coaxed" to attend; a low turnout is not an excuse to try harder to "round up a few more patients." (5) Evening meetings are less likely to be interrupted for medical procedures and physician visits. (6) Patients should be allowed to return to a few subsequent meetings after discharge. (7) Patients should be encouraged to report "adverse effects" as well as "beneficial effects" of the meetings. A neutral person, one who is uninvolved with planning or facilitating, should be the contact person for this feedback.

F. Insurance Issues

Health insurance in the United States remains in a chaotic transition between being dominantly traditional private insurance (pay for service; no restrictions on access to physician or treatment) to one of many types of systems that restrict the patient's choices and impose increased surveillance and economic restraints on physician activities. Many patients have been cut from insurance rolls and others have seen their insurance costs skyrocket while their coverage has been dramatically reduced. Any patient or family whose insurance is not absolutely secure should be referred to social service on admission.

Regardless of what "system" emerges, some general guidelines will probably remain useful: (1) The indication for hospitalization should be apparent from the admission note. Diagnosis-related groups and other insurance considerations may dictate which of many possible diagnoses should be emphasized. (2) The indication for continued hospitalization should be stated, at least intermittently (for some insurance carriers, daily), in the progress notes. (3) If the patient requires a leave of absence (LOA), from the hospital, the reason should be one that transcends medical considerations such as life-threatening illness, death or funeral of a relative, or required attendance at a court proceeding), and that reason should be documented in the patient's chart. (4) If the patient has a problem for which treatment should not be interrupted and the patient is on a drug that is not included in the hospital formulary, the patient should be instructed to bring enough of the drug to last until the hospital pharmacy can obtain it. Some over-the-counter agents and some prescription drugs (especially for dermatologic problems) may never arrive, and the patient might want to bring enough for the entire hospital stay.

The results of key discussions between the CF physician and insurance company representatives and physicians should be documented in the patient's chart. When the CF physician suspects that such a discussion will be of an adversarial nature, he or she may arrange a conference call to include the patient or family member as well; it is the patient and family who is insured, and the insured individual should have the right to be included on insurance coverage issues that involve health or life. These front-seat opportunities to see an insurance company in action may also help families decide whether to renew their contract (or to recommend that insurance company to friends, relatives, and employers.)

G. Interpersonal Interactions

For patients who are hospitalized repeatedly and for sustained periods of time, social aspects of hospital life become important. The physical and emotional stress of illness, the lifting of some parent-imposed restriction, the necessity to fend for oneself to some degree when parents are not around, a wide array of new "role models," good and bad, and a host of other factors combine to set the stage for the emergence of abnormal interpersonal interactions or the aggravation of previous problems.

Irritability

The tendency to "snap" at friends and family (and familiar members of the health care team), crying for no apparent reason or over a seemingly trivial incident, and similar symptoms should be accepted as part of the illness and not necessarily as a new problem that requires psychotherapeutic intervention. Medical personnel who receive the brunt of these verbal attacks should be reassured that most irritable patients save their worst outbursts for those people with whom they feel the most secure. Being "snapped at" is a compliment of sorts. Parents and spouses should be reassured that the behavior is normal, that the medical staff has been through it before with other patients, and that they should not take these outbursts personally. The key diagnostic question is, Does the patient recognize this irritability, realize it is a manifestation of illness, and feel bad for what he or she has said? If so, every effort should be made to do nothing about it, except to give reassurance.

Unreasonable Demands and Abuse of Hospital Personnel

Generally, irritability can be easily differentiated from overtly pathological behavior, such as persistent cursing, screaming, and throwing of objects with no particular target and with no remorse or insight. The patient (and family if appropriate) should be advised that this behavior will not be tolerated, and it may justify restrictions on movement within the hospital or even premature discharge. The physician or nurse coordinator should point out that aggressive behavior is rarely productive and tends to make therapists less likely to perform well. It also discourages people from even entering the patient's room. Psychiatric consultation may be reasonable for some of these patients.

Reasonable Demands

Occasionally, otherwise compliant and nondemanding patients and families request that a specific nurse or therapist not be assigned to them. I believe that every effort should be made to accommodate these requests, even if the patient does not supply a logical reason for the request. Ironically, the physician is the only member of the hospital health care team who is ever chosen by the patient and family, and, in many cases, even the physician is not actually chosen. All other workers are imposed by the system. The system should be flexible.

Similarly, children who are admitted or transferred to two-bed rooms or four-bed wards can be exposed to a disruptive roommate (one who is out of control or one who, because of illness or neurologic disease, causes continuous commotion, particularly at night). If the patient is frightened or is likely to be adversely affected by loss of sleep, the medical staff should not be surprised or offended if the family requests that "something be done about it."

Interactions with Other Patients

Bad Company

Many parents are worried about their children acquiring "bad habits" while in the hospital by, for example, staying up too late, neglecting personal hygiene, or eating too much "junk food," and they tend to blame these problems on other children. For the most part, these parents should be advised to just "cool it!" There is nothing much that can be done about inpatient interactions, and most of the behaviors that they are worrying about are not terribly important. Parental restrictions can be reimposed when the child returns home, and it is rare that a long-lasting discipline problem ensues.

Exposure to "Dangerous Patients"

Parents' concerns that another patient (or family) represents a physical threat (of violence) to their child are quite different, and these complaints must be taken seriously. Some corrective action is almost always necessary.

H. Continuation of Normal Home Activities and Anticipation of Resumption of "Career"

Gentle insistence that school-aged children keep up with homework (or a requirement that the patient attend school in the hospital), work on scouting badge requirements, or help in planning family vacations or other upcoming events is reassuring in that it helps convey the medical establishment's judgment that the acute problem for which the patient is hospitalized will be overcome, allowing resumption of normal activities.

I. Public Relations

Physicians (and other health care workers) may seem to be scary people. Children may be told that what the doctor says, goes. Period, no questions asked, implying that this infrequently seen and somewhat mysterious person has power that transcends that of even their otherwise all-powerful parents. Physicians do procedures that can hurt the patient (many invasive procedures) or cause considerable inconvenience or deprivation (e.g., recommend a back brace or a cast, prevent participation in athletics, or recommend hospital admission); they can poke and prod into places even a parent does not go; they ask questions about things no one else talks about. They can predict the child's future health, growth, even life expectancy (and knowing the future often seems like control over the future). Clearly, the physician is a person who needs a successful public relations (PR) campaign. Good rapport is useful if the doctor must perform a difficult physical examination (e.g., palpate a painful abdomen); rapport helps compliance. Rapport is a critical component of the patient's and family's choice of physician.

Parents should be aware of the tremendous importance of physician–patient rapport and that the quality of this rapport is generated to a considerable degree by the parent. Family conversations that praise or condemn the medical system or the child's physician have far-reaching consequences. Children who repeatedly hear home discussions about perceived medical errors that supposedly injured one or another family member are much less likely to become cooperative or compliant patients. The family should use reasonable self-assertion and appropriate questioning of the need for particular procedures or treatment, while still maintaining reasonable respect for and trust in the physician. How they do that is up to them, but they should understand that their actions have important consequences.

Opportunity for good PR exists at every physician–patient interaction. The only way to get some of the patient's "PR points"; into the physician's "bank" is for the physician to "earn them" personally. The physician gets no PR credit when the child is given a prize by the receptionist or is taken to a favorite fast-food outlet after the physician visit. The physician does earn valuable points by being as kind and gentle as possible at all times and by including the patient in treatment discussions.

The physician can also earn points by giving the patient the most valuable PR currency of all—time for play and fun. What the physician actually does is all part of the physician's style, but it is important to occasionally do something that is purely fun—perform (or teach) a magic trick, tell a joke, discuss a common interest (e.g., sports, movies), take a personal interest in the patient's nonmedical life. So fool around, clown around, and have some fun. PR activities need not take long to pay big dividends in the long run. The same philosophy also applies to teenagers and adults. Any member of the CF team who has a little extra time before lunch or before a meeting would be well advised to go shopping for PR points at a patient's bedside.

J. Depression

Clinically important depression is less common in patients with CF than other chronic medical conditions, such as inflammatory bowel disease; nonetheless, it does occur, especially in adults, and can be debilitating. In addition to the stress of confronting mortality, the patient may also have to deal with mounting disability, abandonment by spouse (or other important family members) and friends, insurance (and other financial) problems, and changing self-image as weight loss, clubbing, and other externally obvious manifestations of life-threatening illness increase. When such a patient complains of being depressed, the CF physician is unlikely to be surprised. Even so, it does not automatically lessen its severity, and antidepressants may be indicated. Relief of depression, in addition to being a worthwhile goal in itself, can also contribute to general CF treatment by increasing optimism, and, perhaps, increasing enthusiasm for other facets of the therapeutic program.

Clinically significant depression (with or without suicidal ideation) may also be a manifestation of endogenous psychiatric disease. Thus, serious depression in patients with relatively mild CF-related symptoms must be taken seriously, and consultation with a psychiatrist or other mental health professional may be indicated.

Finally, "depression" and sadness may not be the depressed patient's chief complaint. Insomnia or abnormal sleep, "lack of energy," and inability to concentrate (and other symptoms) can all stem from depression. The patient may think that these other symptoms are causing the depression and therefore may not report the depression itself.

If depression is a major clinical problem, whatever its cause, pharmacological intervention is often indicated. For some psychoactive drugs, preliminary laboratory tests may be needed (e.g., electrocardiogram for the tricyclic antidepressants). The initiation of treatment and the choice of therapeutic agent may be supervised by a psychiatrist. Despite the theoretical toxicity of the commonly used antidepressant drugs, notably drying of secretions and sleepiness, CF patients often tolerate them well. In most patients, the improved sense of well being, improved sleep pattern, and increased energy level more than make up for whatever minor toxicity does occur.

III. Medical Issues

A. Contagion

Some pathogens are transmitted from CF to non-CF patients. The protection of non-CF patients from CF pathogens is always a consideration when the CF patient harbors methicillin-resistant *Staphylococcus aureus* (MRSA) in pulmonary secretions. These patients should be isolated according to the hospital's routine for that organism. However, transmission of other common CF pathogens (e.g., *Pseudomonas aeruginosa, Burkholderia cepacia, Xanthomonas maltophilia*) has not seemed to be a problem, even when CF patients have been on the same hospital ward as immunosuppressed patients (e.g., patients with malignancy, human immunodeficiency virus infection.) However, it is prudent to avoid having these patients share a room. Pathogens are also transmitted from non-CF patients to CF patients. CF patients are not known to be more susceptible than normal to the common respiratory viruses. However, some viruses, particularly respiratory syncytial virus, parainfluenza, and influenza, pose a major threat to CF patients, and every effort should be made to protect them from unnecessary exposure. Acquisition of bacterial pathogens from non-CF patients is rarely an issue, and no isolation beyond that indicated for normal children is needed.

Transmission of pathogens among CF patients has become a subject of considerable interest since the demonstration that *B. cepacia*, an often aggressive pathogen, is transmissible among hospitalized CF patients. Ideally, patients who harbor this organism should be housed on a separate ward. At many centers, however, separate rooms with isolation techniques is the only practical approach.

Protection of CF patients who do not harbor *P. aeruginosa* from those who do has long been thought to be unnecessary, but, with the advent of very resistant strains of *P. aeruginosa* (including some resistant to all presently available antimicrobial agents), this issue has been reconsidered recently. Although it is impossible to ensure protection of every CF patient from every strain of *P. aeruginosa* or other potential gram-negative pathogen that is more resistant than his or her own, it is prudent to take reasonable safeguards. In addition, patients who have never been colonised with *P. aeruginosa* (especially newly diagnosed infants) should probably be protected from colonized or infected patients.

B. Painful Procedures

Gaining and Preserving Venous Access

The "quality of life" in the hospital for many CF patients depends heavily on the ease of achieving venous access, the ongoing comfort of the IV infusions, and the length of time each new IV lasts. Quality of hospital life also depends on the patient's mind set about the trauma of IV insertion and the nuisance of having an IV at all. It is usually worthwhile to make a general assessment of the patient's IV status on admission. This assessment is the responsibility of the CF center physician or nurse. House staff and hospital IV teams are unlikely to think about the long-range treatment implications of inserting an IV line. Quality of hospital life partially determines patient compliance with advice to initiate IV antibiotic treatment or to enter the hospital.

There is some difference of opinion concerning details, but it is important that a CF center develop some policy concerning the technique and logistics of IV treatment. A reasonable policy is as follows:

Preservation of Venipuncture Sites

Other than a "seconds-are-important" life-threatening emergency, the antecubital veins, which are needed for blood sampling for the rest of the patient's life, should never be used for IV access. There are no exceptions, not even for infants and toddlers, not even for central line access. Fibrosing thromboses and phlebitis eventually develop in antecubital veins even if they are spared exposure to schlerosing drugs. Once antecubital veins have been scarred and lost, the quality of the patient's life in the hospital is dramatically compromised. Furthermore, the high flow through antecubital veins may partially resurrect superficial veins in the upper arm after they are used for central line access. Loss of the antecubital veins also prevents recovery of proximal "pipelines" (i.e., the basilic and cephalic veins), which can then be used for central catheter insertion (see Appendix 1).

To optimize the patient's attitude:

1. Avoid any implication that IV insertion is such a terrible event that it must be delayed or circumvented at all costs. Consider the following two statements made by nurse or physician after IV insertion: (1) "Now, be very careful with that IV or they [OR I] will have to put another one in." (2) "OK, you're all set. You can do whatever you want—if the IV comes out [the only thing that will happen is that I'll [OR they'll] put another one in.

2. Allow older patients (if they wish) the option of having their friends come into the treatment room (or watch at the bedside) when IVs are inserted. Involve the patient (and friends) in the procedure. The patient or a friend (fellow patient) can stretch the skin over the vein or help immobilize the hand and wrist during insertion. An added benefit is that a nurse or other assistant may not be necessary. Patients gain mental strength from numbers, and the fact that the physician and nurse permit the conversion of IV insertion from a dreaded lonely trip to treatment room to a social event implies that the procedure is not that terrible.

3. Encourage patients to watch the procedure (i.e., avoid any type of distraction by parents, such as the "don't look at it" approach or the "think of something nice; what do you want for dinner" approach). The real message of "don't watch" or "don't think about it" is "something so terrible is going to happen to your arm that I don't think you'll be able to stand looking at it." That message is not exactly likely to engender calm.

4. Use local anaesthesia for IV insertion. It is probably true (as skeptics point out) that the pain of injecting lidocaine is often no less than the pain of IV insertion. That is assuming that the insertion is an unevent-

ful "clean hit." If probing is necessary, the anesthetic is worthwhile. Mainly, however, the use of anaesthetic every time virtually guarantees the patient that the procudure will hurt about the same amount each time, and he or she can prepare for it. It is the uncertainty of pain (plus the uncertainty of success) that drives patients crazy. The use of Eutectic Mixture of Local Anaesthetic (EMLA) may be helpful. However, the EMLA cream must be applied 45 minutes before the IV insertion, which also means that the operator must either get the IV on the first try or be willing to come back 45 minutes later (or use EMLA on many potential IV sites initially).

5. Avoid using the upper arm for any IV line other than a central catheter. Even "midline catheters," inserted at or near the antecubital space and extending into the mid-upper arm, although they do tend to last longer than ordinary peripheral catheters, also result in scarring of the large veins of the upper arm, which can be better used later for central line access.

6. For a given course of intravenous antibiotics in a patient with a paucity of peripheral veins, consider the use of a percutaneously inserted central catheter (PICC) preferably via the basilic vein, but the cephalic can sometimes be used as well. [Direct entry into the subclavian vein (at the the clavicle) involves a substantial risk of pneumothorax.] PICCs usually last for the entire treatment course, and can then be removed, eliminating the ongoing risk of a foreign body infection occurring between hospital stays. One easy, quick, and safe method for insertion of a PICC at the bedside is provided in Appendix 1.

7. A Mediport (or other line placed near the subclavian vein) is usually functionally better (although cosmetically less well accepted, especially by women) than a PAS-PORT (or other line with its access port in the arm). The Mediport infection rate may be lower and, in my experience, there is less risk of occlusive thrombosis. Furthersome, the Mediport allows the patient a greater chance for independence because he or she can use both hands to access the line. If upper extremity veins and the subclavian and jugular veins cannot be used, if cosmetic considerations are important, or if patient and physician preference dictates, these ports can also be placed in the upper leg (using the femoral vein).

8. Use PICCs (or central access ports such as Mediport and PAS-PORT) if very corrosive IV antibiotics, such as imipenem, nafcillin, and piperacillin, are needed. There is nothing gained by using peripheral veins first. It is unlikely that treatment can be sustained, and immediate use of a central catheter saves peripheral veins.

9. Tape IV lines flush to the skin; the dressing should be occlusive—no air entry to the insertion site is needed. (No antibiotic ointment should be used, because it results in loosening of tape, it changes spatial relations within the dressing, and it often leads to the loss of the line.) If the line is not over a joint, no arm board or protective "houses" are needed. Furthermore, infection rates are extremely low in IV sites in CF patients, so local antibiotics are not needed. Peripheral IV lines need not be arbitrarily removed after a given time (e.g., 2 or 3 days) as is commonly recommended. Infection and clinically important phlebitis are extremely uncommon.

10. Establish rigid policies regarding who inserts lines and the number of "misses" they are allowed at least for patients with proven paucity of IV sites.

Arterial Blood Sampling

Pain is minimized when arterial puncture is done correctly. In general, I do not use injectable local anaesthesia: (1) the needle used for arterial puncture is small (26 gauge), (2) the wall of the artery can rarely be anesthetized anyway, and (3) the chance for success is reduced by having additional fluid in the subcutaneous tissue above the artery. (I have no experience using EMLA for arterial puncture; it may be worthwhile. However, the pain of arterial puncture should be minimal enough that even EMLA is unnecessary in most older patients.) The operator must feel and aim for the artery (not the pulse). They are not the same. The pulse is a nonspecific throbbing blob of tissue; the artery is a cylindrical three-dimensional structure. Pain is minimized by using the smallest possible (usually 26-gauge) needle and keeping the needle at a minimal (i.e., approximately 20°–30°) angle to the skin. There is no need to enter the skin at a 90° angle and impale the artery against the bone. The radial artery is very close to the surface of the body at the wrist.

C. Continuation of Well Child Care

Despite the CF center's intention to leave routine care to the patient's general pediatrician or family physician. I believe that only a true medical contraindication should prevent the continuation of routine immunization in hospital. These immunizations are important for psychosocial reasons (by reinforcing the fact that the necessity for hospitalization does not mean that the medical establishment believes that all hope for a normal childhood has been lost), medical reasons (some preventable diseases such as measles or severe *Haemophilus influenzae* infections have substantial implication for the lungs), and logistic, reasons (there are so many immunizations needed during infancy that it is getting difficult to find the opportunity to give all of them). The patient's primary physician can be informed of the immunizations given in the hospital, together with an explanation of why they were continued in hospital.

D. Addressing the Patient's Non-CF Medical Problems

The CF specialist tends to categorize the inpatient's medical problems as either "CF-related" or "CF-unrelated." In all likelihood, the patient does not. Patients just have "medical problems," all of which are consuming their energy and that of their parents. Important non-CF problems should not be ignored. Every issue that is successfully addressed allows the patient and family to devote more energy to the CF problem that necessitated hospitalization. For example, benign hemangiomas and other minor congenital anomalies in infants are unlikely to require treatment, but will probably require the reassurance of a specialist or surgeon; other examples are hyperactivity in elementary school–aged children, acne in teenagers, and, in patients of any age, orthopedic problems, suspected hernia, developmental delay, headache, suspicious heart murmur, and failure-to-grow beyond that expected from CF alone.

Systemic complaints that may or may not be related to CF such as fever and headache (see Chapter 4) should also be addressed. Fever can be a particularly vexing problem. Some features of CF that are important to consider in febrile patients are as follows:

1. Many CF patients, particularly those with advanced pulmonary disease, have consistently low central body temperature (35.5°C–36.5°C) Patients who say they feel feverish but have temperatures in the 37°C–38°C range may warrant some workup, particularly if their present temperatures are consistently above their previous baseline.
2. Newly colonized or infected patients with *B. cepacia* and *X. maltophilia* are occasionally febrile; these organisms should be sought in newly febrile patients. Occasionally, a new pulmonary complication (e.g., lung abscess or empyema) can cause fever without a new organism being present on culture.
3. Mycobacterial and fungal infections should be sought. Atypical mycobacteria occasionally cause disease (see Chapter 4).
4. Brain abscess, usually caused by alpha-streptococci, has a slightly increased incidence in CF. This diagnosis should be seriously considered in febrile CF patients, especially those with substantial complaint of headache.
5. The patient with a percutaneously inserted central catheter or semipermanent central venous access device (whether it is being used or not) should have appropriate blood cultures (obtained from the line if

possible). *Staphylococcus epidermidis* is the most common infecting organism, but the alpha-streptococcus and *B. cepacia* are occasionally found in these lines. For *S. epidermidis* and alpha-streptococcus infections, depending on the number of previous line infections and the importance of maintaining the line, an attempt can be made to save it by treatment with vancomycin. If *B. cepacia* is found, the line should be removed.

6. Inflammatory bowel disease is always in the differential diagnosis of fever of unknown origin, but diagnosis is often delayed in CF patient's because the symptoms (e.g., diarrhea and abdominal pain), physical findings (e.g., clubbing and abdominal tenderness), and laboratory findings (e.g., elevated erythrocyte sedimentation rate and anemia) are likely to be dismissed as CF related.

E. Addressing All the Patient's CF Problems

Whatever the chief complaint or primary reason for hospitalization of a CF patient, the physician must begin addressing all CF-related problems immediately. This is particularly true for patients with substantial pulmonary problems who are admitted for a nonpulmonary indication. A decision concerning the need for antibiotics should be made on admission. It is often prudent to start IV antibiotic treatment immediately. If the primary problem is resolved quickly, the treatment can be interrupted and the patient discharged. However, if the primary problem is serious (perhaps requiring surgery), the patient will be in better condition for surgery if his or her lungs are already in or near optimal condition. Minor CF problems (e.g., joint pain (see Chapter 4), chronic headache (See Chapter 4), and chronic abdominal pain (see Chapter 5) are also best addressed early, simultaneous with the chief complaint.

F. Confidentiality Issues

Several factors contribute to making confidentiality more of a problem among CF patients and their caretakers than it is for almost any other patient group: (1) patients are admitted often and thus form friendships with many other CF patients, (2) CF patients have a relatively long "hospital career," often spanning many years, (3) CF is one of the few pediatric chronic illnesses that necessitate frequent hospitalizations for teenagers, 4) CF patients' interactions with caretakers (e.g., respiratory therapists during chest physiotherapy) are often lengthy, (5) despite their ongoing illness, many CF patients often have a relatively normal appearance and have relatively normal social interests and activities, and (6) CF patients vary widely in their views of what medical and nonmedical information is confidential.

A reasonable approach to some aspects of confidentiality follows:

1. All members of the CF team should be educated with regard to the importance of confidentiality, and the center policy should be reemphasized at intervals.
2. All patient information is confidential, that is, it is not transmitted to any nonmedical person and is transmitted only to those medical personnel who need it to help them take care of the patient involved. If such information is to be disseminated for education, the identity of the patient should not be revealed unnecesarily unless the information in question was conveyed to the caretaker in public coversation, the patient (or primary CF physician) says that the information need not be kept confidential, or the information is available from a public source (e.g., published engagement or marriage announcement).
3. Patients and families should be informed of the center's confidentiality policy.
4. Unless parents have given approval (at least verbally) to the contrary, complex medical information should not be released to other family members (including siblings and grandparents) or to family friends and neighbors.
5. All personnel, but particularly physicians, must be aware of "who else is listening" in multipatient hospital rooms, waiting rooms, corridors, and elevators. A family speaking among themselves in a foreign language may understand English; a retarded child may be able to repeat what is said.
6. Nonphysicians should never make an advance commitment to withhold information from the physician.
7. Demographic information (e.g., addresses and telephone numbers; address lists) should not be released without consent.
8. Patients and families should be told that all laboratory results, including culture results, are confidential. The physician cannot tell one patient to "beware" of another because that patient has had MRSA or *B. cepacia* recovered from cultures. Therefore, all patients must make their own decisions with regard to exposure to other people with CF.
9. Certain information (e.g., genetics data) will not be released unless the patient or legal guardian gives witnessed written consent.

When a patient relates information in confidence, but the caregiver thinks the information should be transmitted to a parent, the matter should be discussed with the center physician or nurse coordinator. One of these two individuals may already have dealt with the same issue, and even if they have not, they are still in the best position to resolve the problem.

G. Noncompliance and Denial

The recommended home regimen for most patients with CF is more complicated than for virtually any other long-lasting illness. It involves attention to several organ systems, requires multiple medications administered by different routes, entails several different treatment modalities (e.g., oral medications, aerosols, physiotherapy, dietary restrictions or supplements, and environmental precautions such as avoiding prolonged hear exposure), and may require the assistance of another person (e.g., for postural drainage). It is time consuming. It may require modification depending on present health (e.g., bronchodilators for wheezing) and other variables (e.g., weather or illness in other family members). Compliance with medical advice is extremely variable among patients and for the same patient at different times. Some of the inpatient issues and recommendations discussed in this chapter can be extended to the outpatient. In addition, the patient brings to the hospital personal experience with whatever degree of compliance (and its apparent success or failure) that had been habit at home.

Superficially, the issue of compliance with hospital treatment would seem to be less of of a problem: the doctor writes orders and the hospital personnel carry them out. But, it is not that simple. Even though the IV antibiotic doses are rarely missed, just about everything else can be sabotaged by noncompliance (intentional omission of oral drug doses, lackadaisical participation in airway clearance, or avoidance of follow-up laboratory tests such as failure to supply urine specimens or omission of interval blood glucose determinations for diabetes management).

The physician's ability to prevent and to deal with noncompliance is considerably enhanced by continuity of care (see Section II.A, Continuity of Care). In one approach, all patients, regardless of medical assessment of degree of compliance, can be told:

1. What the physician's policy is regarding compliance.
2. That the physician is, to some extent, emotionally invested in how the patient feels, but not at all emotionally invested in whether the physician's advise is followed. In other words, the physician would rather the patient do well (while ignoring the physician's advice) than do poorly while being completely compliant. However, the physician will not lose any sleep about a patient's noncompliance.
3. That the physician expects that the patient and family will tell the physician what is actually happening with regard to the patient's adherence to medical advice (not what the patient or family thinks the doctor wants to hear). In return, the physician will not berate the patient for noncompliance.
4. That the physician believes that CF is always a threat to health and life and that compliant patients usually do better. However, that does not mean that noncompliance guarantees worsening (and death) or

that compliance guarantees improvement, loss or absence of symptoms, and longevity. However, the individual patient usually does better if he or she is compliant.

5. That the physician believes that patients and families often have a legitimate reason for being noncompliant (e.g., drug side effects, a family member who had a severe reaction to the same drug, no time for treatment, or no money for drugs) and that there may be another approach to treatment that is acceptable, but finding an alternative is impossible if the patient does not relate what is actually happening.

6. That if the patient falsely claims compliance and the physician thinks that health is deteriorating, more dangerous treatment may be prescribed instead of simply reemphasizing what is already recommended.

7. That continued failure to accept a given hospital treatment (e.g., mucus clearance) will result in its being discontinued. In other words, there is no reason for a therapist to come if the patient is not going to cooperate. This does not mean that the physician will immediately "kick the patient out of the hospital" if one of many types of treatments is refused. The physician must weigh many factors before deciding whether to discontinue hospital treatment.

8. That no one will make judgmental or derogatory comments if a compliant patient becomes noncompliant (except to reemphasize some of the above points). No one will make, "I told you so" statements if a noncompliant patient gets sicker and then becomes compliant.

9. That not everyone in the hospital is a member of the CF team and that not everyone has the same approach to noncompliance.

10. That compliance is not necessarily "all-or-none." Some components of the treatment plan are effective, at least to some extent, without the others.

Therapeutic approaches to noncompliance include the following:

1. Offer opportunity to discuss issues with patients who are "lifetime compliers" or "born-again compliers."

2. Be sure the patient and family understands the rationale of the treatment in question.

3. Be sympathetic to the trials and tribulations of CF care and to the most common reasons for noncompliance: (1) Compliance may be a nuisance and time consuming, (2) each time treatment is done or drug is taken, the patient is forced to think momentarily about the fact that he or she has CF, (3) there is an overwhelming need to be normal (even supernormal) especially during the teenage years, (4) treatment is expensive, (5) for some components of therapy, there is a lack of an immediate "pay-off" for compliance, that is, the patient does not feel

better right away, and (6) the patient is curious about the consequences of omission of treatment.

4. Be amenable to "compromise" so the patient and family can have the feeling of being in compliance with the physician's advice (and be doing at least some of it), rather than being secretly and totally noncompliant.

5. Have occasional short notices in the center's newsletter about noncompliance; this may encourage the patient to raise the issue at the next appointment. Compliance issues raised by patients are likely to be more easily addressed than those unexpectedly raised by the doctor or other CF team member.

Noncompliance is not synonymous with denial, and not all denial is bad. Denial can cause noncompliance (e.g., a teenager may suddenly claim that his or her diagnosis was an error and stop taking pancreatic enzyme replacement). On the other hand, the patient with intractable heart failure who "refuses to believe" that the statistics relative to survival after overt heart failure apply to him or her also has denial. However, if the patient is still following all physician recommendations, the prognosis may be better than for the patient who has totally accepted imminent death and stopped all treatment because it is "futile."

H. Participation in Research Studies: The Center's Obligation to CF Patients

Cystic fibrosis patients are in great demand as research volunteers. Center physicians have an obligation to recruit their patients (and the patients have a vested interest in volunteering) for studies that promise to elucidate important features of pathogenesis or that propose to test a promising new treatment. However, these patients are also popular subjects for other research projects, including some that are not likely to help CF research at all and others that are local "curiosity projects" in which data are used for administrative or educational purposes with no chance of peer review publication. The center physician must balance the advantages and disadvantages of participation in these studies and protect the patients from scientific (and pseudoscientific) exploitation. Whenever "main line" CF research is competing for material or volunteers with a mutually exclusive non-CF reaserch, the CF center physician should attempt to complete recruitment for the CF project first.

Laboratory studies of patient samples (e.g., urine, sputum, saliva, or hair), which can be obtained without an invasive procedure, are rarely a problem. Questionnaire studies that do not subject the patient to psychological stress should also be supported (as long as the individual patient is not overused). For older patients, studies that require samples or information that can be obtained using mildly invasive procedures and entailing minimal risk (e.g., venipuncture, sweat collection, and pulmonary function testing) should almost always be encouraged, unless there is a specific patient problem (e.g., poor peripheral veins). However, every effort should be made to minimize patient discomfort such as by coordinating venipunctures for research and clinically needed samples.

Cystic fibrosis patients are ideal control subjects for some non-CF studies (e.g., on another chronic illness) or for studies on more peripheral issues (involving, for example, psychology, medical cost analyses, or medical education studies). CF patients have a disease for which definitive diagnosis is possible, and they are frequently hospitalized. Disease severity can be quantified by a variety of scoring systems, and many CF patients are amenable to medical research in general. Cystic fibrosis center policy should require that the patient's primary CF physician (1) approve participation in any study, CF related or not (2) consider possible adverse interactions of different studies or potentially adverse restrictions imposed on study participants (e.g., an unreasonable number of total blood samples is requested or the study requires that the patient take a certain class of drugs such as antihistamines or beta-adrenergic blocking agents that might otherwise be contraindicated), (3) ensure the patient's ability to refuse because some patients cannot say "no" to study requests and need an advocate.

At the other end of the spectrum, as modern medical research zeroes in on the fundamental pathophysiology of the disease and as geneticists begin tests on gene transfer, there will be increased demand for patient participation in exceedingly complicated research projects of long duration (months or years). The greater the potential benefit, the more inconvenience, risk, and pain that patients can be legitimately requested to accept. Aggressive patient recruitment can then be justified. At the same time, however, CF patients should be more carefully protected from extraneous (non-CF) research projects.

I. Presentation of Medical Information to Patients and Families

Communicating medical information is one of the most important of the fundamental skills necessary for medical practice. Physicians should continue to improve at this all-important component of the art of medicine throughout their careers. There is no one best method. Physicians vary greatly in "style" and are greatly influenced by their own past experience and errors. General points regarding factors that are crucial to successful communication with very sick or very worried people follow. These suggestions are not intended to imply that this is the only correct way of communicating but they may be helpful. Some of the ideas are obvious, but commonly ignored.

1. **If possible, communication should occur when the patient or family is most likely to be receptive and capable of concentrating**. The physician or nurse is then optimally effective, the information

communicated faster and the patient or family remembering it better. The best time for discussion can often be predicted. In my opinion, the general explanation of CF, its treatment, and its prognosis, that is, the "overview," to the family of a newly diagnosed patient is almost always best done as soon as possible after the responsible center physician has seen the patient and met the family. On the other hand, discussion of a serious change in prognosis (e.g., after onset of overt heart failure) is best done when the patient is "on the road" toward improvement (e.g., after oxygen therapy has been optimized and diuretics have had some effect).

2. **Medical information of any complexity cannot be communicated unless the participants are seated and the patient and family believe that the physician is not distracted by the need to get to another appointment.** Sitting down allows the patient and family to concentrate on the message, rather than on how they will be able to squeeze in their questions before the physician escapes. In the long run, sitting down saves time.

3. **Pathophysiology and rationale of treatment cannot be presented unless the patient and family understand the pertinent aspects of the affected organ's normal physiology.** Explanation or review of the basic physiology of the lung or pancreas should take no more than 2 minutes. The physician will do better starting with a blank sheet of paper and drawing diagrams. When presented with preprinted diagrams, however simple they may be, the patient and family may feel that the physician is "ahead of them already" and that they will never "catch up." Having a preprinted diagram of the major airways or of the gastrointestinal tract saves at most 30 seconds. It is 30 seconds well spent for the physician to draw and label the crucial features. Similarly, a three-dimensional model (e.g., of the lung) deprives the patient and family of something they can take home with them to help illustrate what they learned at the hospital. At the least, the drawing, which the physician made especially for them, sends a message that the CF team is interested in them as individuals and is willing to spend time with them.

4. **The "universal questions" must be answered somewhere along the way.** What do I have and how sure are you that I have it? How bad is it and is there any treatment? What will happen if it is not treated at all? What is your recommendation? How expensive is the treatment, how long will it be necessary, how much will it cost, how much will it hurt, and how sure are you that it will help or work? Why did I get sick? (The answer to the last question must include attention to patient and family guilt, even if it is unjustified guilt, as well as to the scien-

tific explanation of what went wrong that led to the present problem i.e., the "proximate cause.")

5. **No unexplained medical or scientific word can slip by without being defined.** This is more important than it seems. For some patients and families, not understanding even a single word early in the session—even if the word is not at all important to the main message—results in sufficient loss of rapport to make it impossible to convey the important points. For example, the patient and family cannot be assumed to understand the following words and phrases: ventilation, air exchange, rales, rhonchi, perfusion, and alveolus. They cannot be expected to know the difference between bacteria and viruses (or even fungi), or between allergy and toxicity.

6. If the patient is an infant or a child who is too young to participate, discussions go more smoothly if the patient is not present. The family may wish to bring another relative to act as baby-sitter for a long meeting. If this is not feasible, perhaps a volunteer, a child life worker, or a nurse can stay with the patient.

7. Even patients who seem to have an extensive medical vocabulary may use a word (e.g., "croupy cough," "wheezing," or "scarring") to mean something quite different from what the physician intended. Common terms (e.g., "severe" or "scarring") can be misconstrued with heavy emotional toll.

Precision in the use of medical terms is a major step toward elimination of confusion. A proposed hospitalization for "clean out" could suggest a bronchoscopic washout to one patient and IV antibiotic treatment to another. Why not say the medically correct (and unambiguous) phrase, "admission for intravenous antibiotic treatment of lung infection"? Patients and families may talk about "clean-outs" (or any other phrases), but center personnel should be as precise as possible. A patient whose increased symptons started after a typical upper respiratory tract infection and is told that he or she has to be admitted because of exacerbation of CF lung infection secondary to "the flu" will be understandably resistant to receiving influenza vaccine again the next year (when it has obviously "failed" this year). Why not reserve "the flu" for "influenza" and use "viral illness" or "a cold" otherwise?

On the other hand, the use of the technically correct, "pneumonia" to describe findings on a CF radiograph can cause unnecessary confusion because "pneumonia" has worrisome connotations to many lay persons. In this case, "CF changes," "mucus retention," or "scarring" would transmit more precise and useful information.

8. Cystic fibrosis patients receive progress reports and advice, some solicited and some not, from many people during each hospital stay. There are few hospital incidents more unnerving to patients and families than receiving apparently contradictory information on treatment or prognosis of a potentially fatal illness from different members of the health care team. In addition, even when professionals have the same opinion, the patient and family members may be confused and hear conflict when none was intended. Furthermore, patients receive information from individuals who are not primary members of the CF team and who therefore may not have even heard the "party line" on a given issue. Some inconsistency is unavoidable (perhaps the professionals really do disagree), but the final arbiter is the patient's center physician (and, for some issues, the nurse coordinator). Physicians and nurses should coordinate their presentations on key topics.

Appendix 1:   A Method for Insertion of Central Venous Catheter via the Basilic or Cephalic Vein

1. The basilic vein is preferable to the cephalic; the route the catheter must take is straighter and movement of the shoulder joint does not disturb the line much. The vein can be entered anywhere in the upper arm, but it is generally optimal to enter the vein about one-fourth to one-third of the way down from the axilla toward the elbow.
2. The entire procedure is done with the patient lying on his or her back and with the arm fully extended toward the operator (at 90° from the body). After the vein is located and the site cleaned with alcohol, local anesthesia is given with 1% or 2% lidocaine. A 16-GA 2-in. Medicut (Catalog number 8888-100222; Sherwood Medical; Tullamore, Ireland) is then inserted.
3. The stylet of the Medicut is removed and the central catheter [12-in. Intracath (17-GA needle, 19-GA catheter; catalog number 3831741) Becton Dickinson; Sandy, UT] is inserted through the introducer. The needle included with the Intracath is not used at all; it should be discarded **before** the catheter is used. The stylet of the Intracath is not inserted—only the plastic catheter is fed into the introducer. Note: some large adults may need a catheter that is longer than 12 in.—this can be fashioned by trimming a 24-in. catheter (catalog number 3831841). If the introducer must be inserted more distally in the upper arm, a somewhat longer catheter (e.g., approximately 15 in.) may also be better.

4. When the catheter is fully inserted, its hub fits into the introducer. A T-connector is then attached to the central catheter, and the whole system is flushed with heparinized saline.

5. **The introducer is left in the vein.** The introducer–catheter is then securely taped in place such that the apparatus at the insertion site is not easily wiggled. No sutures are needed. The line is taped occlusively (no air access). Antibiotic ointment *is not* used. The dressing should not be changed unless absolutely necessary. Routine dressing changes are not needed. Occasionally, there is bleeding from the insertion site, with some blood accumulating under the tape. If this is not enough to actually loosen the tape, no action is needed.

6. Radiologic confirmation of position is then obtained. If position is not acceptable, the central catheter is removed and a new catheter inserted through the same introducer with the patient's head and neck in a different position. This process is repeated until positioning is acceptable. Correct position is almost always attained with the first catheter, but occasionally two or more attempts are needed.

7. The line is flushed with heparinized saline each time the patient is "unhooked" (i.e., before disconnecting the patient between doses).

8. If the central line becomes occluded and cannot be cleared with a small amount (0.05 mL) of heparinized saline in a tuberculin syringe inserted directly into the hub of the central catheter, then the central catheter can be removed and a new line inserted via the same introducer (which has been left in place). (Radiologic confirmation of position should be repeated.) If the introducer kinks, the central line can occasionally be used as a guide wire for insertion of a new introducer (and central catheter), but this would probably take some (telephone) consultation with someone experienced in this technique.

Acknowledgment

Supported in part by Grant DK 27651 from the National Institutes of Health and by grants from the Cystic Fibrosis Foundation and United Way Services of Greater Cleveland.

4

Inpatient Treatment of Cystic Fibrosis Pulmonary Disease

ROBERT C. STERN

Case Western Reserve University School of Medicine
Cleveland, Ohio

I. Pulmonary Indications for Hospitalization of CF Patients

Exacerbations of infection that have not responded to intensification of home treatment and other complications of pulmonary disease are the most common reasons for hospitalization of cystic fibrosis (CF) patients. In addition, many patients who are hospitalized for nonpulmonary indications have clinically important pulmonary disease that must be addressed during their stay. The vast majority of hospital days for cystic fibrosis are a direct consequence of pulmonary disease. Examples of pulmonary indications for hospitalization and continued hospitalization of CF patients are listed in Tables 1 and 2. Details on many of the items listed are included in specific topics discussed in this chapter.

II. Admission Laboratory Tests

Although there are many pulmonary indications for hospitalization in CF, antibiotic treatment of airway infection (involving antimicrobial agents directed against *Staphylococcus aureus* or *Pseudomonas aeruginosa* or other gram-negative pathogen) is almost always instituted. See Table 3 for a suggested list

Table 1 Pulmonary Indications for Hospital Admission in Patients with Cystic Fibrosis[a]

Indications Related to an Uncomplicated Pulmonary Exacerbation
    Progressive or persistent symptoms despite intervention
    Dyspnea
    Increased cough or paroxysmal cough
    Fever (especially in a patient who is colonized with *Burkholderia cepacia*)
    Deteriorating pulmonary physical examination
    Deteriorating pulmonary function text (including blood gas values)
    Deteriorating chest film appearance
    Anorexia or weight loss
    Initiate home intravenous treatment
Specific Pulmonary Complications
    Lobar or segmental atelectasis
    Right heart failure
    Massive or persistent hemoptysis
    Hypoxemia or initiation of oxygen treatment
    Chest pain, e.g., from rib fracture, pleurisy, pneumothorax
    Pneumothorax
    Intractable and severe hypercapnic respiratory failure
    Syndrome of inappropriate antidiuretic hormone secretion
Superimposed Respiratory Illness[a]
    Influenza
    Respiratory syncytial virus infection
    Aspergillosis
    Legionnaire's disease
    Status asthmaticus
Miscellaneous (Selected Examples)
    New onset *Pseudomonas aeruginosa* colonization
    Initiate treatment for methicillin-resistant *Staphylococcus* aureus
    Preparation for elective surgery for a patient with moderately severe disease
    Initiation of comprehensive pulmonary treatment in newly diagnosed patient

[a]A truly comprehensive list of every possible superimposed illness and miscellaneous indication for hospitalization is obviously not possible.

Table 2 Pulmonary Indications for Continued Hospital Stay in Patients with Cystic Fibrosis[a]

Concern About Imminent Worsening or Dangerous Drug Reaction
    Hypoxemia uncontrolled with supplemental oxygen
    Pneumothorax: observation for tension or recurrence or worsening
    Hemoptysis: observation for recurrence
    Use of dangerous drug (e.g., colistin) or drug to which patient has had an
        acute serious allergic or toxic reaction
    Overt right heart failure
    Severe or unstable respiratory failure especially with edema
    Continued deterioration (symptoms, chest film, or pulmonary function)
    Continuing uncontrolled dyspnea
    Undiagnosed or unresolving high fever

Table 2 Continued

Home Care Criteria Not Reached or Home Care Impossible or Unlikely to be Done
    Correct drug levels not achieved
    Patient or family unwilling or unable to give home intravenous medications
    Patient or family unable to cope with illness at home (social chaos)
    Patient or family's previous attempts at home care suggest certain failure
    Patient who lives alone is unable to cope at home (too sick)
    Inadequate venous access would prevent uninterrupted drug administration
    Wheezing infant, e.g., too sick to eat
    Failure to show initial improvement on treatment
    Ongoing chest tube drainage

[a]Common examples of indications for prolongations of hospital stay.

Table 3 Suggested Initial Routine Laboratory Studies for All Cystic Fibrosis Patients Hospitalized for a Pulmonary Indication[a]

Recommended test	Justification for inclusion
Complete blood count with differential count	• Assess white blood cell count as an indicator of infection and as baseline to follow hematological toxicity of antibiotics and other drugs. • Assess eosinophil count as indicator of allergic disease or allergic bronchopulmonary aspergillosis. • Assess hemoglobin level and hematocrit to ensure adequate capacity for oxygen transport, to help rule out iron deficiency and, possibly, vitamin E deficiency, and to follow up drug toxicity. • Help rule out hypersplenism complicating portal hypertension from CF-related cirrhosis.
Wide spectrum serum chemistry screen (e.g., Chem-20 or Chem-23)	Almost all tests are pertinent to cystic fibrosis or to toxicity of the drugs used for its treatment. For example: • Electrolytes (e.g., hyponatremia or hypochloremia complicating sweat losses, SIADH, diuretic treatment; hypokalemia complicating aminoglycoside treatment; hypochloremia reflecting hypercapnia). • Serum glucose (diabetes is common complication). • Blood urea nitrogen and creatinine as baseline before starting potentially nephrotoxic drugs (e.g., aminoglycosides, colistin); renal toxicity from ibuprofen should be excluded in those patients taking the drug prophylactically. • Liver function studies (bilirubin; alkaline phosphatase; SGOT, SGPT, and other enzymes indicating hepatic cellular injury; serum albumin) to assess hepatic status for possible CF-related cirrhosis, and as baseline before use of potentially hepatotoxic drug (e.g., cefalosporins). • Magnesium to assess for hypomagnesemia (secondary to chronic steatorrhea) and as baseline for drug-induced hypomagnesemia (e.g., aminoglycosides).

Table 3 Continued

Recommended test	Justification for inclusion
	• Total protein and albumin to assess nutrition status (albumin) and degree of hypergammaglobulinemia (as prognostic finding).
	• Uric acid [hyperuricemia complicates treatment with pancreatic replacement enzymes (high purine content)].
Coagulation screen (prothrombin and accelerated partial thromboplastin times)	• Assess synthetic function of liver as index of CF-related cirrhosis.
	• Assess for vitamin K deficiency.
Glycohemoglobin	• Help rule out prediabetic state.
Serum IgE	• Help rule out allergic bronchopulmonary aspergillosis or the presence of another major pulmonary allergy.
Urinalysis	• Baseline before administration of nephrotoxic drugs.
	• Assess for glucosuria (to help rule out diabetes).
Chest radiograph (if not obtained before admission	• Baseline before treatment of pulmonary indication for admission.
	• Assess heart size for possible right heart failure secondary to cor pulmonale.
	• Assess for unexpected pulmonary complication (e.g., atelectasis, pneumothorax, pneumomediastinum, "fungal ball").
Sputum culture (standard method for CF patient)	• Ensure availability of up-to-date in vitro susceptibilities on present pathogens.
	• Identify unexpected bacterial pathogens (e.g., *Burkholderia cepacia, Klebsiella pneumoniae*).
Sputum culture (mycobacterial with acid fast smear)	• Help rule out active pulmonary tuberculosis or colonization with atypical mycobacteria.
	• PPD may be unreliable in patients who are on or have recently taken corticosteroids.
Sputum culture (fungal with smear for fungal elements)	• Help rule out aspergillosis or infection with other fungus or yeast.
Erythrocyte sedimentation rate and C-reactive protein (ESR/CRP)	• ESR to help rule out a clinically significant second illness.
	• ESR and CRP can be used to follow up course of exacerbation under treatment.
Pregnancy test	• Pregnancy would change risk to benefit ratio for certain antibiotics.
	• Pregnancy requires its own treatment follow-up, and physicians.

[a]Some of these tests could be omitted for a patient who is admitted frequently and has thus had them performed recently. Tests that are not pertinent (e.g., pregnancy for patient who has had tubal ligation) should be omitted.
SIADH, syndrome of inappropriate antidiuretic hormone secretion; SGPT, serum glutamic pyruvic transaminase; SGOT, serum glutamic oxaloacetic transaminase; PPD, purified protein derivative.

of routine admission laboratory tests. Many of the screening laboratory studies should also be obtained on CF patients who are admitted for a nonpulmonary indication. Additional laboratory tests that are often useful but are not necessary for every patient are listed in Table 4.

III. Routine Pulmonary Treatment

Regardless of the specific reason for hospitalization, virtually all CF patients with a primarily pulmonary indication for admission should receive airway clearance treatment and antibiotics in addition to whatever specific treatment is needed (e.g., surgical procedure for pneumothorax or bronchoscopic investigation of atelectasis).

A. Overview of Antimicrobial Treatment

Whether antimicrobials are really beneficial when used as treatment for CF patients who are in the midst of a pulmonary exacerbation is reviewed elsewhere. Considerable evidence supports the view that infection plays an important role in CF-related pulmonary exacerbations (1), and virtually all CF centers use antibiotics as part of hospital pulmonary treatment.

The choice of antimicrobials is based on a variety of clinical criteria including in vitro susceptibility studies, the patient's present condition, the history of previous drug response and intolerance, and the urgency of the clinical situation. Organisms recovered from sputum are certain to represent lung flora (2). Pathogens recovered from throat cultures may also indicate pulmonary bacteriology status (3). Throat swabs and sputum samples should be clearly labeled as being CF samples so that the laboratory proceeds with identification and bacterial susceptibility studies for all potential pathogens. The aerosol route and the systemic route each has advantages and disadvantages. The decision cascade for the choice of systemic treatment should take into account the following factors (listed in approximate order of importance):

1. The drugs should have a high likelihood of efficacy.
2. Safe treatment should be used in preference to risky treatment, even if it is expected to take longer.
3. When more than one antibiotic is used, it is usually preferable to choose agents whose most frequent serious toxicities affect different organs (e.g., one antibiotic that usually causes hepatic toxicity and one that usually causes renal toxicity).
4. It is desirable to use the fewest different drugs necessary to ensure that each gram-negative pathogen is covered (i.e., is susceptible in vitro) by at least two drugs; one agent is usually sufficient for *S. aureus*.

Table 4 Additional Laboratory Tests to Be Considered for Cystic Fibrosis Patients Hospitalized for a Pulmonary Indication

Laboratory test	Justification for obtaining test
Serum prealbumin	• Acute measure of nutrition status; can be used to follow course.
Arterial blood gas analysis	• Provide valuable data on lung function that cannot be obtained any other way. • Helps in assessment of need for oxygen treatment and allows accurate adjustment of oxygen dose. • Diagnosis of hypercapnia has prognostic and therapeutic implications. • Allows assessment of acid–base status. • Can be used as baseline to evaluate subsequent course. *Note:* Because the test has some risk (e.g., induction of arterial spasm; creation of A-V fistula), it is not prudent to perform one on every patient. It should be obtained for a specific purpose, e.g., to help determine prognosis or to initiate oxygen therapy. When done correctly, the pain of doing the test should be negligible.
Pulmonary function tests	• Provides valuable data on lung function that cannot be obtained any other way. • Can be used as baseline to evaluate subsequent course. • Can be critical in assessment of therapeutic response to bronchodilator (which, on occasion, can cause paradoxical worsening). *Note:* This test is not needed in every patient. It may be contraindicated (e.g., in some patients with pneumothorax or hemoptysis). It is also expensive and some patients can be managed without admission test, as long as one is obtained later. Patients who are very sick and very stable (previous tests performed before and after clinical improvement are usually not substantially different so that the test is not useful to judge efficacy of treatment or need for more treatment) probably do not need the test every hospitalization, and certainly do not need one on admission.
Sinus computed tomography scan (coronal view)	• May be useful for patient with unusually severe sinus symptoms to assess integrity of sinus walls.
Purified protein derivative	• Could be considered in patients who are about to be given systemic corticosteroids. • Could be considered in patients with known atypical mycobacteria (in whom culture for *Mycobacterium tuberculosis* may be difficult) to help in deciding if *M. tuberculosis* infection is also present.
Respiratory viral antigen panel; viral culture; acute phase serum	• Useful to establish precipitating event for deterioration in patients who are acutely ill. • Useful for prognosis (e.g., respiratory syncytial virus, influenza may have worse outcome)

Table 4 Continued

Laboratory test	Justification for obtaining test
	• Could affect treatment (e.g., amantidine for influenza-A) of other patients.
	• Could help determine need for anticontagion measures. *Note:* These tests are usually not necessary in patients who are in midst of uncomplicated exacerbations of CF pulmonary disease.
Specific tests for non-CF bacterial infections	• Includes *Legionella* and *Mycoplasma* *Note:* These tests are not necessary in patients who are in midst of usual exacerbation of CF pulmonary disease.
Serum and urine osmolality	• Should be considered in all very sick patients and in severely hyponatremic adults who have not been given diuretics (test must be obtained before first dose of any diuretic) to help rule out the syndrome of inappropriate antidiuretic hormone secretion. *Note*: Not needed in most patients
Audiometry	• For patients who have complaint of hearing loss and may need aminoglycoside treatment. *Note:* This test is too expensive to be repeated on a regular basis for CF patients who receive many courses of aminoglycosides. However, for CF patients who complain of hearing loss before ever receiving an ototoxic drug, the test is worthwhile to document pre-treatment status.

5. A drug that is known to be tolerated by the patient (or that the patient has never received) is used before drugs that are known to have caused a clinically important allergic or toxic reaction.
6. Drugs that can be monitored by serum drug levels and thus permit a more rational approach to dosing are preferable.
7. Antimicrobials with other medical advantages (e.g., less irritating to veins) are used preferentially.
8. Less expensive agents are chosen over more expensive agents.
9. Other considerations being equal, antibiotics that are more convenient to use (e.g., can be infused faster or can be given at wider time intervals) are chosen whenever possible.

Cystic fibrosis physicians should limit unnecessary risks when prescribing antibiotics. However, in patients with health-threatening (and life-threatening) pulmonary infection, risk-free therapy is not always possible. Similarly, there are long-standing theoretical arguments concerning antibiotic use that have not always proven true. These and other factors that should be considered, but should not preclude the use of a specific antibiotic, are listed in Table 5.

Table 5 Factors that Do Not Preclude Antibiotic Use in Hospitalized Patients with Cystic Fibrosis

Reason for concern	Comment
History of allergic reaction to this drug or class of drug	The patient's history may not be correct. The patient may have had some other toxicity that would currently be of no concern. The rash that was the basis of the allergy history may have been due to another problem.
	Unless the patient has a history of anaphylaxis (or documentation of anaphylaxis can be found in the chart), the drug can almost always be given safely. Appropriate emergency drugs and materials should be available, but need for them is rare.
	Even with a good history of anaphylaxis, the patient can often be desensitized if the drug is essential.
History of toxic reaction (e.g., hepatotoxicity) to this agent or class	The toxic reaction may have been due to something else.
	Not infrequently, hepatic toxicity does not recur (e.g., to piperacillin) or may subside even if the drug is continued (e.g., ceftazidime).
	The severity of the toxicity, even if it does occur, may be acceptable in view of the clinical situation.
Patient is receiving another drug that may produce additive toxicity (e.g., colistin plus aminoglycosides result in additive, possibly synergistic, renal toxicity)	It may still be possible to give both drugs by proper spacing and meticulous monitoring.
Theoretical argument proposed for adverse drug interactions	Theoretical arguments come and go, but clinical experience is more important and often reveals efficacy rather than interference, e.g., the penicillin ("cidal") plus chloramphenicol ("static") argument of the past, which did not pan out in clinical practice, has been replaced by the beta-lactamase induction arguments of the present. Is it valid? Only clinical experience will tell.
Known in vitro resistance	In CF treatment, clinical usefulness of antimicrobials to which all recovered pathogens are apparently resistant is as old as antibiotics are (e.g., tetracycline, chloramphenicol, trimethoprim-sulfa).
Target organism not a common human pathogen	Not a valid argument in CF.
Target organism no longer recovered (or was never present) in sputum or not a recognized human pathogen	Wide clinical experience does not support this as an absolute criterion for withholding an antibiotic, e.g., empirical antistaphylococcal therapy in the absence of *Staphylococcus aureus* on culture, and empirical antianaerobe therapy (e.g., with clindamycin or metronidazole) is frequently effective.

Concern about the emergence of resistance should not play much of a role in the selection of antimicrobial agents for hospitalized CF patients. Many patients remain susceptible to antimicrobial agents despite many years of heavy exposure. On the other hand, all too often, patients who have never been exposed to a given antimicrobial acquire resistant organisms anyway and, therefore, in effect, were denied the benefit of receiving the drug while their organisms were fully susceptible.

Efficacy

The bottom line of efficacy is clinical success. In vitro susceptibility suggests that the antibiotic will have clinical efficacy. However, optimal treatment depends heavily on empirical clinical experience, both with CF patients in general and the specific patient in particular. In general, antimicrobials that show in vitro efficacy should be used first, especially for treating *S. aureus* and *P. aeruginosa,* but if an antimicrobial combination fails, empirical trials of other agents (occasionally including those to which the organism shows in vitro resistance) can be successful. It is not feasible to try every known antimicrobial agent in every possible combination. A reasonable decision cascade for efficacy is given in Table 6. For very resistant organisms, in vitro testing for antibiotic additive or synergistic effect, available from specialized laboratories, may be helpful (4). Antibiotics that are ineffective in vitro are occasionally effective clinically. This is well known with, for example, tetracycline and chloramphenicol. Whether this benefit derives from a true "antimicrobial" effect that cannot be detected on in vitro testing or from another (nonantibiotic) effect of the drug is not known, but the possibility of successful empirical use of antibiotics is widely recognized among CF physicians (see Table 5).

Safety

The main consideration in safety is the possibility that the drug will cause immediate and irreversible toxicity that compromises the function of a vital organ (e.g., renal failure secondary to aminoglycosides or colistin or aplastic anemia caused by chloramphenicol) and how much recovery can be expected if toxicity develops. Acute toxicity (e.g., nausea or irritation of vein is a secondary consideration. The possibility of cumulative toxicity (e.g., the risk of blindness from optic neuritis after a high lifetime dose of chloramphenicol or occurrence of deafness after many courses of aminoglycosides) must also be considered. A suggested decision cascade for safety is given in Table 6.

Nephrotoxic antibiotics (e.g., aminoglycoside plus colistin) are known to cause additive or synergistic toxic effects. A similar phenomenon with hepatotoxicity has not been reported in CF patients, but it is not unreasonable to avoid such a "double exposure" if possible. This concept is reflected in the

Table 6 Decision Cascades for Antibiotic Selection in Hospitalized Cystic Fibrosis Patients[a]

A. Efficacy Considerations Only
  1. *Pseudomonas aeruginosa*
     Drug 1: Ceftazidime → imipenem → mezlo/piperacillin → aztreonam
     Drug 2: colistin → tobramycin → ciprofloxacin → chloramphenicol →
        trimethoprim-sulfa
     Drug 3 (if needed): ceftazidime → colistin → tobramycin → ciprofloxacin →
        imipenem → aztreonam.
  2. *Burkholderia cepacia*
     Drug 1: ceftazidime → imipenem → piperacillin → chloramphenicol →
        aztreonam → ciprofloxacin → trimethoprim-sulfa
     Drug 2 (if needed): chloramphenicol → novobiocin → aztreonam →
        ciprofloxacin → trimethoprim-sulfa
  3. *Staphylococcus aureus*
     Drug 1: vancomycin → nafcillin (or other effective penicillin) → tobramycin
        → ciprofloxacin → chloramphenicol; novobiocin may be useful for
        resistant *S. aureus*, or if the patient is already receiving this antibiotic for
        treatment of *B. cepacia*
     Drug 2: none needed
     Note: This sequence concerns efficacy only; vancomycin is very effective
     against this organism, but should always be held in reserve unless there is
     methicillin resistance or empirical failure of other agents to control the
     infection.
B. Safety Considerations Only (major organ toxicity considered)
   P. aeruginosa and *B. cepacia*
   Drug 1: ceftazidime → mezlo/piperacillin → trimethoprim-sulfa → aztreonam →
      ciprofloxacin → imipenem → tobramycin → chloramphenicol → colistin
   S. aureus
   Drug 1: nafcillin → ciprofloxacin → tobramycin → chloramphenicol →
      vancomycin
C. Other Safety and Logistical Considerations: Examples of antibiotics that present
   minor medical drawbacks or logistical inconvenience
   Imipenem: Venous irritation; relatively frequent administration (every 6 hr) is
                hard to "mesh" with every 8 hr agents; requires slow infusion
   Penicillins: Frequent doses (i.e., every 4–6 hr); high salt load; venous irritation
   Vancomycin: Venous irritation; 12-hour frequency is hard to "mesh" with every 8
                hr agents
D. Cost Considerations
   Expensive antibiotics: ceftazidime, imipenem, vancomycin, aztreonam, colistin,
   ciprofloxacin
E. Drug Levels Available for Clinical Use
   Levels frequently used: aminoglycosides, chloramphenicol, vancomycin
   Levels theoretically available: trimethoprim-sulfa, ciprofloxacin
   Note: The clinical necessity to monitor drug levels for aminoglycosides is being
   challenged by some experts.

[a]Right arrow means that the first antibiotic is probably superior and is at least equal to the second
for the property under consideration.

suggestions for two-drug and three-drug therapy in Table 6. The use of an aminoglycoside plus colistin is occasionally useful and is discussed in subsequent paragraphs.

"Two Antibiotics for Each Pathogen" Therapy

It is usually possible to accomplish dual coverage for each gram-negative pulmonary pathogen present in sputum culture by using only two antibiotics altogether. Adequate (but often single) coverage of *S. aureus* is often achieved by the same (two) antibiotics used to cover gram-negative pathogens. For example, the most common two-drug combination for *P. aeruginosa,* an aminoglycoside (often tobramycin) and ceftazidime, is often adequate to cover *S. aureus* as well. If the *S. aureus* is more resistant, nafcillin or vancomycin may be added. Chloramphenicol is also an excellent antistaphylococcal agent (see Table 6).

Systemic Versus Aerosol Administration

Aerosol administration has the advantage of potentially achieving an extremely high level of the antibiotic in pulmonary secretions, but only in areas that have relatively good ventilation. Systemic administration ensures that at least some drug gets to all areas. Combined treatment combines these benefits (at the expense of additional therapy time and cost). Some clinicians feel that there is at least some additional benefit of aerosol antibiotics even if the patient is receiving the same antibiotic intravenously. A list of antibiotics that can be given by aerosol is given in Table 7.

Dosing Considerations

The infection in CF is primarily endobronchial and therefore is not in a tissue that has a good blood supply. From the topological viewpoint, most of the infecting organisms are literally outside the body. High blood levels in contiguous blood vessels and tissues (and therefore high doses) of antibiotics are necessary to help ensure that meaningful levels are achieved in the purulent secretions. Furthermore, many CF patients demonstrate accelerated drug metabolism and excretion for many antimicrobials (see Chapter 11), which is another reason to give high doses (5). In general, the higher the dose the better (from the efficacy viewpoint). Suggested starting doses, major toxicity, and target serum levels (if commonly used for monitoring) for the most commonly used inpatient antimicrobials are listed in Table 8. Intravenous administration of an aminoglycoside as a single (large) daily dose (6) may be advantageous if the patient is receiving only one intravenously administered antibiotic; however, if more than one agent is used, particularly if both have potential nephrotoxicity, once-a-day dosing may be impractical.

Table 7 Antimicrobials Given by Aerosol Route

1. Antimicrobials safely given by aerosol

Antibiotic class	Solution concentration	Dose
Gentamicin/tobra-mycin/amikacin	Undiluted from drug vial	1–2 vials
Colistin	150 mg in 2 mL diluent	150 mg
Ceftazidime	1 g in 3 mL diluent	1 g
Antistaphylococcal penicillins[a]	1 g in 3 mL diluent	1 g
Amphotericin		

2. Antimicrobials for which aerosol route has not been reported

    Aztreonam
    Trimethoprim-sulfa
    Vancomycin

3. Antimicrobials for which there appears to be a valid theoretical obstacle to aerosol administration

Chloramphenicol:	Exposure of other family members—risk of aplastic anemia; this antibiotic penetrates into all areas very well when given systemically.
Imipenem:	Contains two drugs—one cilistatin to prevent toxicity—if thianamycin is absorbed and cilistatin is destroyed by aerosolization, dangerous toxicity could theoretically result.
Ciprofloxacin:	Aerosolization appears feasible, but its smell and wheezing may prevent its use.
Neomycin:	Risk of deafness.

[a]Theoretically increased risk of sensitization to drugs applied to mucosal surfaces—seldom experienced in practice.

Augmentation of Antibiotic Effect by Other Drugs

Many drugs that do not have intrinsic antibiotic effect have been proposed, on the basis of in vitro data or theoretical arguments, as possibly offering additive or synergistic effect with antibiotics. Combined amiloride and tobramycin for *B. cepacia* is one example (7). Clavulanic acid is one case in which clinical efficacy has been documented. For most, however, convincing demonstration of efficacy has not been presented. Others have failed in reported clinical studies. Some antibiotics (e.g., erythromycin) have direct effects on the immune system that could be beneficial in CF.

Table 8 Suggested Initial Doses for Antimicrobial Agents for Hospitalized Patients with Cystic Fibrosis

Class of antimicrobial individual agents	Principal toxicity for class	Recommended dose for cystic fibrosis patients	Comment
Aminoglycosides Tobramycin Gentamicin Amikacin	Renal otological	Tobramycin 10 mg/kg/day (3 doses) Gentamicin 10 mg/kg/day (3 doses) Amikacin 30 mg/kg/day (3 doses)	Optimal peak serum level: 10–12 mg/L Trough level: <2 mg/L Optimal serum level: 25–40 mg/L Trough level: 5–10 mg/L
Cephalosporins Ceftazidime	Hematological, hepatic, allergic	Adults: 4 g every 8 hr Infants/children: 150 mg/kg/day (1–4 g every 8 hr usually tolerated by older patients)	Levels not monitored; drug has very favorable therapeutic index
Penicillins Piperacillin Mezlocillin Nafcillin	Hematological, allergic rash Allergic rash	450 mg/kg/day (4–6 doses)	Levels not monitored; drugs in this class have very favorable therapeutic index
Polymyxin Colistin	Renal, neurological, neuromuscular, ototoxicity	100–200 mg/kg/day	Serum levels not routinely available
		5–7.5 mg/kg/day (3 doses) Maximum adult dose: 100 mg every 8 hr	
Carbapenems Imipenem	Nausea	Adult: 1 g every 6 hr Children: 90 mg/kg/day up to 1 g every 6 hr	Start with low dose and increase every 2 days
Aztreonam	Nausea "Bloating"	Adult: 1 g every 8 hr Children: 90–120 mg/kg/day (3–4 doses)	Levels is not monitored; drug has very favorable therapeutic index
Chloramphenicol	Hematological, "metallic taste," Antabuse effect	Adult: 1 g every 6 hr Children > 2 months: 50 mg/kg/day	Oral route preferred; optimal serum peak level: 25–30 mg/L Trough: <10 mg/L

Table 8 Continued

Class of antimicrobial individual agents	Principal toxicity for class	Recommended dose for cystic fibrosis patients	Comment
Novobiocin	Jaundice, nausea Allergic rash/serum sickness/arthritis	250–500 mg 4 times per day	Oral capsules No intravenous form available in the United States
Quinolones Ciprofloxacin Norfloxacin Ofloxacin	Nausea, insomnia, photosensitivity	Child: 20–60 mg/kg/day (3–4 doses) Adults: 750 mg 3–4 times per day	Oral or intravenous Levels not monitored
Trimenthoprim-sulfa	Hematological Allergic rash	Adult: 2 ds Cap bid Children: rs Cap qid	Levels not monitored
Clindamycin	Soft stools (*Clostridia difficile*) pseudomembranous colitis	Adult: 1200 mg/day (up to 4800 mg/day has been used in adults) Child: 40 mg/kg/day	Levels not monitored
Metronidazole	Nausea, neuropathy seizures, Antabuse effect	Adult: 500 mg every 6 hr	Levels not monitored
Erythromycin	Nausea	Adult: 250–500 mg 4 times per day Child: 250 mg 3–4 times per day	Levels not monitored
Vancomycin	Renal	Adult: 1 g every 12 hr Child: 10–20 mg/kg/dose (every 8 hr)	Optimal peak serum level: 35–40 mg/L Trough: 5–10 mg/L

B. Airway Clearance

Overview

Whereas considerable controversy exists about how best to clear pulmonary secretions in patients with obstructive pulmonary diseases, the desirability of doing so does not appear to be in doubt. Secretions clearly block air flow, thus aggravating whatever other mechanisms of obstruction are present. In addition, secretions may precipitate or worsen reactive bronchospasm, again increasing obstruction. Equally important, in CF, the secretions are thought to contain corrosive materials (e.g., elastase, oxygen radicals, cytokines, and leukotrienes), which are derived from the pulmonary defense system but are produced in such quantities that they cannot be neutralized by normal mechanisms (e.g., by antiproteases). These unopposed cytotoxic chemicals then become the main vehicle of destruction of airways and pulmonary parenchyma.

Theoretically, every therapeutic measure directed at lung disease can be construed to be part of airway clearance. For example, by reducing infection, antibiotics decrease bacterial load and the reaction of the lung to it, thus contributing to airway clearance. Systemic bronchodilators (albuterol; aminophylline) and systemic corticosteroids are used frequently by CF patients and do play a somewhat more direct role in airway clearance. However, only rapidly acting aerosolized drugs, physiotherapy, and breathing techniques are discussed here. A systemically administered expectorant could be useful, but no convincing evidence has been presented for the efficacy of any of the commonly used agents, including SSKI (saturated solution of potassium iodide), guaifenesin, and intravenous fluid given in excess of the amount necessary to prevent dehydration. Although systemic dehydration results in dehydrated (and therefore viscous) secretions, neither intravenous nor oral "overhydration" appears to increase water content of bronchial secretions in the euhydrated patient.

A comprehensive approach to airway clearance treatment includes a combination of the following: (1) enlarging the bronchial lumen as much as possible by minimizing inflammatory obstruction and reducing bronchospasm, (2) using mucolytic agents to reduce sputum viscosity, (3) using chest physiotherapy to separate the sticky secretions from the airway walls, and (4) using gravity drainage, voluntary cough, or other type of final clearance maneuver to complete the physical removal of the secretions from the lung. After airway clearance treatment, a variety of medications such as antiinflammatory drugs (e.g., corticosteroids and cromolyn) and antibiotics can be given by aerosol to take advantage of the optimally open airways. These aerosols, which are not components of the airway clearance procedure per se, are discussed elsewhere in this chapter.

Airway clearance has received considerable attention recently, both from CF physicians and respiratory therapists (8) as well as from inventors and distributors of related equipment. The variety of drugs and equipment available is summarized in Table 9. The final coordinated prescription for airway clearance should be individualized, based on patient preferences and the observations of the patient and the respiratory therapists. An enthusiastic and dedicated respiratory therapist with a specific interest in this area is a key member of the CF team.

Reducing Inflammatory Obstruction and Bronchospasm

Bronchodilators are effective in many patients. Aerosolized phenylephrine has been used to reduce inflammatory airway edema. There are no data supporting its use, however, and it seems likely that airway tachyphylaxis would develop as rapidly as it does in the nose. Only smooth muscle relaxants (i.e., bronchodilators) can be recommended; however, a paradoxical worsening occasionally develops in a patient after inhaling beta-adrenergic agents, and this must be considered in patients who deteriorate unexpectedly or who do not show expected improvement with intensive airway clearance procedures.

Mucolytic Agents

Until recently, *N*-acetylcysteine (Mucomyst) was the only mucolytic agent available. It is effective in vitro. Its mucolytic effect is rapid and easily demonstrable in a test tube or petri dish. Unfortunately, it has the unpleasant odor of rotten eggs and can cause mucosal irritation, which can result in bronchospasm and, theoretically, aggravation of a preexisting hypersecretory state. Thus, the use of this agent must be carefully monitored and it cannot be assumed to be useful for all patients. It seems likely that *N*-acetylcysteine will be largely replaced by hrDNase; however, for patients who do not tolerate hrDNase, *N*-acetylcysteine can be an effective alternative. The usual dose of *N*-acetylcysteine is 2–3 cc of a 10% or 20% solution before chest physiotherapy 1–3 times a day.

Cystic fibrosis endobronchial mucus contains many substances, including neutrophil DNA, which accounts for much of the viscosity of the secretions. The recently approved (December 1993) hrDNase (Pulmozyme) offers the advantage of potency (in vitro, DNase causes quick and dramatic liquification of CF sputum) with no disagreeable odor. Anaphylaxis, which can occur with other forms of DNase, has not been reported. Preliminary studies suggest its usefulness as an adjunct to airway clearance (9). Forced expiratory volume in 1 second (FEV_1) improved acutely (albeit only modestly) in human efficacy trials. However, long-term human toxicity studies have not been done, and the drug should therefore be used with caution until physicians acquire more experience with it in everyday practice. Nonhydrolyzed DNA probably binds elastase and some other destructive chemicals, and it is not clear whether DNA hydrolysis will result in the remaining (uncleared) secretions, becoming even

Table 9 Overview of Mucus Clearance Techniques for Hospitalized Patients with Cystic Fibrosis

Optimization of airway diameter during Rx	Pharmacologic/physical mucolysis or reduction in viscosity	Separation of mucus from airway wall	Final evacuation of secretions from airway
Traditional approach			
Bronchodilator aerosol	N-Acetyl cysteine (Mucomyst®)	Chest physiotherapy (clapping/vibration)	Chest physiotherapy (clapping/vibration)
Decongestant aerosol[a] (e.g., phenylephrine)	(Bovine) DNase (Dornase®)[b]	Voluntary cough	Electric percussor
Systemic bronchodilator	Hypertonic urea[c]		Electric vibrator
Aerosolized/systemic corticosteroid	Expectorants[d], Guaifenesin[a], SSKI[a]		Voluntary cough
	IV hydration[a]		Suction catheter
Pursed-lips breathing		Bronchoalveolar lavage[e]	Bronchoalveolar lavage[e]
		Exercise	Exercise
Recent additions			
	rhDNase (Pulmozyme®)	Sonic Percussor®	Sonic Percussor®
	Gelsolin (experimental)	Intrapulmonary percussive ventilation	Intrapulmonary percussive ventilation
Flutter® valve		Flutter® valve	Flutter® valve
Positive expiratory pressure (PEP)		Autogenic breathing	Autogenic breathing
		Chest vest	Chest vest
			FET (forced expiratory technique) maneuver

[a]No convincing evidence of therapeutic effect.
[b]Human preparation no longer available.
[c]Not in common use.
[d]No good evidence exists for the existence of any systemically administered drug which has clinically important expectorant effect in the human.
[e]Not widely used for this purpose.

more injurious. At present, the recommended dose (aerosolized by one of several nebulizers) for most patients is 2.5 mg once a day. Because of the concern that sudden liquification of a large amount of mucus could flood the airways with thin secretions, especially in patients with severe disease (i.e., those with FEV_1 of less than 40% of predicted), the official recommendation is for routine airway clearance to be performed before administration of the DNase. It seems likely that DNase will cause some patients with severe airway obstruction to be overwhelmed by newly mobilized airway mucus, whereas others with equally severe obstruction will benefit. As physicians become more experienced, adaptation of DNase treatment to individual patients will probably become easier.

Gelsolin, a new compound that acts on microfibrils, has shown promise in vitro (10), but clinical trials have not been reported (see Chapter 15).

Dislodging Mucus from Airway Walls

Chest percussion, introduced (for CF regimens) in the 1960s (11), was the standard, if not only, "mucus loosening" procedure used in the United States until recently. In the last few years, however, a variety of other modalities has been introduced. The final airway clearance program used by an individual patient may include two or more of the following: manual (12,13) or mechanical chest percussion (14), external oscillatory devices (mechanical percussors, Sonic Percussor), internal oscillatory devices [Flutter valve (15), intrapulmonary percussive ventilation], breathing techniques (autogenic drainage, "huffing"), and physical exercise (16,17). Detailed information on the use of these techniques is available from standard respiratory therapy texts or the product inserts. The efficacy of these newer techniques depends heavily on the quality of the initial instruction sessions and the commitment of the patient.

Expectoration of Mobilized Mucus

This final step in airway clearance can involve voluntary cough, autogenic drainage (18), forced expiratory technique (FET), (19) "huffing," suction, or a combination of these techniques. Positive expiratory pressure (PEP) devices are occasionally used in conjunction with these techniques (20).

IV. Treatment of "Uncomplicated" Pulmonary Exacerbation

The patients included in the category of "uncomplicated" pulmonary exacerbation have one or more of the physical examination findings or laboratory abnormalities listed in Table 10 and no major complication, such as pneumothorax, heart failure, or hemoptysis.

Table 10 Characteristics of Uncomplicated Pulmonary Exacerbations in Patients with Cystic Fibrosis[a]

Symptoms
Increased cough, paroxysmal cough, nocturnal cough
Increased sputum production
New onset or increased dyspnea
Streaky hemoptysis
Loss of appetite
Fatigue
Irritability
Cyanosis
Fever
Physical Findings
Weight loss (or failure to gain weight); growth failure
Increased crackles, localized or diffuse
Decreased air exchange
New onset or increased use of accessory muscles of respiration
Wheezing (infant)
Laboratory Abnormalities
Deterioration in pulmonary functions test (decreased FVC, FEV_1; increased RV, RV/TLC ratio)
Deterioration in chest radiograph (mucus retention, bronchial cuffing, acute infiltrate)
Worsening blood gas: decreased P_{O_2} or increased P_{CO_2}

[a]Most patients will have several of these findings. FVC, forced vital capacity; FEV_1, forced expiratory volume in 1 second; RV, residual volume; TLC, total lung capacity.

A. Overview

The goal is to initiate treatment that, when completed in the hospital or at home, will result in returning the patient to his or her best recent pulmonary status. Most patients achieve this goal. Those who do not are discussed in subsequent paragraphs.

Antibiotic Treatment

Initial treatment usually includes the continuation of most of the prehospital home regimen with the exception of antibiotics. Oral antibiotics are usually discontinued and replaced with the safest intravenous (IV) antimicrobials that have a high likelihood of success (see Tables 6 and 7). For many uncomplicated patients, ceftazidime and tobramycin emerge as the ideal combination. Determination of the proper tobramycin dose is detailed in Appendix 1. Aerosol antibiotic treatment (often tobramycin, occasionally colistin; see Table 7) may be continued or added.

If the initial workup (including appropriate laboratory data from tests listed in Tables 3 and 4) does not show an unexpected problem, the patient may be ready to undertake home treatment as soon as adequate doses are established and shown to be tolerated. For many patients, however, it is appropriate for the entire course of treatment to be completed in the hospital (see Table 2). Although home antibiotic treatment has been reported to be as effective as inpatient treatment for a variety of infections (21), results with CF patients have been mixed (22,23). Furthermore, the selection criteria for patients to be included in some studies of home care were quite restrictive (24) and would exclude many patients for whom home care is presently being considered (or even mandated by insurance carriers). Some reasons for the failure of home treatment with some CF patients (especially adults who live alone) are that CF patients require considerable home treatment in addition to IV infusions and they may not have the time to get it all done and that CF patients are more likely to have ongoing disease-related fatigue and other obstacles to their performing IV drug administration every 6 or 8 hours. Conversely, patients with osteo-myelitis, endocarditis, and similar infections may be virtually asymptomatic by the time they are discharged to home care. There are other considerations, but it is clear that home care is not optimal treatment for every CF patient.

Patients who are experiencing truly uncomplicated pulmonary exacerba-tions have such a high likelihood of rapid improvement that the systemic symptoms of the exacerbation (e.g., irritability, anorexia or weight loss, and fatigue) often do not need specific attention. Anorexia, in particular, resolves quickly and weight gain follows.

Pulmonary symptoms and signs, such as dyspnea, cough and chest pain (see Appendix 2), hypoxemia and cyanosis, and bronchospasm may merit specific treatment. However, even these symptoms and signs may not need specific attention if they are not particularly bothersome, if the patient prefers to wait, and if rapid improvement is anticipated.

Other Routine Treatment

The patient should be encouraged to be as active as possible. Ideally, this includes walking around the hospital corridors, using the stairs, and perhaps participating in an organized exercise program (with appropriate attention to the prevention of desaturation in patients with more marginal pulmonary status) (25). All students should be encouraged to stay current with their schoolwork.

Concurrent Preventive Pulmonary Treatment

High-dose ibuprofen (peak serum levels between 50 and 100 μg/mL) was recently shown to be effective in slowing the progression of CF-related pulmonary disease, particularly in children between 5 and 14 years of age (26). Hospitalized patients may already be taking prophylactic ibuprofen before admission or may be started on treatment while they are hospitalized. Ibuprofen can contribute to the severity of hemoptysis (by interfering with platelet function and clotting) and should be discontinued, at least temporarily, when substantial pulmonary bleeding develops. Ibuprofen, particularly in high dose, can also cause renal failure and must be considered in all CF patients who enter the hospital with abnormal serum tests of kidney function or show deterioration during their stay. Whether the drug will alter aminoglycoside pharmacokinetics to a clinically important degree or will cause additive or synergistic renal toxicity is unknown, but would not be surprising. Other toxic effects of long-term high-dose ibuprofen in CF patients will likely become apparent within the next few years.

If long-term treatment with ibuprofen is started in the hospital, the dose should be established by a pharmacokinetic study that is sufficiently accurate to ensure that the blood levels are never higher than 100 μg/mL but do achieve at least 50 μg/mL. After the dose is established, the patient must continue using the same brand of ibuprofen used for the pharmacokinetic study. The details of this testing and treatment can be found elsewhere.

Common Problems

Hypoxemia and Hypercapnia

Supplemental oxygen may be needed during airway clearance treatments, especially traditional postural drainage (to facilitate cough and to allow the patient to lie in a head-down position). Oxygen is usually given by nasal cannulae (masks interfere with coughing and expectorating) in a dose of 2–3 L/M and can be discontinued immediately after the conclusion of the treatment. The correct dose should be determined by the functional outcome—the patient's ability to participate appropriately in airway clearance procedures—rather than by a preset goal for the arterial Po_2. Arterial blood gas (ABG) measurements are not even necessary for this use of oxygen. Some patients who require nasal oxygen during treatments may benefit from the availability of a mask with 40% oxygen, which then can be used for brief periods in addition to the nasal oxygen to relieve dyspnea during or after meals or if airway clearance treatment precipitates severe coughing spells. Removal of the elastic straps from the 40% mask helps prevent the patient from falling asleep with the mask in use.

Although hemoglobin saturation, as measured by pulse oximetry, is commonly used to guide oxygen therapy (and this is acceptable practice), it is the actual oxygen tension that is correlated to pulmonary arteriolar spasm and thus the severity of cor pulmonale. For that reason, oxygen tensions are discussed in this section. For patients with arterial Po_2 values of more than 50 mm Hg, continuous supplemental oxygen is not usually an absolute necessity if the patient prefers to go without it. Overt heart failure secondary to cor pulmonale is unusual in such patients (27). Some patients with long-standing hypoxemia tolerate even lower arterial Po_2 levels without development of any of the major complications of hypoxemia. For most patients whose arterial oxygen tension is less than 50 mm Hg and for other patients whose ABG measurements are better but who are overtly symptomatic (e.g., morning headache is relieved by oxygen), continuous oxygen may also be needed. A reasonable approach is to give the lowest dose of oxygen needed to bring the arterial oxygen tension to approximately 55 mm Hg.

Oxygen therapy is not without controversy. In one view, too much supplemental oxygen, although it relieves dyspnea, can reduce the work of breathing to such an extent that the muscles or respiration begin to atrophy, and weaning off oxygen becomes difficult. Patients worry about "getting addicted to oxygen" and they immediately understand the concept behind the statement, "I want to ensure that you have the best chance for 'getting off oxygen,' so I want to maintain the strength of your respiratory muscles." In other words, "I don't want to make you too comfortable by giving too much oxygen!" The more widely held view of this issue is that insufficient oxygen directly compromises diaphragmatic function or causes systemic acidosis, and these events outweigh the risk of incurring some diaphragmatic atrophy caused by unnecessary "rest."

Wheezing and Bronchospasm

Symptomatic bronchospasm can precede hospital admission, but it can also be a complication of treatment. If the patient has not experienced bronchospasm previously or if it is unusually severe, additional workup may be indicated. If a serum IgE test was not obtained on admission (see Table 3) to screen for allergic bronchopulmonary aspergillosis, then the test should be ordered if wheezing and bronchospasm become a significant clinical problem. Additional workup including a fungal precipitin panel, *Aspergillus* skin testing, and a specific anti-*Aspergillus*–IgE level may be needed. All medications should be reviewed to help ensure that one with potential to cause bronchospasm (e.g., beta-adrenergic blocking agent) has not been ordered for another reason (e.g., hypertension) or that ongoing treatment for allergic disease has not been inadvertently stopped on admission. The patient and hospital personnel should be questioned about the use of sprays (e.g., "air fresheners" or germicidal agents). The patient and the patient's roommate should be asked whether they have received flowers or tried each other's cosmetics. If the patient is a toddler, the possibility of foreign body aspiration should be considered. Dynamic collapse of bronchiectatic airways occurs in response to beta-adrenergic agents in approximately 10% of patients with CF (28), and this should be considered as a possible cause for wheezing, even if the patient has previously had a beneficial or neutral response to these agents (29). Aerosolized colistin can also cause bronchospasm, particularly in adults (30).

Use of aerosolized bronchodilators, especially before airway clearance, is often helpful. It may be necessary to add a beta-adrenergic agent to an aerosolized drug that is producing bronchospasm (e.g., colistin or amphotericin B). Persistent or worsening bronchospasm may respond to the addition of aerosolized cromolyn or aerosolized or systemic corticosteroid treatment.

F. Monitoring Progress and Terminating Treatment

Treatment of an uncomplicated exacerbation, depending on a variety of factors (see Table 2), may be completed at home or in the hospital. Nonmedical considerations (e.g., financial limitations and career or school obligation) may necessitate an arbitrary end to IV therapy, but substantial additional improvement after premature cessation of intensive treatment is unlikely (31). Therefore, although the physician may have to accept an early termination of treatment, he or she should not recommend it unless it is unlikely that additional improvement will occur.

Estimation of progress includes assessment of one or more of the items listed in Table 11.

Table 11 Monitoring Progress in a Cystic Fibrosis Patient Hospitalized for an Uncomplicated Pulmonary Exacerbation[a]

Clinical parameter	Therapeutic goal
Vital signs T/P/R	Patients remains afebrile
	Sleeping pulse and respiration to baseline status or stop improving
Physical examination	No crackles and good air exchange—or return to baseline
Chest radiograph	Baseline status
ABGs/pulse oximetry	Adequate arterial P_{O_2}—or return to baseline status
PFTs	Return to baseline
Exercise testing	Return to baseline
Cardinal symptoms/signs of lung disease: dyspnea, cough, sputum production, etc.	Resolved or returned to baseline
Systemic manifestations of lung disease, including reduced energy/exercise intolerance, anorexia, irritability	Resolved or returned to baseline
CRP/ESR/serum elastase	Return to normal or baseline
Bronchoscopy	Best variables for monitoring still under investigation

[a]If these criteria cannot be met, the hospitalization is, by definition, not uncomplicated.

V. Complications and Problems

A. Failure to Improve

Cystic fibrosis patients who are undergoing treatment for an uncomplicated pulmonary exacerbation may report subjective improvement by the end of the third treatment day (earlier improvement is usually due to change in environment, for asthma, or other non-treatment–related reason) and should be expected to show some subjective and objective improvement by the end of the fifth treatment day. Once improvement begins, steady subjective and objective improvement should be discernible, usually over 3-day intervals (the patient should confirm that he or she feels "better than I did 3 days ago"). If these milestone events do not occur, immediate "trouble-shooting" should be undertaken (Table 12).

Even if the patient appears to be receiving optimal therapy based on previous course and microbiology data, an empirical switch in antibiotic coverage may be effective (see Table 6). The following antibiotics are especially likely to be effective as second-line agents, even if in vitro susceptibility cannot be demonstrated: ceftazidime, chloramphenicol, Imipenem, ciprofloxacin, norfloxacin, or ofloxacin. The following antibiotics may be effective even if others are equally effective in vitro: tobramycin, colistin, and ceftazidime. For patients who have not improved on ceftazidime and tobramycin, the ceftazidime can be replaced with, for example, Imipenem or aztreonam; tobramycin can be replaced with colistin. If the patient still does not improve, both colistin and tobramycin can be given together with the other antibiotic already in progress. In general, a new antibiotic combination deserves a 5-day trial to ensure that a potentially useful drug or drug combination is not abandoned too early.

Simultaneous Administration of Tobramycin and Colistin

Both tobramycin and colistin are nephrotoxic and both have been reported to cause neuromuscular blockade. Because tobramycin is rapidly excreted, the infusion of colistin is begun 3 hours after (and therefore 5 hours before) tobramycin. This minimizes the chance that high levels of both agents will be in the circulation at one time. This probably reduces the risk of nephrotoxicity and it seems reasonable to assume that it reduces the risk of neuromuscular blockade as well. Tobramycin (and other aminoglycosides) also have substantial ototoxicity, but this toxicity is not a major problem with colistin. Patients who are receiving tobramycin and colistin should receive sufficient supplemental oxygen to optimize arterial oxygenation; hypoxemia causes additive nephrotoxicity with each of these antibiotics and is even more dangerous if both are being given.

Table 12 Trouble-Shooting for Cystic Fibrosis Patients with Uncomplicated Pulmonary Exacerbation Who Do Not Show Improvement or Are Deteriorating by the End of the 5th Treatment Day

Possible explanation	Possible investigation/corrective action
Inadequate antibiotic coverage	Check results of admission culture; recheck previous culture; change antibiotics if appropriate; empirical addition of antistaphylococcal coverage even if *Staphylococcus aureus* not recovered from culture; addition of empirical gram-negative coverage if not included in original regimen. Consider mycobacterial or fungal disease.
Inadequate antibiotic dose	Review drug doses and blood levels (see Table 8); possibly raise doses.
New onset of CF pulmonary complication	Evaluate for possible pneumothorax (repeat chest film); allergic bronchopulmonary aspergillosis (check admission IgE level); heart failure (recheck heart size on chest film, check for peripheral edema and excess weight gain, inquire about change in dietary salt intake); consider empirical trial of intravenous diuretic; hypoxemia (check arterial blood gas and pulse oximetry, offer supplemental oxygen).
Patient has a second pulmonary problem	Perform specific diagnostic tests and empirical treatment for second infectious disease: *Mycoplasma* (perform appropriate serology); *Legionella* infection (sputum cytology, serology). Consider empirical addition of erythromycin or clarithromycin. Test for mycobacterial or fungal infection (be sure cultures have been obtained); consider empirical treatment for yeast). Evaluate for asthma and reactive airway disease. Also review differential diagnosis for asthma. Consider empirical addition of bronchodilator or corticosteroid. Evaluate for possible aggravation of gastroesophageal reflux by bronchodilators or institution or intensification of postural drainage. Consider adding ranitidine or cimetidine, perhaps omeprazole.
Paradoxical worsened obstruction from beta-adrenergic drugs	Measure flow rates before and after aerosolized beta-adrenergic aerosol. If paradoxical worsening is documented, use other pharmacological approach to bronchospasm.
Inadequate airway clearance treatment	Reevaluate method of airway clearance used and patient cooperation. Consider instituting another treatment modality (see Table 9); offer supplemental oxygen with treatments. Consider mucolytic agents.
Noncompliance and patient sabotage	Review respiratory therapy and nursing notes; investigate possible unsatisfactory social situation. Consider psychotherapeutic intervention.

Table 12 Continued

Possible explanation	Possible investigation/corrective action
Depression	Ask about depression and suicide ideation and related symptoms. Consider psychiatry consultation and treatment.
Maximum improvement has been achieved	Determine whether patient has returned to his or her subjective and objective baseline. Consider terminating treatment and discharge.
Munchausen's syndrome by proxy	See Chapter 3

If a potent intravenous diuretic is needed, it should be given *instead* of one of the colistin doses. Furosemide and Bumex increase both the excretion and the toxicity of nephrotoxic antibiotics.

When a patient who has had a series of uneventful and successful courses of intravenous antibiotics for uncomplicated pulmonary exacerbations fails to respond adequately, it seems reasonable to treat aggressively for up to 4–5 weeks as described before accepting that a return to baseline status is not possible. However, once such extended treatment has failed, the new status should be accepted as the patient's baseline and the patient should not necessarily be subjected to another prolonged treatment course with potentially toxic drug combinations the next time pulmonary status deteriorates.

Hypoxemia and Oxygen Treatment

Some specific issues unique (or particularly important) to CF inpatients are addressed in this section.

Oxygen treatment is used for one or more of the following indications: (1) to treat or prevent a complication of hypoxemia (e.g., hypoxemia-induced pulmonary arterial hypertension with right heart failure or additive nephrotoxicity of hypoxemia with other nephrotoxic agents such as diuretics or aminoglycosides, (2) to relieve dyspnea, (3) to improve function such as exercise capability (32), ability to cooperate with or perform airway clearance procedures, (4) to help compensate for the increased oxygen requirement and compromised diaphragmatic expansion associated with eating, and (5) to relieve another symptom of hypoxemia (e.g., headache). The dose of oxygen and the method of administration may vary with these different goals.

Treatment and Prevention of Hypoxemia-Related Complications

For the initial treatment of very sick patients, see Special Problems. The minimum initial goal is usually to raise the arterial Po_2 above 50 mm Hg, preferably as close to 60 mm Hg as possible. (If pulse oximetry is used, the goal should be

88% hemoglobin saturation.) For most patients, nasal cannulae are preferable, because they do not interfere with coughing, expectorating, or eating. If the arterial PCO_2 is not elevated, the FiO_2 can be raised in 1-L/M increments (at 30-min intervals), until the pulse oximetry increases to more than 88%. At that point, an ABG can be repeated to confirm adequate arterial PO_2. If the initial arterial PCO_2 was elevated, the same procedure is followed except that arterial punctures are necessary every 30 minutes. Alternatively, end-tidal CO_2 measurements could be monitored. The arterial PCO_2 can be expected to increase and the physician must decide how high a "CO_2 price" he or she is willing to pay for the achieved PO_2. Generally, PCO_2 in the 60s or 70s are not cause for much concern. Occasionally, the FiO_2 will have to be increased slowly over a couple of days to allow time for compensation for respiratory acidosis. If the PCO_2 elevates into the 80s, it may be necessary to settle for a lower PO_2 or pulse oximetry reading. (In very sick patients with initial arterial PO_2 values in the 30s, occasionally PO_2 values as low as 45 mm Hg may be the best that can be achieved initially.) It is not uncommon for the PCO_2 to remain constant or even decrease with oxygen supplementation. In these cases, the hypoventilation was probably a result of fatigued hypoxic ventilatory muscles and not inadequate drive to breathe.

Nocturnal oxygen has been useful in the treatment and prevention of right heart failure due to cor pulmonale in adult patients with non-CF pulmonary disease (33,34). Such an effect could not be demonstrated in CF patients over the course of one 3-year study (35), but those patients did not receive the same duration of oxygen treatment daily which was shown effective in adults with non-CF chronic obstructive pulmonary disease (32,33). Although this controversy is not particularly germane for inpatients because there would be little reason not to give continuous oxygen, it does have to be considered for discharge planning.

Treatment of Dyspnea (see also Appendix 2)

FiO_2 is raised by 1-L/M increments until dyspnea is sufficiently relieved but not necessarily eliminated. As discussed, there is controversy concerning the possibility that oxygen administration, in excess of the minimum dose necessary to prevent the complications of chronic hypoxemia, could greatly complicate weaning from oxygen later (by allowing the patient's respiratory muscles to decondition).

Treatment of Functional Impairment

To help facilitate airway clearance treatments, if the patient cannot lie in head-down positions. Nasal cannula oxygen at the lowest flow needed to allow treatment is acceptable. An increase in PCO_2 is not an issue and blood gas monitoring is unnecessary. The patient is not going to become dangerously hypercapnic while participating in airway clearance procedures. The oxygen (or the increased oxygen) is stopped at the end of the treatment. Patients who are afraid to cough or resist coughing because of associated dyspnea (whether they are already using nasal cannula oxygen or not) often do well with an oxygen mask (at 40%) that they can hold in their hand and use (or add to nasal oxygen) during coughing spells. This allows them to cough while breathing oxygen, move the mask away to expectorate, and then replace it until the paroxysm is over. If patients delay or do not finish eating because of the dyspnea caused by the work of eating, the distention of the stomach, or the oxygen requirement of digestion, oxygen therapy is indicated.

To improve exercise ability, the ideal oxygen dose can be precisely determined by performing sequential ABGs via an indwelling arterial catheter while the patient walks on a treadmill and breathes various concentrations of supplemental oxygen. The oxygen requirement can also be determined empirically (and less invasively) by gradually increasing the oxygen dose, ending at the lowest dose that allows the patient to perform the necessary activity with reasonable comfort. Patients whose resting arterial Po_2 is in the range of 60 mm Hg will probably do acceptably well with an empirical oxygen dose of 30% (36). Chronically hypercapnic patients may need to be warned to remove (or reduce) the oxygen after each exercise session.

B. Right Heart Failure Secondary to Cor Pulmonale

Right heart failure, defined clinically as an increase in the cardiac silhouette (by 1 cm from a reasonably recent standard posteroanterior chest film, that is, not a portable film), together with evidence of fluid retention (peripheral edema or hepatic enlargement and tenderness), is an ominous event in any patient with obstructive pulmonary disease. Hepatic tenderness in CF patients often involves primarily the left lobe and often manifests as midline tenderness to light percussion, rather than classical right upper quadrant tenderness. Also, the increase in cardiac silhouette is an essential part of the diagnostic criteria (but is not always easy to document because increased air trapping, common with a pulmonary exacerbation, often makes the heart appear smaller). Severe hypercapnia alone can cause fluid retention because of the obligate "saving" of sodium that occurs when bicarbonate is conserved to compensate for respiratory acidosis.

Initial laboratory workup should include the studies described for the uncomplicated pulmonary exacerbation (see Table 3). In addition, if the patient was not taking any diuretics before hospital admission, urine osmolality and serum osmolality should be measured initially to help rule out the syndrome of inappropriate antidiuretic hormone (ADH) secretion (SIADH). Echocardiography can supply valuable information, especially if visualization of the pulmonary valve allows measurement of systolic ejection intervals to help assess the pulmonary systolic pressure. A standard electrocardiogram can occasionally be helpful in estimating the degree of right ventricular hypertrophy.

Arterial blood gases should be obtained to assess the degree of hypercapnia and to help adjust oxygen dose. Radionuclide studies can provide more precise data about cardiac performance, but this information does not seem to be essential for routine patient care.

Treatment is directed at relieving acute manifestations of heart failure and reversing the underlying pulmonary disease that has caused sufficient cor pulmonale and increased pulmonary vascular resistance (primarily as a consequence of hypoxia) to cause heart failure. The mainstays of treatment are oxygen and salt restriction and diuretics. Oxygen relieves hypoxia, the prime stimulus for pulmonary vasospasm. See Treatment and Prevention of Hypoxia-Related Complications. Every effort should be made to elevate the arterial Po_2 to 50 mm Hg and, if possible, to 60 mm Hg or more (or to achieve pulse oximetry readings of at least 89% and preferably $\geq 93\%$).

Diuretics reduce right atrial pressure (37) and should be given on the admission day (or soon after the onset of heart failure if it develops in a hospitalized patient). To minimize the risk of renal injury, the IV diuretic should be given after the institution of oxygen therapy and not within 3 hours of an intravenous nephrotoxic antibiotic. (See Simultaneous Administration of Tobramycin and Colistin). Adults should receive 40 mg of furosemide as the first dose; an appropriately reduced dose (1 mg/kg) should be used for children. It may be helpful to have the patient measure urine output for 3 hours after IV diuretics, but prolonged measurements of intake and output (I & O) are rarely necessary. Similarly, daily weighing of the patient, although less of a nuisance, is also rarely necessary. If the 3-hour diuresis is unexpectedly low, a double dose of furosemide (or one IV dose of Bumex 0.5–1.0 mg, perhaps following metolazone) can be given. Most patients should then begin a daily potassium-sparing oral diuretic (e.g., aldactone, 75–100 mg/day, or triampterene, 100 mg/day). All patients should have some degree of salt restriction, ranging from 0.5 g/day to "no added salt," depending on the patient's prior salt intake (which can be as much as 20 g/day in CF patients who are accustomed to compensating for sweat losses) and the severity of the heart failure.

Digitalis is rarely useful for uncomplicated right heart failure due to cor pulmonale. In general, it adds potential toxicity (especially arrhythmia) without benefit. However, occasional CF patients have left heart failure as well (from hypoxia or because dilatation of the right ventricle compromises left ventricular function), and these patients may benefit from digitalis.

Unloaders (e.g., prazosin) are occasionally useful, but need not be instituted immediately. Tolazoline and other agents touted as specific pulmonary vasodilators have not lived up to early hopes. The effect of inhaled nitric oxide has not been reported in CF patients. It may prove useful in some patients, but it will not be easy to administer safely, and safe continuation of nitric oxide treatment at home is virtually impossible. Hydralazine, nifedipine, and phentolamine have not been extensively tested but do not appear to have clinically useful pulmonary vasodilation activity in CF patients with advanced pulmonary disease (38).

Intravenous albumin should rarely be used even if serum albumin is low. Heart failure is often worsened by increased intravascular volume, before reduction of edema and subsequent diuresis results from the increased osmotic pressure.

Elevation of the legs, tight fitting hose, and other physical measures aimed at mobilizing fluid can be helpful (and nontoxic) adjunctive treatments.

Treatment of Underlying Pulmonary Disease

Pulmonary infection should be addressed as described for the uncomplicated pulmonary exacerbation with the following additions:

1. Antipseudomonal penicillins, in the doses used for CF, may contribute a substantial sodium load and should be used cautiously. If possible, other antibiotics (see Tables 6 and 8) should be given.
2. The intravenous fluid used to deliver antibiotics should be 5% D/W unless the antibiotic must be given in saline. In any case, the smallest possible amount of IV fluid should be used.
3. New onset or uncontrolled diabetes should not be tightly controlled so that sudden reduction of osmotic diuresis does not further aggravate heart failure.
4. Participation in an exercise program should be delayed and, if instituted after the patient improves, monitored closely with pulse oximetry or ABG analysis to ensure that sudden extreme drops in arterial oxygen saturation are avoided (25).
5. The patient may not tolerate head-down positions for airway clearance and these treatments may have to be modified accordingly. Other techniques for airway clearance may also require modification. For example, autogenic drainage and "huffing" may not be possible because of dyspnea. The patient's inability to perform a full forced expiratory maneuver may compromise the effectiveness of the Flutter. (See also Treatment of Functional Impairment.)

Follow-up and Prognosis

If the patient emerges from heart failure with resolution of peripheral edema and diminution in the transverse cardiac silhouette on chest film, and goes on to reachieve baseline status, then specific cardiac treatment (e.g., diuretics, salt restriction, or tight hose) may no longer be necessary. This depends almost entirely on the degree of improvement in pulmonary status. In general, however, clinically important right heart failure due to cor pulmonale is not likely to recur as long as the arterial Po_2 exceeds 55 mm Hg.

Long-term prognosis depends on the rapidity of progression of the pulmonary deterioration that led to heart failure. An acute event such as influenza may eventually resolve and leave the patient virtually unscathed. However, the patient who slowly worsens and slips gradually into right heart failure has a much more ominous prognosis, with the outlook for survival usually being less than 2 years (27).

C. Chest Pain (See also Appendix 2)

Bilateral symmetric chest pain is usually of musculoskeletal origin and rarely originates in the lung or pleura. It can be related to lung disease. For example, the pain of muscle strain can occur because of sudden increase in work of breathing, and therefore can vary with breathing. Often, no laboratory workup is necessary and analgesics and antiinflammatory drugs are usually all that is needed.

Unilateral or midline chest pain, especially if its onset occurred with an acute increase in dyspnea, is often of pulmonary origin (e.g., pneumothorax, pneumomediastinum, sudden onset of lobar atelectasis, pleurisy, or large lung abscess) and deserves workup with chest film and perhaps other tests. Duration of pain before the patient sought medical attention is rarely diagnostically help-ful. The chest pain associated with air leaks, pleurisy, and, occasionally, atelec-tasis is often rather sudden in onset. Patients with pleurisy often lie on the affected side (to restrict its excursion with breathing); a friction rub can occa-sionally be found. Rib fracture, which can occur with strenuous cough, and costochondritis can usually be strongly suspected or ruled out on the basis of the presence or absence of point tenderness. Unilaterally reduced breath sounds that were not heard previously or subcutaneous air is strongly suggestive of an air leak.

Cystic fibrosis patients with severe new-onset unilateral chest pain almost always require a chest radiograph (preferably not a portable film) for evaluation. In some patients, chest pain develops at the onset of an air leak, but they have sufficient adhesions to hold the lung in place until after the first chest film, only to experience clinically important collapse later; another film obtained 24 hours later may be helpful. Patients with persistent pain may need follow-up rib films several days later to detect the callus of a healing fracture. Patients with esophagitis often have midline (retrosternal) pain, but their pain is occasionally localized by the patient slightly lateral to the midline. Empirical treatment with antacids or antiyeast agents can help with diagnosis.

D. Pneumothorax and Pneumomediastinum

Pneumothorax may require specific intervention if one or more of the following apply:

1. Breathing is acutely impaired (e.g., with dyspnea or hypoxemia).
2. Cough is impaired or less effective (e.g., with chest pain or partially atelectatic areas).
3. Chest pain is intolerable.
4. The patient must travel or be transported by airplane or helicopter.
5. The large size of the pneumothorax indicates that substantial resolution will take a long time even if there is no longer an active air leak. Estimation of the size of the pneumothorax (e.g., "15%") is not very accurate in CF patients, because the CF lung is so stiff that it may not collapse or compress very much. A relatively small volume of extra-pulmonary air may actually be under a good deal of tension.
6. Tension pneumothorax (theoretically included in numbers 1 and 5) often requires immediate emergency treatment (e.g., tube thoracostomy, occasionally preceded by needle insertion to relieve tension).

Treatment

Whatever specific treatment for pneumothorax is undertaken, antibiotic treatment of pulmonary infection should be instituted (See Treatment of Uncomplicated Pulmonary Exacerbation and Special Problems.)

The ideal specific treatment for pneumothorax complicating CF would have the following characteristics: result in prompt resolution and totally prevent recurrence, be noninvasive or minimally invasive and painless, have no toxicity or risk, not result in any pulmonary function sequelae, and not adversely affect the patient's future options and prognosis with regard to lung transplant. Such a treatment does not exist (and probably never will) and, therefore, the treatment of pneumothorax involves considerable judgment and compromise.

A small asymptomatic leak usually does not require any specific intervention. Ongoing treatment (including airway clearance procedures) can continue. High-concentration oxygen may hasten resolution slightly, but can cause other problems (e.g., it can aggravate hypercapnia) and is rarely indicated.

Larger leaks, particularly if recurrent, usually deserve surgical intervention. Tube thoracostomy alone, even if it achieves prompt resolution, is relatively ineffective in preventing recurrence. Therefore, for all practical purposes, the main treatment options are surgical pleurectomy and pleural abrasion (39,40) (which is often the preferred treatment) and chemical pleurodesis.

If surgical pleurectomy is chosen it should be done as soon as possible (preferably on admission or the next morning). Waiting to "get the patient in better condition" for surgery is rarely successful; instead, ongoing chest pain and interference with airway clearance, caused by the pneumothorax or chest tube, contribute to slow deterioration. Prolonged tube thoracostomy is associated with a very high mortality rate (41). Surgery can be successfully accomplished even if the patient has very compromised pulmonary function (as demonstrated on a prepneumothorax test), but if the patient is desperately sick such as with severe respiratory failure or right heart failure, then chemical pleurodesis, Heimlich valves, or more prolonged observation may be a better initial approach. In any case, it is important that the surgeon has substantial experience with thoracic surgery in CF patients.

Apical blebectomy with oversewing (42) has been suggested (43) as an alternative to surgical pleurectomy because it would have little impact on the patient's future candidacy for transplantation, while still offering a reasonable chance of quick resolution and prevention of recurrence. Furthermore, this procedure might be possible, at least in some patients, with thoracoscopy (44), thus sparing the very sick patient a thoracotomy.

Chemical pleurodesis (the instillation of a sclerosing agent into the chest tube) requires one to three daily treatments (depending on the agent used). Quinacrine (Atabrine) is a good choice (45); it causes sufficient inflammation, but not so much that a "frozen diaphragm" develops. However, the parenteral form of quinacrine is no longer widely available. Use of the oral form for intrapleural instillation has been reported but is not in widespread use. Tetracycline does not produce adequate adhesions. Talc is effective; it virtually always achieves resolution and has a high success rate in preventing recurrence, but it causes such extensive fibrosis that it is likely to cause a frozen diaphragm. Silver nitrate causes a severe burn of the pleura; it is effective but very painful (instillation often requires general anesthesia) and may result in a long-lasting effusion. Overall, there is not much to recommend silver nitrate over surgical pleurectomy. Pleurodesis with either talc or silver nitrate, because of their tendency to cause frozen diaphragm, reduce the chance that a lung transplant will be successful.

Once resolution is achieved, recovery from acute pneumothorax (whether after surgery, pleurodesis, or observation) is usually fairly rapid, and the patient can be discharged as for uncomplicated pulmonary exacerbation, except that pulmonary function tests are probably best omitted for several weeks.

E. Hemoptysis

Minor episodes of hemoptysis (small amounts of blood–specks, streaks, or small clumps mixed with sputum) are frequent in CF patients, even when the patient is not in the midst of an acute exacerbation. They probably originate from "feeder vessels," which serve the airways themselves. Bleeding usually stops spontaneously. These episodes rarely require specific treatment and do not affect long-term prognosis. However, these patients probably deserve:

1. A coagulation screen with the next regularly scheduled venepuncture.
2. An oral dose of vitamin K (if the patient is not receiving it already).

3. A review of the present medications to determine whether any interfere with clotting. Common examples are aspirin, ibuprofen, or other nonsteroidal antiinflammatory agent, antipseudomonal penicillin, occasionally cephalosporin, and excessive doses of heparin for maintaining patency of VI line.

4. If the bleeding is more than minimal, temporary discontinuation of chest percussion, Flutter, and some other forms of airway clearance (e.g., intrapulmonary percussive ventilation) until an arbitrary time (perhaps 6–12 hours) after the bleeding has stooped. On the other hand, although positioning for postural drainage may precipitate a recurrence of bleeding, this is often detectable by the patient ("I feel a gurgling when I go right-side down"). In the absence of an obvious correlation between these maneuvers and bleeding episodes, a good case can be made for continuing airway clearance practices in that infection helps initate bleeding and airway clearance helps control infection, blood is ciliatoxic, and blood is a good culture medium and therefore should be moved from the airways.

5. Explanation of the pathophysiology of hemoptysis, the therapeutic plan, and the prognosis.

Major hemoptysis including massive hemoptysis (variously defined as greater than 300 mL or 500 mL or enough blood to cause postural blood pressure changes), usually originates in a systemic pressure vessel (a large pulmonary artery tributary in a patient with cor pulmonale or, more likely, a vessel of bronchial artery origin). The approach to some patients who do not have one major episode, but whose combined daily bleeding causes progressive anemia, is very similar and these patients are discussed together. Although acute exsanguination was not uncommon in early reports (46), most episodes stop before clinically significant hypotension occurs (47). Treatment is the same whether hemoptysis is the reason for admission or occurs in the course of hospitalization for another indication. The actions suggested for minor hemoptysis apply to major hemoptysis as well (administration of vitamin K should be oral or intramuscular; IV administration can cause anaphylaxis). In addition, contingency plans should be made (if none already exist as standard CF center practice) for treatment if hemoptysis continues and leads to severe anemia or hypotension and shock. Emergency treatment with volume expanders (e.g., saline and blood) should be used with caution and only if hypotension is severe enough to threaten life. Bleeding may be perpetuated by artificially maintaining the blood pressure above the point at which elastic recoil and clot formation can successfully stop the bleeding. This concept, although not specifically demonstrated for massive hemoptysis, has been implicated in penetrating torso injuries (48). The following are major therapeutic options for severe or continuing bleeding.

1. Procrastinate: None of the following choices is entirely benign or guaranteed successful. If the bleeding is not overwhelming, waiting, perhaps while giving a few (one to three) blood transfusions over a several day period, may be the best choice. Primum non nocere.

2. Vasopressin: Control of hemoptysis has been reported (in adults) with use of vasopressin (49). (Initial dose is 20 units over 15 minutes, followed by 0.2 units/min for 36 hours.) Concomitant use of nitroglycerin may be indicated to minimize the effect of vasopressin on cardiac blood flow. Even if this treatment is successful, serious consideration should be given to proceeding to bronchial artery embolization, as soon as possible.

3. Tamponade of bronchus serving the site of bleeding: This tamponade requires bronchoscopy, localization of the bleeding site, insertion of balloon (e.g., Foley catheter) into the relevant airway, inflation of balloon, and fixing catheter's position while removing the bronchoscope, and then maintaining the catheter and balloon in place—all in a dyspneic bleeding patient. This approach can be successful (50), but it is very difficult to accomplish and is rarely needed.

4. Bronchial artery embolization (51,52): In this procedure, the descending aorta is catheterized, usually via the femoral artery, and the bronchial artery origins are located and entered. An arteriogram is performed to ensure that the artery to the lung can be embolized with little danger of causing a functional transection of the spinal cord by the inadvertent embolization of a spinal artery, which can occasionally arise from the bronchial artery. The bronchial artery is then embolized with, for example, 250–590 μm particles of polyvinyl alcohol foam and adsorbable gelatin pledgets. The size is important; the particles must be large enough to tamponade the vessel without gaining access, by collaterals, to the pulmonary artery circulation, but small enough to get into the bronchial artery orifice. The procedure is repeated until all bronchial arteries that can be located have been embolized. Arteries that seem to supply only the nonbleeding lung often send branches back to the other side. If the embolization cannot be completed because the maximum allowable 24-hour dose of contrast material has been used, the remaining vessels are addressed in a repeat procedure, usually the next day. These procedures should be carried out by an interventional radiologist who has had experience with CF patients. These procedures are tedious and require the patient to remain in a recumbent position for up to 5 hours. Some patients require sedation. Even after successful procedures, tortuous recanalizing vessels may form, accounting for the frequent recurrence of clinically important bleeding 2–5 years later.

Table 13 Check List for Evaluating a Cystic Fibrosis Patient for Lobectomy

1. Is the patient and family willing to incur the pain and expense of surgery despite the knowledge that the procedure might not be dramatically successful and involves substantial immediate and short-term risks?
2. Is the patient free of nonpulmonary contraindications to major surgery?
3. Does the patient have distinctly worse parenchymal disease (severe bronchiectasis, intractable atelectasis or abscess) in one lobe than in the rest of both lungs?
4. Does the patient have systemic symptoms, such as fever, anorexia, or fatigue, suggesting that the localized disease is "active?"
5. Does control of the localized disease, for example, after a course of intravenous antibiotics, result in the patient's having a substantially improved functional level with regard to decreased morbidity (e.g., disappearance of fever) and exercise capability?
6. Do computed tomography scans confirm the lack of advanced disease in the remaining pulmonary parenchyma?
7. Do ventilation or perfusion scans suggest that there has already been substantial shunting of blood away from the proposed target for lobectomy?
8. If the lobe being considered for resection still has substantial blood flow, do cardiac catheterization data indicate that pulmonary hypertension will not be unacceptably worsened by the loss of the vascular bed in the area targeted for removal?

5. Emergent and semiemergent lobectomy: Lobectomy is rarely necessary because there are other treatment options available. However, if all else fails and the site of bleeding has been unequivocally demonstrated, lobectomy can be life saving (53). Although not all the criteria may apply (and the situation under discussion here is life, death, and urgent), Table 13 may be helpful with the final decision about lobectomy.

F. Allergic Bronchopulmonary Aspergillosis

Screening for allergic bronchopulmonary aspergillosis (ABPA) (IgE, sputum culture for fungus) should be done for every CF patient who is admitted for a pulmonary indication. Very high IgE levels (defined by local standards) should trigger more detailed testing (*Aspergillus* skin test, fungal hypersensitivity pneumonitis panel, and perhaps measurements of anti-aspergillus specific IgG and IgE). Unfortunately, the diagnosis of ABPA (and particularly separating ABPA from simple *Aspergillus* allergy or clinically unimportant *Aspergillus* colonization of the airway) is often difficult, because CF patients who do not have ABPA often have many of the component findings (e.g., fleeting infiltrates, wheezing) by which the disease is defined in non-CF patients (54). *Aspergillus* skin tests were positive in 56% of CF patients in one study, but at least 50% of these patients did not reach even liberal criteria for the diagnosis of ABPA (55). *Aspergillus fumigatus* was recovered from respiratory secretions of 60% of the patients in another center; only 25% of these were thought to have

ABPA (56). Even *Aspergillus*-specific IgE (and IgG) levels can fluctuate (and even disappear) spontaneously (or at least without corticosteroid treatment) (57). Elevated *Aspergillus*-specific IgE has been reported in up to 50% of CF patients (58): either this test is not as specific as would be hoped or a huge percentage of CF patients have ABPA. The incidence of ABPA may be higher in CF patients who live in rural areas, which may partially account for the variable incidence of ABPA in different CF centers (59). The bottom line is that each CF center must develop its own criteria for this diagnosis, and even then the physicians should recognize that absolute certainty regarding the diagnosis of ABPA is often impossible in CF patients.

Cystic fibrosis patients whose ABPA goes unrecognized are at risk for development of ABPA-related central bronchiectasis; patients who have simple *Aspergillus* allergy but are incorrectly diagnosed as having ABPA may unnecessarily be exposed to the major complications of corticosteroid therapy. There is no good test to exclude ABPA in CF patients whose IgE level is in excess of 5 times the local (asthmatic patient) average. More specific tests would be useful but, in all likelihood, the diagnosis of ABPA will continue to be difficult for most CF patients.

The treatment of ABPA in CF patients is much the same as it is for other patient populations. Systemic corticosteroid is still the mainstay of treatment. Oral prednisone (0.5–1.0 mg/kg/day as a starting dose) should be given until the total IgE (*Aspergillus*-specific IgE can be used if the test is available) has reentered the normal range or at least until it has stopped decreasing. The prednisone can then be tapered and eventually maintained at a very low (or alternate day) dose or discontinued altogether. The patient is then followed up for regular IgE levels. Although the diagnosis is often made on inpatients, this treatment will still be in progress at discharge. Aerosolized corticosteroids are frequently used in patients who are intolerant of systemic treatment (e.g., those in whom diabetes or pseudotumor cerebri develop or those who refuse treatment because of cosmetic effects of drug, fear of diabetes, or some other reason); however, there is no good evidence that aerosolized corticosteroids are effective. Systemic antifungal agents (e.g., amphotericin-B) have been thought ineffective, but with less toxic agents now available (e.g., itraconazole), this approach is being used more often (60). Aerosolized amphotericin B (5 mg in 3 cc) is also thought effective by some CF physicians.

G. Edema

Unilateral edema (one leg; one arm) is almost always due to compromised venous return secondary to an unusual sleeping position or prolonged maintenance of an unusual posture to facilitate breathing.

The differential diagnosis of generalized edema is presented in Table 14. Initial laboratory workup should include (1) a standard (i.e., not a portable)

Table 14 Differential Diagnosis of Generalized Edema in Patients with Cystic Fibrosis[a]

Etiology	Diagnostic clues
Heart failure	Severe pulmonary disease, distended neck veins, tender hepatomegaly (especially toward epigastrium), gallop rhythm, increase in transverse cardiac dimension by 1 cm or more in standard posteroanterior projection compared with previous film
Hypoalbuminemia	Albumin <2.0 and usually <1.8 g/dL; history of liver disease; generalized edema; in infant, breast feeding or use of soy-based formula
Syndrome of inappropriate antidiuretic hormone section	Very sick patient; hyponatremia; concentrated urine with hypoosmolar serum (in patient who has not been treated with diuretics)
Severe respiratory Failure	Markedly elevated arterial P_{CO_2} and serum bicarbonate
Compromise of venous return from legs	Very dyspneic patient who sits leaning forward almost to the point that the upper body is parallel to the legs; only legs are edematous

[a]More than one may apply in any given patient.

chest film to help rule out right heart failure secondary to cor pulmonale, (2) serum chemistry panel to detect dilutional hyponatremia that would suggest SIADH, detect very high serum bicarbonate (as compensation for hypercapnia), which would imply an obligate retention of sodium, and detect very low serum albumin secondary to poor nutrition, renal loss (e.g., from drug-induced nephropathy), or decreased synthesis due to liver disease, and (3) in any CF patient who presents with generalized edema and who has not been treated with diuretics for at least 48 hours simultaneous measurements of urine and serum osmolality (also to help rule out SIADH).

Treatment of SIADH is by fluid restriction. Details on this syndrome and its treatment are available elsewhere. For other causes of edema (see Table 14), treatment directed at the underlying cause of the edema should be initiated as promptly as possible but often will not result in prompt resolution of edema.

H. Pulmonary Hypertrophic Osteoarthropathy

Pulmonary hypertrophic osteoarthropathy (PHOA) is probably pathophysiologically related to clubbing, but the exact mechanism of either of these clinical manifestations of pulmonary disease is unknown. The arthropathy primarily affects the large joints (knee, ankle, wrists—in that order) and can cause considerable pain and disability (primarily by interference with walking). Small (finger) joints are occasionally affected (61). It is uncommon before age 12 years (62). The diagnosis is made by the presence of clubbing (virtually universal in CF children and adults); generally symmetrical joint involvement, including arthralgia, stiffness, joint swelling and effusions; warmth or tenderness of affected joints; and subperiosteal bone formation, especially of the distal tibia, fibula, ulna, and radius. The various signs and symptoms may not occur simultaneously, and all usually vary in intensity, usually in some relation to the activity of the pulmonary disease. Fever or erythema nodosum may be present. However, a variety of other forms of arthritis may develop in CF patients as well, and the differential diagnosis can be tricky. Other entities to be considered include a nonspecific episodic arthritis (63) commonly seen in CF patients, classical juvenile rheumatoid arthritis, sarcoid-associated arthritis (64), and arthropathy associated with gastrointestinal disease, including "blind loop syndrome (65), Crohn's disease (66), and pancreatitis.

Acute treatment with antiinflammatory agents, such as ibuprofen, is often extremely effective. However, some CF patients either do not respond to these agents or are intolerant of them (e.g., they have gastrointestinal toxicity or aggravation of hemoptysis) and must be treated with corticosteroids. The long-range prognosis rests primarily with successful treatment of the underlying CF-related pulmonary disease.

I. Diabetes

Diabetes (see Chapter 7) complicating the pancreatic lesion of CF is uncommon until the mid-teenage years, after which it becomes increasingly prevalent. Although the onset can be abrupt with a classical history of recent polyuria, polydipsia, and weight loss, most patients have a more insidious course and complain only of some nocturia and weight loss. In any case, insulin treatment is almost always necessary. The goal of treatment for most patients should be tight control (as it is with most modern diabetes treatment programs), and most patients do best with a program that allows them virtually unlimited diet (e.g., as with a multiple daily injection regimen). This recommendation is based on the following: (1) the life expectancy of most of these CF patients is long enough so that they can be expected to be at risk for long-term vascular complications of uncontrolled diabetes, and (2) the pulmonary disease may be adversely affected if the glucose gradient is high enough to facilitate bacterial growth. Hospitalized diabetic CF patients should usually receive their IV antibiotics in saline instead of glucose; the actual sugar load of the glucose infusion is not quantitatively great, but it seems to cause considerable problems with diabetes control. As discussed, newly diagnosed diabetes in patients with new-onset overt right heart failure and fluid retention should be controlled slowly to avoid suddenly increasing vascular volume by reducing the osmotic diuretic effect of hyperglycemia and glucosuria.

Other Types and Causes of Diabetes

Diabetes induced by systemic corticosteroids (e.g., for ABPA) almost always requires insulin treatment as well. Some patients lose their insulin requirement after discontinuation of corticosteroids, but many continue to be insulin dependent, suggesting that diabetes would have occurred eventually anyway. Diabetes of any cause is more difficult to control during corticosteroid therapy. Alternate day corticosteroid therapy is particularly difficult; some CF patients are able to maintain good glycemic control with alternate day insulin therapy. Occasional CF patients are sufficiently overweight for weight loss to be used as a primary approach to treatment.

Very early onset diabetes (in patients younger than age 12 years) is unlikely to be pathophysiologically related to CF and is more likely to be common-variety juvenile diabetes mellitus. Ketoacidosis, which is very rare in the typical diabetes of CF that develops later in life, is more likely to develop in these patients. It is much more "brittle" and harder to control, even with diligent patient effort. These patients should not be "automatically" chastised if their glycohemoglobin levels are persistently abnormal. Similarly, achieving tight control in these patients while they are hospitalized is unrealistic and probably not worthwhile because their insulin requirements will be totally different after they return home.

The long-term implications of diabetes for the pulmonary lesion are not clear. There is no convincing evidence that these patients have more rapid progression of lung infection.

J. Anemia

Unlike most other patients who have chronic hypoxemia (e.g., cyanotic congenital heart disease in children; severe noninfectious pulmonary disease in adults), polycythemia does not usually develop in patients with CF. In fact, many CF patients with severe pulmonary disease are overtly anemic. The anemia is attributable to several factors, including nutritional deficiencies (e.g., lack of iron and perhaps vitamin E) and chronic blood loss from minor episodes of hemoptysis. For patients with marginal pulmonary function and substantially compromised arterial Po_2, this deficiency in oxygen-carrying capacity can be of great importance, because of its effect on the patient's dyspnea, cachexia, and fatigue.

Whatever its cause, the anemia is often a sufficiently important abnormality to justify specific treatment. Furthermore, even patients whose hemoglobin level and hematocrit are within the normal range may actually have a relative anemia, that is, they would have more hemoglobin if nutritional deficiencies and chronic illness were not interfering with appropriate compensation for hypoxemia. Some suggestions for dealing with this problem follow.

1. Diagnostic studies include complete blood count with red blood cell indices and reticulocyte count, iron studies (serum iron and total iron binding capacity with calculated percent saturation), and serum ferritin. A serum vitamin E level may be worthwhile, but only if the patient is newly admitted and has not received a water-soluble vitamin E preparation in the hospital. (Even patients who are not compliant with vitamin E treatment or who have not been taking a water-soluble form can demonstrate a rapid elevation in the serum vitamin E after initiation of supplementation.) Other vitamin studies may also be worthwhile. Although red cell survival studies may help clinch vitamin E deficiency anemia, supplementation is so easy (and inexpensive) that these studies are rarely done. Bone marrow examination is rarely necessary. If the explanation of the anemia is not certain, the stool should be tested for occult blood and the patient and family should be closely questioned about other sources of blood loss (e.g., epistaxis), which could require specific treatment (e.g., cautery or discontinuation of nonsteroidal antiinflammatory agents).

2. Despite the theoretical advantages of correcting anemia, transfusion can often be avoided, even for patients whose hematocrit and hemoglobin are quite low after hemoptysis. As a general rule, for patients who are no longer actively bleeding (and are not desperately hypoxemic or air hungry), transfusion is rarely necessary if the hemoglobin level and hematocrit are at or above 7.5 g/dL and 21%, respectively. However, every other available measure to optimize hemoglobin and red cell production should be pursued.

3. A water-soluble supplement of vitamin E should be given in adequate dose (correct dose is controversial, but at least 400 IU a day is justified in anemic patients).

4. Iron replacement should be instituted in all patients with significant anemia who are iron deficient (that is most of them). Oral iron is theoretically adequate, but it fails in many patients. Cystic fibrosis patients often do not tolerate oral iron, and, even then, rarely more than one dose per day (because of gastrointestinal toxicity, mainly abdominal pain and nausea), and few continue to take it because the beneficial results are slow and many patients will not accept any toxicity. Intravenous iron dextran should be considered in any patient with a substantial iron deficit (dose can be obtained from the *Physician's Desk Reference*). After the recommended IV test dose (0.5 mL), the balance of the recommended dose is infused in 250 mL of normal saline over 3–4 hours. The drug should be given by an infusion pump with a slow (e.g., 20 mL/hr) starting rate, and the patient must be closely monitored for anaphylaxis (mainly hypotension), especially

during the first 30–60 minutes of treatment. The dose can be increased gradually to 70 mL/hr if hypotension does not develop. Anaphylaxis is treated by stopping the infusion and administering IV Benadryl and corticosteroid (e.g., hydrocortisone); vasopressors are rarely needed. Despite the theoretical danger in this approach (which should be explained to the patient and family before starting), successful infusion of the total dose obviates the need for prolonged (usually toxic) oral iron and it produces a much quicker initial response (usually in less than 1 week).

5. The clinical effectiveness of erythropoietin has not been reported in CF. At least some CF patients would probably benefit from erythropoietin treatment, and it is possible that it could become a valuable therapeutic agent for all anemic CF patients (and possibly for some nonanemic patients as well if it could produce mild polycythemia).

K. Sinusitis

In virtually all CF patients, radiological examination shows opacification of all the paranasal sinuses (67), except for the frontal sinuses, which may be very small or undeveloped. However, classical symptoms of sinusitis (obstruction of nasal air flow, rhinorrhea or purulent nasal discharge, facial pain or headache, postnasal drip and sore throat) are surprisingly uncommon. Even when these symptoms are present, sinusitis may not be the cause. Furthermore, although worsening pulmonary status may be ascribed to sinus disease by patients and families and physicians, such an association has been difficult to prove, both in the individual patient and in CF in general. Fortunately, antibiotic treatment directed at the pulmonary lesion is probably all that is needed for the sinus disease in most inpatients, so establishing conclusive proof that the sinus disease is clinically important is rarely necessary if the patient is being treated for pulmonary disease.

If sinuses do cause pulmonary disease in some patients, they deserve specific (usually surgical) treatment. In addition, serious complications of sinusitis have been reported in CF patients; these definitely require specific, and often urgent, attention. Mucopyocele with erosion of a wall of the sinus (thus endangering the orbit or the central nervous system) usually occurs with severe, often unrelenting, headache, and worrisome ophthalmological symptoms, including visual disturbance (e.g., double vision) and proptosis (68,69). Fever is usually low-grade or absent.

For CF patients in whom sinusitis is thought to be clinically important in precipitating exacerbations of pulmonary disease (70) and in whom traditional sinus surgery (71) has failed, or for those who have had frequently recurrent nasal polyps, a new treatment approach has recently been proposed (70). After removal of infected secretions at surgery, maxillary drainage windows are created as usual, but then a small catheter (fashioned from the tubing of a butter-fly IV needle) is inserted through the nose into each sinus and taped to the cheek. Tobramycin (40 mg) is instilled into each catheter twice daily for up to 10 days, and then the catheters are removed. The patient returns for a repeat outpatient instillation (using a syringe and soft catheter and local anesthesia) once a month. Reduced morbidity from sinus symptoms, reduced frequency of polyp recurrence, and perhaps some improvement in pulmonary disease have been reported. The computed tomography appearance of the sinuses improved noticeably (or cleared) in all patients.

L. Atelectasis

Lobar and segmental atelectasis can result from either complete obstruction of the related airway or gradual destruction of the pulmonary parenchyma, which eventually loses volume and becomes nearly airless. For patients in the latter group, substantial reexpansion is unlikely and, at best, is transient. Treatment directed at resurrecting the atelectatic area is futile. The best outcome is for the entire involved area to become fibrotic. This area would then not be functional, but would no longer pose a threat to the remainder of the lung. At worst, the involved area becomes an abscess and causes systemic symptoms, including fever, anorexia, and malaise, as well as classical pulmonary symptoms of cough and sputum production. Rarely, a patient who meets these criteria improves substantially after lobectomy (see Table 13). The best candidates for surgical intervention have substantial systemic symptoms but relatively minimal parenchymal disease elsewhere.

Patients whose atelectasis appears to be due to intrinsic airway obstruction (by thick secretions) of a lobe or segment that has relatively normal parenchyma should be evaluated by bronchoscopy and then given intensive treatment, beginning with bronchoscopic lavage and suctioning, but also including intravenous antibiotic and other treatment, perhaps including mucolytic agents and intensive and frequent local drainage and percussion. The prognosis for complete and sustained recovery has never been good (72,73), but surgical treatment is not indicated in the absence of systemic symptoms. In an occasional patient who does not respond to aggressive treatment initially, the area does reexpand spontaneously several months later.

M. Headache

Severe headache is a common complaint among CF patients who are hospital-ized during a pulmonary exacerbation. Headache, in addition to causing substantial morbidity, interferes with other aspects of treatment (e.g., cough and airway clearance). Diagnosis and specific treatment (e.g., discontinuation of drug or correction of hypoxemia) is essential. The principal entities to be

Table 15 Differential Diagnosis of Headache Related to Pulmonary Disease or Its Treatment in Hospitalized Cystic Fibrosis Patients

Etiology	Diagnostic Clues/Tests
Hypercapnia	Headache is worst (or is present only) when patient awakens; diminishes or disappears over first half-hour of wakefulness. Oxygen (or increased oxygen) has no immediate effect. Arterial blood gas (ABG) shows compensated hypercapnia with P_{CO_2} levels while awake above 60 mm Hg.
Hypoxemia	Headache is worst (or is present only) when patient awakens; diminishes or disappears over first hour or so that patient is awake. Oxygen (or increased oxygen) provides immediate relief of headache. ABG with patient using present oxygen prescription shows hypoxemia (P_{O_2} below 60 mmHg) at rest.
Drug toxicity (especially colistin)	Very severe headache, temporally related to administration of drug; no response to oxygen and often minimal or no response to analgesics. Headache not present before use of intravenous antibiotics. Patient may have history of headache during previous hospitalization.
Neuromuscular headache	Occipital headache. Recent increase in respiratory distress with patient using accessory muscles of respiration. Patient may be sleeping in unusual position (i.e., a change from previous pattern) and often sleep with head at unusual angle from body (i.e, putting stress on neck muscles.
Sinus disease	Frontal headache, facial pain, or pain in upper jaw may be present, along with other common symptoms of sinus disease. Ophthalmological symptoms (visual disturbance including diplopia and proptosis) may indicate serious complication of chronic sinusitis with erosion of wall of sinus.
Electrolyte disturbance	Very severe pulmonary disease. Serum chemistries show substantial hyponatremia or hypochloremia. Patient may have laboratory data supporting diagnosis of syndrome of inappropriate antidiuretic hormone secretion.
Migraine/atypical Migraine	Family history of migraine. Previous history of headache. Pain may be atypical i.e., occurring daily, bilateral, not associated with photophobia or vomiting. Migraine may be precipitated by increased hypoxemia.
Caffeine withdrawal	Relatively recent discontinuation or markedly decreased use of coffee, tea, or certain soft drinks (caffeine-containing colas or Mountain Dew.

included in the differential diagnosis are listed in Table 15. Treatment with mild analgesics may be indicated, especially if this treatment allows continuation of a critical drug. However, treatment with opioid analgesics is fraught with problems. Because the pain is not likely to be transient (and patients get considerable relief of anxiety and dyspnea in addition to pain relief from opioids), physiological and chemical dependence may occur quickly. At that point, withdrawal and dependency symptoms (including headache) may dominate the clinical picture and make evaluation of the original symptom virtually impossible (see Chapter 3).

VI. Special Problems

A. Slowly Progressive, Severe Illness

Children and young adults are capable of remarkable physiological compensation to severe chronic illness. As pulmonary status deteriorates and the patient drifts into more severe respiratory failure, worsening hypoxemia and hypercapnia (and their respective symptoms and metabolic consequences and symptoms) result in a variety of physiological adaptations. Renal compensation for acidosis results in extremely high bicarbonate levels (up to 55 mEq/L), allowing the patient to cope with chronic arterial Pco_2 values as high as 100 mm Hg; hematological compensation (polycythemia and increased erythrocyte diphosphoglycerate (DPG) for diminished oxygen tension) allow the patient to survive prolonged periods during which the arterial Po_2 does not exceed 40 mm Hg; cardiac hypertrophy allows the patient to cope with pulmonary hypertension); hypertrophy of the respiratory muscles allows the patient to cope with the additional work of breathing; and neuroendocrine adjustments, including weight loss or failure to grow, keep body mass to a minimum. These changes circumvent the failure of the weakest link in the patient's homeostatic chain, the lungs. All these secondary adjustments, in combination, optimize the patient's gradually diminishing ability to maintain the conditions necessary for life.

Furthermore, many CF patients, after a life of coping with chronic illness, have found that, to keep up with their peers, they must persevere with normal activities to the last possible moment. Eventually, however, even the most stoic psyche and most physiologically resourceful body surrenders and agrees to hospitalization. At that point, the patient is often in severe distress and, as initially evaluated, desperately ill.

For these very sick patients, who have drifted slowly into their present condition, a multisystem aggressive therapy approach involving the initiation (or major change of dose) of many potent drugs is often not what the doctor should order. Delicate physiological compensations can be undone, and the patient may worsen precipitously. There is less of a need to take drastic emergency actions than might seem to be the case. These patients are not much sicker than they had been the day before admission. Left alone, they would not be much worse the next day. A comprehensive diagnostic evaluation (as discussed earlier) should be initiated, but a sequential therapeutic approach, beginning with the least toxic and most immediately helpful measures. An example of this approach as applied for the first 2 days after admission of an 18-

Table 16 Treatment of a Cystic Fibrosis Patient Who Has Slowly Developed Very Severe Multisystem Symptoms and Signs

Elapsed time (hours: minutes)	Diagnostic and therapeutic measures

Example: An 18-year-old patient with chronic respiratory failure and severe hypoxemia, nutritional deficiency, cor pulmonale, and right heart failure.

Admission	Obtain admission laboratory work, including CBC, serum electrolytes and (if patient has not been taking diuretics) urine and serum osmolality, and sputum cultures (routine, mycobacteria, fungus). SIADH, if present, may necessitate changes in the management of edema. Make every effort to obtain a standard chest film (i.e., not a portable) so that heart size can be assessed and followed. Initiate intravenous correction of hypokalemia if present. Obtain ABG. If patient is anemic, serum iron studies could be added to original laboratory request. Obtain standard ECG. Ignore nutrition status; however, advise patient about avoiding high salt foods.
00:15	Take no specific (direct) measures to correct acidosis. Begin partial correction of hypoxemia but do not necessarily attempt to elevate arterial Po_2 to completely "safe" levels. The patient has been hypoxic for quite a while. Simply raising the Fio_2 by 1 L/M by nasal cannulae will result in substantial improvement in the arterial Po_2 and will not usually have much adverse effect on Pco_2 (and pH). Additional adjustment of Fio_2 can be done at a later time. On the first day, achieving an arterial Po_2 of 50 mm Hg would be quite acceptable. In some patients, an improvement by 5–10 mm Hg may be all that can be safely achieved on the first day. No additional adjustments of Fio_2 for the least 1 day.
01:30	Begin to treat edema. Establish that renal function is reasonably good. Then, administer one dose of a potent intravenous diuretic (e.g., 1 mg/kg of furosemide). Measure urinary output for 3 hr after the dose. The use of tight-fitting hose (e.g., TEDS) to facilitate additional diuresis is controversial; other forms of leg compression may be better at least for some patients. If tight-fitting hose is used, begin by applying the hose to one leg only for very edematous patients. Begin daily spironolactone (Aldactone) at 75–100 mg per day.
04:15	Begin intravenous (4–5 m $MgSO_4$ in 250 mL D5W over 3–4 hr) correction of hypomagnesemia if serum Mg^{2+} is ≤1.30 mEq/L.
04:30	End of peak action of intravenous diuretic and period of rapid diuresis. Begin to treat pulmonary infection. Start intravenous antibiotics 3 hr after intravenous diuretic to avoid additive/synergistic nephrotoxicity and to avoid increased urinary loss of antibiotic caused by diuresis).
04:30–24:00	Initiate airway clearance procedures as tolerated and deemed effective by patient. Consider use of ThAIRapy Vest or similar device that requires the least patient effort to be effective.

Table 16 Continued

Elapsed time (hours: minutes)	Diagnostic and therapeutic measures
24:00	Make additional adjustments in FIO_2 based on repeat ABGs. For some patients, the "CO_2 price" of achieving an arterial Po_2 of 60 mm Hg is not worth the security of the slightly greater oxygen saturation. There is still no need for direct treatment of acidosis.
24:00	Repeat measurements of serum electrolytes and other chemistries. The patient may need a repeat dose of intravenous magnesium sulfate. Potassium dose may have to be changed. If the patient is anemic, obtain serum iron studies (if not obtained previously; if serum iron is low, consider treating iron deficiency with intravenous iron as outlined in this chapter, but this should not be done yet).
24:00	Many patients would benefit from an additional dose of intravenous diuretic (if ordered, dose should be given midway between every 8 hr doses of nephrotoxic antibiotics).
24:00	Suggest that the patient drink calories (i.e., supplements) instead of eating solid food. Drinking is easier and quicker. The slightly lower CO_2 production, which is achievable with Pulmocare or other low-carbohydrate supplement, does not offer sufficient advantage to justify depriving the patient of a supplement that tastes better. However, some attention to salt content is important.
24:00	Discuss (with patient) possibilities of increased vigor of airway clearance treatments.
48:00	If clinically significant edema is still present, consider addition of oral hydrochlorthiazide so that daily doses of nephrotoxic intravenous diuretics can be stopped or given less frequently.
48:00	Check routine (CF) culture for unexpected organisms (e.g., *Staphylococcus aureus*; *Klebsiella pneumoniae*), which might necessitate change of antibiotics.

CBC, complete blood count; SIADH, syndrome of inappropriate antidiuretic hormone secretion; ABG, arterial blood gas; ECG, electrocardiogram

year-old patient with severe pulmonary disease and new-onset right heart failure is presented in Table 16. In essence, a slow sequential attack on a few fronts is usually safer than a precipitous attempt at total or near-total correction of all biochemical and blood gas abnormalities.

B. Pregnancy

Pregnancy, labor, delivery, and the immediate postpartum period are usually uneventful if pulmonary function is normal or only mildly impaired before conception, especially in patients with some preservation of exocrine pancreatic function (74,75). These patients may not even require hospitalization until delivery.

Table 17 Impact of Pregnancy on Inpatient Treatment of Pulmonary Disease in Cystic Fibrosis Patients

Area of concern	Management
Radiographic examinations	Limit chest films (especially on admission) and particularly during first trimester) to those needed to rule out an immediately treatable condition, e.g., pneumothorax, heart failure. Delay contrast and computed tomography evaluation of any chronic abdominal complaint until after pregnancy or until the third trimester.
Teratogenic effect of antibiotics and other drugs	Attempt to limit treatment to antibiotics for which there is no reported teratogenic effect. Antibiotics with no data either way should be considered acceptable unless a proven-safe agent with in vitro activity is available. Other (nonantibiotic) drugs with either known teratogenic effect or unknown teratogenic effect status should be avoided if possible.
Interference with mucus clearance	Consider replacing conventional postural drainage or clapping (which is made more difficult by the increasing uterine size) with one or more of the newer modalities e.g., Flutter, autogenic drainage, positive expiratory pressure devices). However, there is no information on the safety of any of these treatment modalities or with the ThAIRapy Vest during pregnancy. DNase could be useful, but has also not been approved for use during pregnancy.
Compromise of lung expansion	If lobar atelectasis is suspected by physical examination (e.g., localized reduction in breath sounds) or history (sudden onset of localized chest pain), especially in a patient with a previous episode of atelectasis, a radiograph should be done because lobar atelectasis may justify diagnostic or therapeutic bronchoscopy. Intensified local clapping may also be helpful. However, as with lobar atelectasis in nonpregnant CF patients, the prognosis for sustained reexpansion (especially during pregnancy) is not good.
Hyperemesis gravidarum, "fatigue of pregnancy," "anemia of pregnancy," progesterone-induced dyspnea	Management is the same as for non-CF, but these complications can interfere with usual hospital treatment. It may not be easy to distinguish hyperemesis from drug toxicity. It may not be easy to differentiate "fatigue of pregnancy" or "anemia of pregnancy" from similar symptoms and signs due directly to CF or to drug toxicity. The gravid state itself, especially if associated with substantial anemia, may predispose the patient to heart failure in patients whose cardiac function is already compromised by cor pulmonale and systemic hypoxemia.
Weight loss and inadequate caloric intake	The patient may be too anorectic from chronic illness to eat enough calories to maintain normal fetal development. Circumvention of appetite (by jejunal feeding or intravenous alimentation) may be justified.

Some patients with mild to moderate pulmonary disease also do surprisingly well, but others require at least one course of IV antibiotics, especially during the third trimester. However, pregnancy in women with moderately severe or severe CF-related lung disease carries a substantial risk of increased morbidity or even death (76). Patients whose immediate pregravid state was already complicated by frequent hospitalizations for pulmonary exacerbations or who have moderate to moderately severe impairment of pulmonary function, particularly if associated with hypoxemia or hypercapnia, should be advised of these risks and offered therapeutic abortion. Those who choose to continue with the pregnancy must expect frequent and prolonged hospitalization, as well as early delivery (perhaps by cesarean section) of a premature infant.

The major areas of impact of pregnancy on the management of CF-related pulmonary disease are summarized in Table 17. Most experts on high-risk pregnancies agree that preserving the overall health of the mother supersedes concerns about drugs with unknown teratogenicity potential, and, therefore, most patients should receive the antibiotics and others drugs that they really need, unless case reports indicate danger of the drug or class of drugs to the fetus.

Appendix 1: Regulation of Tobramycin Dose* in Cystic Fibrosis Patients

The initial dose is empirical (see Table 8).

Method 1 (Initial Drug Pharmacokinetics): On admission, the patient is given a single intravenous (IV) dose of tobramycin (approximately 3.3 mg/kg) over 30 minutes. At least three accurately timed serum levels are drawn, beginning approximately 1 hour after the start of the drug infusion. Pharmacokinetic analysis can then be used to predict the dose necessary to achieve the target peak level (which, in CF, should be 10–12 mg/L).

Method 2 (Peak-Level Method): This method assumes that renal, function, independently tested, is normal. After 4–5 dose intervals, a peak level is obtained (peak levels are always drawn 1 hour after the start of the drug infusion, which ideally should take 30 minutes; if infusion is not exactly 30 minutes, the level is still drawn 1 hour after the start). The dose is adjusted until the peak level is 10–12 mg/L. At that point, a trough level is drawn for the first time—if it is less than 2 mg/L, no further levels are needed if routine renal function tests remain normal.

NOTE: Cystic fibrosis patients often require doses of 12–15 mg/kg/day to achieve adequate levels. If the final predicted dose is below 10 mg/kg/day or if

---

*Other aminoglycosides can be handled in a similar way. Tobramycin is the most commonly used agent in this class for patients with cystic fibrosis.

the predicted dose interval is greater than 8 hours, the methodology (especially sample timing) should be carefully reviewed. A common error is not timing the sample from the start of the infusion and not knowing to the minute when the infusion began and when each sample was obtained.

Appendix 2: Symptomatic Treatment of Pulmonary Symptoms

1. *Chest Pain:* Assuming that physical examination and/or appropriate studies have ruled out a complication, such as pneumothorax, pleural effusion, pneumomediastinum, rib fracture, or esophagitis, which would justify specific intervention, chest pain related to cystic fibrosis pulmonary disease (whether pleuritic or not) probably originates from musculoskeletal injury or stress, pleural disease, or blood vessels. Analgesics and antiinflammatory agents can be very effective. Adequate analgesia, in addition to being a worthwhile goal in itself, also can speed overall recovery by improving cooperation with airway clearance, improving sleep, and contributing to an optimistic outlook. Generally, nonsteroidal antiinflammatory agents should be tried first. They are excellent analgesics and may directly affect the inflammatory process that is causing the pain. The possibility that these agents could aggravate or precipitate hemoptysis should be considered, but this does not appear to be a frequent problem in practice. If nonsteroidal antiinflammatory agents fail, opioids may be necessary, but the physician should (1) obtain a "toxicology screen" to help ensure that the complaint is not a manifestation of drug-seeking behavior—a problem worthy of special attention (see Chapter 3) and (2) consider the possibility of physical dependency (if opioid analgesic is going to be required for a prolonged time) and discuss this with the patient and family either before starting treatment or shortly thereafter. Codeine (usually with acetaminophen) is often effective; if not, oral meperidine or Dilaudid can be used. Chest pain in terminally ill patients is discussed elsewhere.

2. *Dyspnea (see also Chapter 14):* The neurological basis for dyspnea remains unknown. In obstructive pulmonary disease, it seems related, at least in part, to work of breathing. Symptomatic treatment includes: (1) reducing work of breathing, such as by positioning to maximize leverage of the accessory muscles of respiration, usually involving the patient sitting up and leaning forward (in the extreme, some patients lean so far forward that their upper body is almost parallel to their legs), continuous positive airway pressure, including high-flow nasal oxygen, supplemental oxygen, and bronchodilators; (2) exposure, especially of the face, to moving cool air (e.g., from an open window

or fan); and (3) relief of anxiety. Morphine is extremely effective, but drawbacks generally preclude its use in patients who are not terminally ill. Caffeine-containing beverages are occasionally helpful, perhaps by increasing efficiency or strength of diaphragm.

3. *Cough:* Although spontaneous cough is an important component of airway clearance, cough suppression may be indicated on occasion. If the patient has severe pleuritic pain and is voluntarily suppressing cough intensity, cough suppression may be helpful in allowing sleep. If coughing paroxysms are interfering with sleep, a cough suppressant given before sleep may be well worth the therapeutic tradeoff (a short period of diminished airway clearance). Clinically meaningful cough suppression can probably be accomplished only with codeine or a similar drug (for codeine, dose for school-aged children and adults is 15–30 mg at bedtime; repeat one to three times a day) or aerosolized local anaesthetic (e.g., Lidocaine 2 mL of 2% solution at 4-hr intervals). Airway clearance and expectorants are discussed in the chapter.

Acknowledgments

Supported in part by Grant DK 27651 from the National Institutes of Health and by grants from the Cystic Fibrosis Foundation and United Way Services of Greater Cleveland.

References

1. Regelmann WE, Elliott GR, Warwick WJ, Clawson CC. Reduction of sputum *Pseudomonas aeruginosa* density by antibiotics improves lung function in cystic fibrosis more than do bronchodilators and chest physiotherapy alone. Am Rev Respir Dis 1990; 141:914–921.
2. Thomassen MJ, Klinger JD, Badger SJ, van Heeckeren DW, Stern RC. Cultures of thoracotomy specimens confirm usefulness of sputum cultures in cystic fibrosis. J Pediatr 1984; 104:352–356.
3. Ramsey BW, Wentz KR, Smith AL, Richardson M, Williams-Warren J, Hedges DL, Gibson R, Redding GJ, Lent K, Harris K. Predictive value of oropharyngeal cultures for identifying lower airway bacteria in cystic fibrosis patients. Am Rev Respir Dis 1991; 144:331–337.
4. Saiman L, Niu WW, Prince A, Neu HG. A referral center to study multi-resistant *Pseudomonas aeruginosa*. Pediatr Pulmonol 1991; S6:279.
5. Prandota J. Drug disposition in cystic fibrosis: progress in understanding pathophysiology and pharmacokinetics. Pediatr Infect Dis J 1987; 6:1111–1126.
6. Powell SH, Thompson WL, Luthe MA, Stern RC, Grossniklaus DA, Bloxham DD, Groden DL, Jacobs MR, DiScenna AO, Cash HA, Klinger KD. Once-daily vs continuous aminoglycoside dosing: efficacy and toxicity in animal and clinical

studies of gentamicin, netilmicin, and tobramycin. J Infect Dis 1983; 147:918–931.

7. Cohn RC, Rudzienski L. Observations on amiloride-tobramycin synergy in *Pseudomonas cepacia*. Curr Therapeutic Res 1991; 50:786–793.

8. Hardy KA. A review of airway clearance: new techniques, indications, and recommendations. Respir Care 1994; 39:440–452.

9. Fuchs HJ, Borowitz DS, Christiansen DH, Morris EM, Nash ML, Ramsay BW, Rosenstein BJ, Smith AL, Wohl ME, et al: Effect of aerosolized recombinant human DNase on exacerbations of respiratory symptoms and on pulmonary function in patients with cystic fibrosis. N Engl J Med 1994; 331:637–642.

10. Vasconcellos CA, Allen PG, Wohl ME, Drazen JM, Janmey PA, Stossel TP. Reduction in viscosity of cystic fibrosis sputum in vitro by gelsolin. Science 1994; 263:969–971.

11. Matthews LW, Doershuk CF, Wise M, Eddy G, Nudelman H, Spector S. A therapeutic regimen for patients with cystic fibrosis. J Pediatr 1964; 65:558–575.

12. Reisman JJ, Rivinaton-Law B, Corey M, Marcotte J, Wannamaker E, Harcourt D, Levison H. Role of conventional physiotherapy in cystic fibrosis. J Pediatr 1988; 113:632–636.

13. Desmond KJ, Schwenk WF, Thomas E, Beaudry PH, Coates AL. Immediate and long-term effects of chest physiotherapy in patients with cystic fibrosis. J Pediatr 1983; 103:538–542.

14. Warwick WJ, Hansen LG. The long-term effect of high-frequency chest compression therapy on pulmonary complications of cystic fibrosis. Pediatr Pulmonol 1991; 11:265–271.

15. Konstan MW, Stern RC, Doershuk CF. Efficacy of the Flutter in airway mucus clearance in cystic fibrosis patients. J Pediatr 1994; 124:689–6934.

16. Zach MS, Purrer B, Oberwaldner B. Effect of swimming on forced expiration and sputum clearance in cystic fibrosis. Lancet 1981; 2:1201–1203.

17. Zach M, Oberwaldner B, Hausler F. Cystic fibrosis: physical exercise versus chest physiotherapy. Arch Dis Child 1982; 57:587–589.

18. McIlwaine M, Davidson AGF, Wong LTK, Pirie G: The effect of chest physiotherapy by postural drainage and autogenic drainage on oxygen saturation in cystic fibrosis (Abstract). Pediatr Pulmonol Suppl 1991; 6:291.

19. Oberwaldner B. Evans JC, Zach MS. Forced expirations against a variable resistance: a new chest physiotherapy method in cystic fibrosis. Chest 1991; 100:1350–1357.

20. Mahlmeister MJ, Fink JB, Hoffman GL, Fifer LF: Positive-expiratory-pressure mask therapy: theoretical and practical considerations and a review of the literature. Respir Care 1991; 36:1218–1229.

21. Brown RB. Outpatient parenteral antibiotic treatment: selecting the patient. Hosp Pract 1993; 28 (suppl 1):11–15.

22. Donati MA, Guenette G, Auerbach H. Prospective controlled study of home and hospital therapy of cystic fibrosis pulmonary disease. J Pediatr 1987; 111:28–33.

23. Bosworth D, Nielson DW. Home treatment of *Pseudomonas* pneumonia in cystic fibrosis is not as effective as in-hospital treatment. Am Rev Respir Crit Care Med 1993; 147:A580.

24. Gilbert J, Robinson T, Littlewood JM. Home intravenous antibiotic treatment in cystic fibrosis. Arch Dis Child 1988; 63:512–517.

25. Henke KG, Orenstein DM. Oxygen saturation during exercise in cystic fibrosis. Am Rev Respir Dis 1984; 129:708–711.
26. Konstan MW, Byard PJ, Hoppel CL, Davis PB. Effect of high-dose ibuprofen in patients with cystic fibrosis. N Engl J Med 1995; 332:848–854.
27. Stern RC, Borkat G, Hirschfeld SS, Boat TF, Matthews LW, Liebman J, Doershuk CF. Heart failure in cystic fibrosis: treatment and prognosis of cor pulmonale with failure of the right side of the heart. Am J Dis Child 1980; 134:267–272.
28. Landau LI, Phelan PD. The variable effect of a bronchodilating agent on pulmonary function in cystic fibrosis. J Pediatr 1973; 82:863–868.
29. Pattishall EN. Longitudinal response of pulmonary function to bronchodilators in cystic fibrosis. Pediatr Pulmonol 1990; 9:80–85.
30. Maddison J, Dodd M, Webb AK. Nebulized colistin causes chest tightness in adults with cystic fibrosis. Respir Med 1994; 88:145–147.
31. Redding GJ, Restuccia R, Cotton EK, Brooks JG. Serial changes in pulmonary functions in children hospitalized for cystic fibrosis. Am Rev Respir Dis 1982; 126:31–35.
32. Nixon PA, Orenstein DM, Curtis SE, Ross EA. Oxygen supplementation during exercise in cystic fibrosis. Am Rev Respir Dis 1990; 142:807–811.
33. Nocturnal Oxygen Therapy Trial Group. Continuous or nocturnal oxygen therapy in hypoxemic chronic obstructive lung disease: a clinical trial. Ann Intern Med 1980; 93:391–398.
34. Medical Research Council Working Party. Long-term domiciliary oxygen therapy in chronic hypoxic cor pulmonale complicating chronic bronchitis and emphysema. Lancet 1981; 1:681–686.
35. Zinman R, Corey M, Coates AL, Canny GJ, Connolly J, Levison H, Beaudry PH. Nocturnal home oxygen in the treatment of hypoxemic cystic fibrosis patients. J Pediatr 1989; 114:368–377.
36. Marcus CL, Bader D, Stabile MW, Wang C-I, Osher AB, Keens TG. Supplemental oxygen and exercise performance in patients with cystic fibrosis with severe pulmonary disease. Chest 1992; 101:52–57.
37. Whitman V, Stern RC, Bellet P, Doershuk CF, Liebman J, Boat TF, Borkat G, Matthews LW. Studies on cor pulmonale in cystic fibrosis: 1. Effect of diuresis. Pediatrics 1975; 55:83–85.
38. Geggel RL, Dozor AJ, Fyler DC, Reid LM. Effect of vasodilators at rest and during exercise in young adults with cystic fibrosis and chronic cor pulmonale. Am Rev Respir Dis 1985; 131:531–536.
39. Stowe SM, Boat TF, Mendelsohn H, Stern RC, Tucker AS, Doershuk CF, Matthew LW. Open thoracotomy for pneumothorax in cystic fibrosis. Am Rev Respir Dis 1975; 111:611–617.
40. Spector ML, Stern RC. Pneumothorax in cystic fibrosis: a 26 year experience. Ann Thorac Surg 1989; 47:204–207.
41. Penketh A, Knight RK, Hodson ME, Batten JC. Management of pneumothorax in adults with cystic fibrosis. Thorax 1982; 37:850–853.
42. Rich H, Warwick W, Leonard A. Open thoracotomy and pleural abrasion in the treatment of spontaneous pneumothorax in cystic fibrosis. J Pediatr Surg 1978; 13:237–242.
43. Noyes BE, Orenstein DM. Treatment of pneumothorax in cystic fibrosis in the era of lung transplantation. Chest 1992; 101:1187–1188.

44. Wakabayashi A, Brenner M, Wilson A, Tadir Y, Berns M. Thoracoscopic treatment of spontaneous pneumothorax using carbon dioxide laser. Ann Thorac Surg 1990; 50:786–790.
45. McLaughlin FJ, Matthews WJ Jr, Strieder DJ, Khaw KT, Schuster S, Shwachman H. Pneumothorax in cystic fibrosis: management and outcome. J Pediatr 1982; 100:863–869.
46. Holsclaw DS, Grand RJ, Shwachman H. Massive hemoptysis in cystic fibrosis. J Pediatr 1970; 76:829–838.
47. Stern RC, Wood RE, Boat TF, Matthews LW, Tucker AS, Doershuk CF. Treatment and prognosis of massive hemoptysis in cystic fibrosis. Am Rev Respir Dis 1978; 117:825–828.
48. Bickell WH, Wall MJ, Pepe PE, Martin RR, Ginger VF, Allen MK, Mattox KL. Immediate versus delayed fluid resuscitation for hypotensive patients with penetrating torso injuries. N Engl J Med 1994; 331:1105–1109.
49. Bilton D, Webb AK, Foster H, Mulvenna P, Dodd M. Life threatening hemoptysis in cystic fibrosis: an alternative therapeutic approach. Thorax 1990; 45:975–976.
50. Swersky RB, Chang JB, Wisoff BG, et al. Endobronchial balloon tamponade of hemoptysis in patients with cystic fibrosis. Ann Thorac Surg 1979; 27:262–264.
51. Fellows KE, Khaw KT, Schuster S, Shwachman H. Bronchial artery embolization in cystic fibrosis; technique and long-term results. J Pediatr 1979; 95:959–96
52. Cohen AM, Doershuk CF, Stern RC. Bronchial artery embolization to control hemoptysis in cystic fibrosis. Radiology 1990; 175:401–405.
53. Levitsky S, Lapey A, di Sant-Agnese PA. Pulmonary resection for life-threatening hemoptysis in cystic fibrosis. JAMA 1970; 213:125–126.
54. Nelson LA, Callerame ML, Schwartz RH. Aspergillosis and atopy in cystic fibrosis. 1979; 120:863–873.
55. Valletta EA, Braggion C, Mastella G. Sensitization to *Aspergillus* and allergic bronchopulmonary aspergillosis in a cystic fibrosis population. Pediatr Asthma Allergy Immunol 1993; 7:43–49.
56. Mrouch S, Spock A. Allergic bronchopulmonary aspergillosis in patients with cystic fibrosis. Chest 1994; 105:32–36.
57. Hutcheson PS, Rejent AJ, Slavin RG. Variability in parameters of allergic bronchopulmonary aspergillosis in patients with cystic fibrosis. J Allergy Clin Immunol 1991; 88:390–394.
58. Galant SP, Rucker RW, Groncy CE, Wells ID, Novey HS. Incidence of serum antibodies to several *Aspergillus* species and to *Candida albicans* in cystic fibrosis. Am Rev Respir Dis 1976; 114:325–331.
59. Simmonds EJ, Littlewood JM, Hopwood V, Evans EGV. *Aspergillus fumigatus* colonisation and population density of place of residence in cystic fibrosis. Arch Dis Child 1994; 70:139–140.
60. Mannes GPM, van der Heide S, van Aalderen WMC, Gerritsen J. Itraconazole and allergic bronchopulmonary aspergillosis in twin brothers with cystic fibrosis. Lancet 1993; 341:492.
61. Dixey J, Redington AN, Butler RC, Smith MJ, Batchelor JR, Woodrow DF, Hodson ME, Batten JC, Brewerton DA. The arthropathy of cystic fibrosis. Ann Rheum Dis 1988; 47:218–223.
62. Cohen AM, Yulish BS, Wasser KB, Vignos PJ, Jones PK, Sorin SB. Evaluation of pulmonary hypertrophic osteoarthropathy in cystic fibrosis. Am J Dis Child 1986; 140:74–77.

63. Newman AJ, Ansell BM. Episodic arthritis in children with cystic fibrosis. J Pediatr 1979; 94:594–596.
64. Soden M, Tempany E, Bresnihan B. Sarcoid arthropathy in cystic fibrosis: case report. Br J Rheumatol 1989; 28:341–343.
65. Lawrence JM III, Moore Tl, Madson KL, Rejent AJ, Osborn TG. Arthropathies of cystic fibrosis: case reports and review of the literature. J Rheumatol 1993; 20(suppl 38):12–15.
66. Euler AR, Ament MF. Crohn's disease: a cause of arthritis, oxalate stones, and fistulae in cystic fibrosis. West J Med 1976; 125:315–317.
67. Ledesma-Medina J, Osman MZ, Girdany BR. Abnormal paranasal sinuses in patients with cystic fibrosis of the pancreas. Pediatr Radiol 1980; 9:61–64.
68. Levine MR, Kim Y-D, Witt W. Frontal sinus mucopyocele in cystic fibrosis. Ophthal Plastic Reconstr Surg 1988; 4:221–225.
69. Sharma GD, Doershuk CF, Stern RC. Erosion of the wall of the frontal sinus caused by mucopyocele in cystic fibrosis. J Pediatr 1994; 124:745–747.
70. Umetsu DT, Moss RB, King VV, Lewiston NJ. Sinus disease in patients with cystic fibrosis: relation to pulmonary exacerbation, Lancet 1990; 335:1077–1078.
71. Cuyler JP. Follow-up of endoscopic sinus surgery on children with cystic fibrosis. Arch Otolaryngol Head Neck Surg 1992; 118:505–506.
72. di Sant'Agnese PA. Bronchial obstruction with lobar atelectasis and emphysema in cystic fibrosis of the pancreas. Pediatrics 1953; 12:178–190.
73. Stern RC, Boat TF, Orenstein DM, Wood RE, Matthews LW, Doershuk CF. Treatment and prognosis of lobar and segmental atelectasis in cystic fibrosis. Am Rev Respir Dis 1978; 118:821–826.
74. Corkey CWB, Newth CJL, Corey M, Levison H. Pregnancy in cystic fibrosis: a better prognosis in patients with pancreatic function? Am J Obstet Gynecol 1981; 140:737–742.
75. Canny GJ, Corey M, Livingstone RA, et al. Pregnancy and cystic fibrosis. Obstet Gynecol 1991; 77:850–853.
76. Palmer J, Dillon-Baker C, Tecklin JS, Wolfson B, Rosenberg B, Burroughs B, Holsclaw DS Jr, Scanlin TF, Huang NN, Sewell EM. Pregnancy in patients with cystic fibrosis. Ann Intern Med 1953; 99:596–600.

5

Gastrointestinal Complications

ROBERT J. ROTHBAUM

Washington University School of Medicine
and St. Louis Children's Hospital
St. Louis, Missouri

I. Esophagus

A. Gastroesophageal Reflux Disease

Gastroesophageal reflux (GER) is a physiological process occurring in all normal individuals. In some instances, reflux of acid gastric contents or bile into the esophagus leads to complications defined as gastroesophageal reflux disease (GERD), which includes failure to thrive, esophagitis, esophageal stricture, and pulmonary disease (1). Esophagitis may cause dysphagia, odynophagia, or heartburn (2). Infants with esophagitis may be irritable and refuse to eat. Repeated vomiting may indicate GER but not necessarily GERD. Failure to gain weight is uncommon in uncomplicated GER. Different mechanisms can produce a reduction in net energy intake: (1) dysphagia or dysmotility may interfere with ability to eat, (2) feedings may be reduced or manipulated to decrease emesis, and (3) the volume of regurgitated material may be excessive. With GERD, children and adolescents may suffer epigastric or substernal pain after meals. These older patients may report acid brash (reflux of acid gastric contents into the pharynx) or water brash (a sudden increase in saliva production that accompanies acid reflux into the distal esophagus). Dysphagia may occur with disordered esophageal peristalsis or with esophageal stricture.

Pulmonary disease associated with GER may occur as aspiration pneumonia, bronchospasm, or persistent cough (3). Bronchospasm may follow direct acid irritation of the airway or may occur through a vagally mediated reflex following acid irritation of the distal esophagus. A direct relationship between GER or GERD and pulmonary symptoms is often difficult to prove. Continuous pulmonary symptoms do not allow for segregation of symptoms related to GER. Intermittent pulmonary symptoms often do not occur during the time of a particular study [e.g., upper gastrointestinal (GI) series, radionucleotide milk scan, or prolonged pH study] that documents reflux events. Lipid-laden macrophages identified in bronchoalveolar lavage fluid are not specific for aspiration of gastric contents. Such macrophages can be seen with inflammatory or obstructive lung disease alone. Often, the association of GER or GERD with pulmonary symptoms is only strongly suggested by improvement in the pulmonary symptoms after treatment of GER or GERD.

Several small clinical studies document the occurrence of GERD in cystic fibrosis (CF) patients but they do not allow for generalization to the entire population. In 1982, Bending et al. described severe GERD in seven CF patients, aged 8 to 31 years old (4). Scott et al. documented that complaints of regurgitation and heartburn were common in CF patients with significant respiratory disease (5). Feigelson et al. evaluated 49 CF patients by esophagoscopy performed in conjunction with bronchoscopy (6). All patients had "marked" respiratory disease, and 25 of the 49 had "ulcerative" esophagitis. Only 16 of the 25 patients had any symptoms referable to the esophagitis (6). Thus, the influence of the esophagitis on each patient's clinical condition is unclear. In usual clinical practice, evaluation for GERD is performed in CF patients with symptoms or signs directly referable to GERD and on selected CF patients with pulmonary disease refractory to usual therapy.

Because all individuals have periodic acidic gastroesophageal reflux but GERD develops in only a few, several defense mechanisms protect against the development of esophagitis (Table 1) (7). Alterations in any of these defense mechanisms may predispose the individual to the development of acid-induced esophageal injury. In many patients with GERD, inappropriate relaxation of the lower esophageal sphincter (LES) occurs, allowing for more frequent reflux of acid into the distal esophagus. This increased acid exposure presumably produces mucosal damage and inflammation. The usual resting tone of the LES limits spontaneous GER. Medications or foods that reduce LES tone might reduce the effectiveness of this defense mechanism. Changes in the angle of His or in the angle of the esophagus passing through the diaphragmatic crus may occur with pulmonary hyperinflation or with scoliosis, decreasing the overall effectiveness of the LES barrier. Swallowing disorders decrease the initiation of primary esophageal peristalsis, reducing acid clearance from the distal esophagus. With sleep, swallowing and saliva production are both reduced. Thus, acid

Table 1 Factors Preventing Gastroesophageal Reflux Disease

Defense mechanism	Function
Lower esophageal sphincter (LES) barrier, including the LES itself, diaphragmatic crus, and angle of His	Retains acid contents in stomach
Gravity	Keeps gastric contents in stomach when subject is upright or prone
Primary peristalsis with swallowing; secondary peristalsis with reflux	Clears esophagus of acidic material
Saliva	Dilutes and buffers acid reflux
Burping	Decreases gastric volume
Gastric emptying	Reduces volume of acid gastric contents
Esophageal mucosal defense	Helps protect mucosa of esophagus against acid injury

reflux occurring during sleep may lead to prolonged exposure of the distal esophagus to acid. Esophagitis itself may produce a motility disorder that disrupts secondary peristalsis, leading to further retention of acid refluxate on already damaged mucosa. Defects in esophageal mucosa that reduce resistance to acid-induced damage are hypothesized but not proven.

Several features of CF and its treatment may predispose patients to GERD by interfering with the normal esophageal defenses (Table 2). However, no studies have systematically examined the relative importance of these mechanisms in CF patients with GERD.

Diagnosis

1. Barium studies of the upper GI tract delineate anatomical abnormalities, such as gastric outlet obstruction, duodenal narrowing, or malrotation, which predispose the patient to gastric retention and subsequent acid reflux. Visualization of GER during an upper GI examination is common. Its presence does not predict an underlying pathological condition. Its absence does not exclude GERD. The air-contrast barium esophagram is specific but not sensitive for the diagnosis of esophagitis. If mucosal irregularity or "ringed esophagus" is present, then endoscopic or histological esophagitis is likely present. A normal esophagram does not exclude esophagitis or GERD.

2. Esophageal mucosal biopsy with or without upper GI (UGI) endoscopy is the "gold standard" for the documentation of esophagitis. Endoscopy may help define the extent and severity of the inflammation, allow identification of mucosal metaplasia (Barrett's esophagus), or permit diagnosis of coincident candida or vital infection. In infants, blind esophageal suction biopsy provides tissue for excellent histological definition and reduces the need for sedation or general anesthesia. It is not as widely available as endoscopy.

Table 2 Potential Effects of CF or Its Treatment on Esophageal Defense Mechanisms

Defense mechanism	CF-related problem
Lower esophageal sphincter tone	Reduced by theophylline, anticholinergics, beta-agonists, caffeine, chocolate
Gravity	Counteracted by gravity in head-down position
Diaphragm position	Flattened by pulmonary hyperinflation
Thoracoabdominal pressure gradient	Increased intraabdominal pressure with frequent cough
Peristalsis	Unaltered except with established esophagitis
Gastric emptying	Slowed by anticholinergics, vagotomy, nocturnal or high caloric density feeds
Esophageal mucosal defense	Characterized incompletely

3. A prolonged esophageal pH study documents reflux of acid material into the distal esophagus, but the findings do not correlate closely with the presence of esophagitis (8). A pH study may allow the correlation of specific symptoms (e.g., wheezing, apnea, irritability, night awakening) with acid reflux (3). Also, the pH study may permit documentation of medication effect, such as reduction of acid reflux following therapy. The Bernstein test (direct instillation of dilute acid into the distal esophagus) is a provocative test that may elicit symptoms associated with GER. This test must be performed by personnel familiar with the technique and its interpretation.

Therapy of GER

Gastroesophageal reflux usually requires no specific therapy. In infants, time and maturation lead to resolution in 95% of patients by age 18 months. Thickened feedings and positional changes may decrease emesis. Reduction in volume of feedings does not usually affect emesis but may limit overall energy intake and interfere with weight gain.

Therapy of GERD

The following changes in lifestyle or medications represent initial therapy of GERD (7).

1. Assume body positions to avoid reflux. Anatomy and gravity work to reduce the frequency of GER with the prone or right lateral decubitus position. Gastroesophageal reflux occurs more often in the supine or left lateral decubitus positions. In infants, the presence of GERD might necessitate deviating from the recent American Academy of Pediatrics recommendation for supine positioning during sleep.

2. Avoid large meals within 1 to 2 hours of retiring. Large volumes of acidic gastric contents will not then be present in the stomach to reflux while the patient is supine and sleeping.
3. Avoid intake of caffeine and chocolate, which may reduce LES tone.
4. Elevate the head of the bed by 6 inches to use gravity as a force to keep acid contents in the stomach.
5. Attempt to reduce or eliminate medications that reduce LES tone. These medications include anticholinergics, theophylline, and, possibly, beta-adrenergic agonists.

Medications that reduce gastric acid output are mainstays of therapy for esophagitis because most esophagitis is related to acid-induced damage of the distal esophageal mucosa. If the esophagitis has produced a motility disorder of the distal esophagus that impairs acid clearance or the function of the lower esophageal sphincter, treatment of the esophagitis may also improve the motility disorder, improving clearance of acid refluxate from the distal esophagus. Prokinetic agents may increase LES pressure and speed gastric emptying. These dual effects reduce the frequency and severity of acidic GER, thereby protecting the distal esophageal mucosa and promoting healing. See Table 3.

Table 3 Medications for Treatment of Gastroesophageal Reflux Disease

Class of agent	When used	Dose	Comments
Antacid	For periodic symptom relief; initial therapeutic trial	1 mL/kg 1 and 3 h p.c.	Nonadherence limits effect: may block
H_2-receptor antagonists	For moderate or severe esophagitis or if antacids fail	Cimetidine: 10 mg/kg qid Ranitidine: 2–5 mg/kg bid to qid	Higher doses are not officially endorsed, but are often needed.
Proton pump inhibitors	When previous agents fail	Omeprazole in infants: 0.7 mg/kg qd (increase to bid if symptoms are not relieved) Omeprazole in older children and adolescents: 20 mg qd; may be required bid	Most potent inhibition of acid secretion
Coating agents	For resistant esophagitis; bile acid–induced esophagitis		Rarely needed

qid = four times per day; qd = every day; bid = twice a day

Documentation of Effectiveness

In treating esophagitis, therapeutic benefit is usually assessed by diminished heartburn, dysphagia, or odynophagia. Repeated endoscopies and mucosal biopsies are usually not necessary. The necessity of documenting histological resolution of esophagitis in the asymptomatic patient is not clear. Such documentation may be needed in selected patients (e.g., in patients with asymptomatic occult GI bleeding producing anemia or symptoms related only to esophageal stricture). Many children and adults with esophagitis have recurrent symptoms. Presumably, whichever compromised defense mechanism predisposed the patient to esophagitis is not reversed by resolution or improvement of inflammation. Reinstitution of medical therapy is likely to have repeated success.

Fundoplication

Fundoplication to stop acid reflux is not usually required for treatment of GERD. Esophagitis refractory to medical therapy and recurrent symptomatic esophageal stricture are the major indications for fundoplication. Occasional patients merit fundoplication because of excessive calorie loss from vomiting or a high index of suspicion of recurrent aspiration of gastric contents with associated chronic pulmonary disease. Fundoplication reduces acid reflux and its associated problems, but postoperative problems are not unusual. Up to 20% of postfundoplication patients report abdominal pain, bloating, or dysphagia after the surgery (9,10). Approximately 15% of infants and children suffer persistent retching with feeding (11). The symptoms usually improve during the first 6 postoperative months. Ten to 20% of children have recurrence of symptoms of GERD at a mean of 11 months after the original surgery. This period may, however, be long enough for esophagitis to heal and for esophageal clearance or defense mechanisms to improve.

B. Medication-Induced Esophagitis

Erosive esophagitis, or "pill esophagitis," develops in a few individuals who are taking particular medications. Direct mucosal irritation from retained capsules or tablets provides the most plausible mechanism for the esophageal injury. Tetracycline and its derivatives produce well-circumscribed, superficial ulcerations (12). Nonsteroidal antiinflammatory drugs (NSAIDs), aspirin, and potassium chloride are also suspected to cause similar lesions. Odynophagia is a prominent symptom. The esophagitis resolves with discontinuation of the offending medication.

C. Infectious Esophagitis

Esophageal infection is usually due to candida or herpes virus. Patients taking corticosteroids along with medication that reduces gastric acid output are at highest risk for development of candida esophagitis. Odynophagia and dyspha-

Table 4 Treatment of Candida Esophagitis

Medication	Dose
Nystatin	1–3 million units (10–30 mL) swish and swallow four times a day
Clotrimazole	1/2–1 troche (10 mg) by mouth four times a day
Fluconazole	50–200 mg by mouth everyday

gia predominate. Endoscopy demonstrates typical white plaques of candida adherent to underlying superficial ulceration. Biopsy shows invasion of stratified squamous epithelium by candida hyphae. Brushings of plaques are useful for fungal culture (13). Table 4 outlines treatment options. Herpetic esophagitis afflicts immunocompetent or immunodeficient individuals (14). Fever and odynophagia begin suddenly and persist for 5 to 7 days. Diagnosis is by biopsy or culture. Acyclovir therapy (5.0 mg/kg or 250 mg/m^2 intravenously every 8 hours) may shorten the course. Acid-induced esophagitis may be a predisposing factor to this infection. Biopsy would also identify the rare infection with cytomegalovirus.

II. Stomach and Duodenum

A. Gastritis and Ulcer Disease

Although the pH in the duodenum of CF patients is lower than in normal individuals, duodenal ulceration is uncommon. Small series of CF patients with duodenal ulcers have been reported, but the risk within the population is not defined. Barium UGI studies may not be informative because thickened duodenal folds and interfold niches are commonly seen in CF patients. *Helicobacter pylori* infection and gastritis are described in isolated reports (15). This infection may be less common in CF patients than in the general population because two types of medication frequently used in CF regimens (i.e., oral antibiotics and drugs that decrease gastric acid production) are mainstays of treatment.

Nonsteroidal antiinflammatory drugs relieve pain, reduce fever, and may decrease endobronchial inflammation, but may induce esophageal, gastric, or intestinal mucosal damage (16,17). Symptoms of esophagitis, abdominal pain, gastrointestinal bleeding, and mucosal ulceration occur with acute or chronic use (18). Most often, the gastric antrum and prepyloric regions are affected. The frequency of these complaints is difficult to define because most reports describe patient populations with complications rather than a large group of unselected patients taking NSAIDs. Significant gastrointestinal side effects require treatment or change in medication in approximately 1% of patients.

If a CF patient suffers gastrointestinal side effects of NSAIDs, the medication should be interrupted, if possible. If continued NSAID use is required, medications to reduce gastric acid production (see Tables 4 and 6) may ameliorate the distressing symptoms. Theoretically, misoprostol, a prostaglandin agonist, should provide optimal relief of NSAID-related symptoms (19). In practice, however, ranitidine provides equivalent benefit with fewer side effects of abdominal cramps and diarrhea. Misoprostol may also alter the kinetics of indomethacin metabolism, reducing peak serum levels and "area under the curve" (20). Considering the recent report that chronic high-dose ibuprofen delays progression of pulmonary disease in CF, careful titration of serum NSAID concentrations with minimization of side effects may become an important goal in CF care (21).

III. Pancreas

A. Pancreatic Insufficiency

Approximately 85%–90% of individuals with CF have exocrine pancreatic insufficiency (EPI), resulting in steatorrhea and azotorrhea. In a program that identified CF in newborns, approximately 65% of the CF patients had EPI at diagnosis, and EPI developed in at least half of the remainder within the first few years of life (22, 23).

Diagnosis of EPI

Often, caregivers assume that a newly diagnosed CF patient has EPI. The "gold standard" for diagnosing CF-related pancreatic insufficiency is direct measurement of pancreatic enzyme and bicarbonate output into the duodenum. In routine clinical practice, this test is seldom performed (24). The objective criteria commonly used include the following:

1. Poor weight gain or slow growth while on an age-appropriate diet in untreated CF patient
2. Biochemical evidence of malabsorption:
   - Prolonged prothrombin time (PT) and partial thromboplastin time (PTT) due to vitamin K deficiency. Supplemental vitamin K corrects the coagulopathy within 24 hours.
   - Low serum vitamin E level due to vitamin E deficiency. Most often, the patient has no neuropathy.
   - Low serum vitamin A to retinol binding protein ratio due to vitamin A deficiency.
   - Low serum 25-OH-vitamin D level due to vitamin D deficiency. Most often, serum calcium, phosphorus, and alkaline phosphatase are normal and there is no radiological evidence of rickets.
   - Hypoalbuminemia and anemia at 2–4 months of age in untreated infants. These findings represent critical malnutrition. When

originally described in the 1970s, infants with this presentation had a mortality rate of 40% (25). With prompt recognition and therapy, these infants now recover fully.

3. Documentation of undigested fat in a spot stool sample by staining with Sudan III and examination by light microscopy

4. Inability to detect chymotrypsin in a random stoll specimen. Enteric bacteria may, however, produce or digest chymotrypsin, yielding false-positive or -negative results.

5. The bentiramide (Chymex) test involves oral ingestion of para-amino-benzoic acid (PABA) conjugated in a form that is unabsorbable unless split by chymotrypsin. After enzymatic cleavage, the PABA is absorbed, and the serum concentration is measured 1 hour after ingestion. Although the detection of a normal serum PABA level usually excludes exocrine pancreatic insufficiency, failure to detect PABA produces a false-positive rate of approximately 15%–20%.

6. Determination of the coefficient of fat excretion during a 72-hour period provides a direct measure of the efficacy of pancreatic function. A 3-day dietary record and stool collection are obtained simultaneously. The coefficient of fat excretion equals the fat excreted (g) divided by the fat ingested (g). A value of greater than 10% is abnormal in all patients beyond infancy. Outpatients can easily complete these studies. Major GI centers and commercial laboratories perform fecal fat determinations. Samples can be sent through the mail or by special delivery service. These collections represent the only method confirmed accurate in evaluating the efficacy of supplemental pancreatic enzyme therapy. The other methodologies listed have been used only to differentiate pancreatic sufficiency from insufficiency in untreated CF patients.

Treatment with Pancreatic Enzyme Supplements

Enteric-coated enzyme capsules are generally prescribed. These capsules are available in various strengths in numbered preparations. The number refers to the minimum lipase content in thousands of units within the whole capsule. The amounts of protease and amylase increase along with the lipase in high-potency capsules (Table 5).

Many studies validate the effectiveness of these various enzyme preparations, which are manufactured from processed porcine pancreas (26–28). No particular product appears to have a distinct advantage. Clinical efficacy with various preparations varies from patient to patient. Some hospital and health maintenance organization (HMO) pharmacies may restrict their formularies of pancreatic enzyme products, limiting flexibility to change products to increase effectiveness. Generic enzyme supplements are not reliable or effective

Table 5 Pancreatic Enzymes Comparison Guide

Product	Manufacturer	Lipase[a] (IU)	Protease[b] (IU)	Amylase[c] (IU)	Special features
Cotazym	Organon	8,000	3,000	3,000	Capsules, cherry flavor, no enteric coating
Cotazym S	Organon	5,000	20,000	20,000	Capsules, enteric-coated spheres
Creon 5	Solvay	5,000	18,750	16,600	Capsules, enteric-coated minimicrospheres
Creon 10	Solvay	10,000	37,500	33,200	Capsules, enteric-coated minimicrospheres
Creon 20	Solvay	20,000	75,000	66,400	Capsules, enteric-coated minimicrospheres
Pancrease	McNeil	4,000	25,000	20,000	Capsules, enteric-coated microtablets, dye-free
Pancrease MT4	McNeil	4,000	12,000	12,000	Capsules, enteric-coated microtablets, dye-free
Pancrease MT10	McNeil	10,000	30,000	30,000	Capsules, enteric-coated microtablets, dye-free
Pancrease MT16	McNeil	16,000	48,000	48,000	Capsules, enteric-coated microtablets, dye-free
Pancrease 20	McNeil	20,000	40,000	56,000	Capsules, enteric-coated microtablets, dye-free
Ultrase	Scandipharm	4,500	25,000	20,000	Capsules, enteric-coated microspheres
Ultrase MT6	Scandipharm	12,000	37,000	39,000	Capsules, enteric-coated microspheres
Ultrase 12	Scandipharm	12,000	39,000	39,000	Capsules, enteric-coated microspheres
Ultrase 18	Scandipharm	18,000	58,500	58,500	Capsules, enteric-coated microspheres
Ultrase 20	Scandipharm	20,000	65,000	65,000	Capsules, enteric-coated microspheres
Viokase Tablet	Robins	8,000	30,000	30,000	No enteric coating
Viokase Powder	Robins	16,800	70,000	70,000	Amount per teaspoon, no enteric coating
Zymase	Organon	12,000	24,000	24,000	Enteric-coated spheres in capsules

[a]Lipase, fat-digesting enzyme; most important for CF patients; one capsule with 8000 units of lipase is roughly equivalent to two 4000-unit capsules of lipase (if all are enteric coated or all non–enteric coated).
[b]Protease, protein-digesting enzyme.
[c]Amylase, starch-digesting enzyme.

substitutes for name brands. In one study, many generic capsules contained much less active enzyme than advertised (29).

A very limited amount of enzyme is active in the proximal small bowel, the predominant location for fat digestion and absorption (30). Only 10% of normal lipase activity is required to abolish steatorrhea, and this amount of lipase probably becomes available from the supplemental enzymes throughout the length of the small bowel. Approximately 80% of CF patients achieve adequate fat absorption with enzyme supplementation alone; the remaining 20% of patients may require additional measures, particularly a reduction in gastric acid output (31). A persistent acidic environment in the proximal small bowel prevents dissolution of enzyme beads, reduces the activity of released lipase, and limits the formation of intraluminal micelles with bile acids (32). Increasing intraluminal pH by limiting gastric acid production can ameliorate these problems (Table 6) (33,34). No known clinical parameters predict which CF patients will require acid suppression.

Most often, efficacy of treatment is assessed by weight gain, growth, and improvement in gastrointestinal symptoms. In special situations, more exact documentation of effect is necessary. Infants and children whose CF is treated should follow normal growth curves. Diets should usually be unrestricted and appropriate for age.

Enzyme dosing is as follows (35):

1. In infants, offer 2000 to 4000 units of lipase per 120 mL of formula or breast milk. Enzymes capsules are opened, and the beads or microtablets are administered, mixed in small amounts of applesauce or other pureed fruit. Some infants will take the enzymes directly just before staring the liquid feeding. Generally, even very young infants quickly learn to accept the enzyme supplements. Nursing or formula feeding should follow immediately so that the beads are washed out of the mouth, preventing irritation of oral mucous

Table 6 Medications to Increase Intraluminal pH

Medication	Dose	How supplied
Cimetidine	10 mg/kg qid, up to 300 mg per meal	300 mg/5 mL 200 or 300 mg/tab
Ranitidine	2–5 mg/kg bid, up to 150 mg bid	15 mg/mL 150 mg/tab
Famotidine	1 mg/kg bid	40 mg/5 mL 10 or 20 mg/tab
Omeprazole	0.7 mg/kg up to 20 mg per dose; may increase dose to bid	20 mg/cap
Misoprostol	50–100 mcg by mouth qid	100 mcg and 200 mcg/tab

bid = twice per day; qid = four times per day.

membranes. This is particularly important with the powdered (non–enteric-coated) preparations.

2. In children aged 1–4 years, offer 1000 units of lipase per kilogram of body weight per meal. Dosages may be increased gradually to 2500 units/kg/meal if necessary. Provide one-half of the standard dose of enzymes with snacks.

3. In children older than age 4 years, provide approximately 500 units of lipase per kilogram of bodyweight per meal. The dose may be increased up to 1000 units/kg/meal if necessary. Thus, the 30-kg child would take 15,000 to 30,000 units of lipase per meal. Enzyme dosages may be consolidated into higher-dose capsules, for example, three of the 4000-unit capsules may be replaced with one of the 10,000-unit capsules. The exchange of enzymes may not always produce equivalent success. The dissolution characteristics and enzyme survival in the proximal small bowel may vary among enzyme products.

4. In adolescents and adults, follow guidelines similar to those for older children. Avoid gradual and progressive increases in enzyme dosages. If patients have reached the upper limits of enzyme dosages, consider reduction by 50% with subsequent fecal fat collection to document efficacy. The cost savings and increase in adherence can be substantial. Also, consider alternative diagnoses for persistent steatorrhea or gastrointestinal complaints.

5. In any age group, generally, lipase dosages should not exceed 1000–2500 units of lipase per kilogram of body weight per meal. Two recent studies suggested higher enzyme dosages to improve fat digestion and absorption. In both studies, however, the improvement gained was marginal in most patients, and at least half the study patients had adequate fat absorption on doses similar to those recommended in this chapter (36,37). Furthermore, there is recent suggestion that very high enzyme doses may be associated with fibrosing colonopathy.

If the CF patient demonstrates poor weight gain or suboptimal growth, consider the following approach:

1. Ensure that intake is adequate. Most often, poor weight gain or slow growth in CF patients is the result of low energy intake (31). Ascertain whether the diet is not restricted in fat. Identify conditions that may limit intake (e.g., increased pulmonary disease, dysphagia, abdominal pain, vomiting, and anorexia). If a limitation of intake is identified, then attempt to reverse it with dietary advice and nutritional supplements (see Chapter 6).

2. If resistant steatorrhea is suspected, consider the following general measures: (1) change the enzyme product, (2) match enzyme intake to fat intake, or (3) try a new bottle of enzymes. Different enzyme products release enzymes at different rates and at slightly different pH (38). A new product may better match the intraluminal conditions in a particular patient. Some patients

consume large amounts of fat at selected meals. Matching the amount of lipase intake to the fat intake may provide more enzyme when it is needed. Enzymes may lose potency if stored for long periods of time or exposed to high environmental temperature.

3. If resistant steatorrhea is suspected, add medication to reduce gastric acid output and increase pH in the proximal small bowel (Table 6). This increase in pH may allow for greater dissolution of enzyme beads, higher lipase activity in less acidic milieu, and better solubilization of intraluminal bile acids to form micelles for fat digestion and absorption.

4. If these measures are not sufficient, persistent steatorrhea should be confirmed by determining the coefficient of fat excretion with a 72-hour fecal fat collection with simultaneous dietary record. A coefficient of excretion of 10% or less is not likely to improve with further manipulations.

5. If steatorrhea is confirmed, consider additional diagnoses (Table 7).

6. If gastrointestinal symptoms such as abdominal pain, bloating, or increased flatus persist on a particular enzyme regimen, these same steps may be followed for evaluation and therapy. If steatorrhea is not present, then consider additional diagnoses (Table 8).

Problems with Pancreatic Enzyme Supplements

Too little enzyme supplementation results in steatorrhea. Too much enzyme generally causes no signs or symptoms, but occasionally produces diarrhea. High enzyme doses may lead to asymptomatic hyperuricosuria and hyperuricemia. Very high enzyme doses (greater than 6000 units of lipase per kilogram of body weight per meal) are associated with fibrosing colonopathy (35,39).

Table 7 GI Conditions that May Produce Resistant Steatorrhea

Condition	Mechanism
Cholestatic liver disease	Limits bile acid secretion and availability to form micelles to digest and absorb fat
Postoperative short gut	Limits surface area available for absorption
Partial small bowel obstruction with bacterial overgrowth	Produces mucosal damage and dysfunction
Gluten-sensitive enteropathy or postinfectious enteropathy	Causes villous atrophy that reduces surface area
Portal hypertension	Produces lymphatic and venous congestion that may interfere with absorption
Giardiasis	Produces steatorrhea through unknown mechanism

Table 8 GI Conditions that Produce GI Complaints Without Steatorrhea

Condition	Signs and symptoms
Lactose or sucrose intolerance	Watery diarrhea, crampy abdominal pain, and increased flatus
Clostridium difficile infection	Described, but is most often asymptomatic
Irritable bowel syndrome	Crampy abdominal pain; constipation and/or diarrhea
Recurrent abdominal pain of childhood	Periumbilical abdominal pain, pallor, and vomiting
Eating disorders	Abdominal pain and early satiety
Laxative use or abuse	Diarrhea and crampy pains
Constipation	Abdominal pain and infrequent bowel movements
Inflammatory bowel disease	Crampy abdominal pain, watery diarrhea, hematochezia, weight loss

Patients with CF often gradually take more and more enzyme, increasing the dose in response to transient GI symptoms (40). Dosages are seldom reduced. For these patients, even a large enzyme dose reduction (as much as 50%–75%) may be tolerated with no deleterious effect on fat absorption (32). Fecal fat studies may be useful to document the lack of effect of enzyme reduction and continued success of lower enzyme doses in reversing steatorrhea.

B. Pancreatitis

Pancreatitis develops in approximately 1% of CF patients. Pancreatitis may be the presenting problem of previously undiagnosed CF. Initially, clinicians noted only adolescents with CF-related pancreatitis, but more recent reports describe pancreatitis in very young children with CF (41, 42). Patients with CF with pancreatitis retain sufficient exocrine pancreatic function to prevent steatorrhea. Pancreatitis occurs as severe abdominal pain in the epigastrium or left upper quadrant. Pain may radiate through to the back. Vomiting is frequent. Epigastric tenderness may be present.

Diagnosis of Pancreatitis

Characteristic pain (severe midabdominal pain with radiation to the back) initiates evaluation. Serum amylase and lipase concentrations are elevated. In the acute phase of pancreatitis, both these serum enzymes are usually elevated a minimum of 5 times the upper limit of normal. Some caution is necessary before attributing elevated amylase or lipase to pancreatitis, because other conditions (e.g., peptic ulcer, intestinal obstruction, renal failure, diabetes) may also increase serum levels. Most serum amylase assays also detect salivary and other amylases, so elevation of serum amylase alone may occur with injury to salivary glands or ovaries. Lipase elevation is thought to be more specific for pancreatic disorders, but less information is available about how other medical conditions affect serum lipase levels (43).

Imaging studies (abdominal computed tomography (CT) scan or ultrasound) may show pancreatic enlargement or edema, peripancreatic edema, or ascites. It is not unusual, however, for CF patients with pancreatitis to have normal imaging studies even during an attack. Plain abdominal films are useful to exclude bowel obstruction and to identify calcifications within the pancreas or biliary tree. Upper GI fluoroscopy with small bowel follow through is helpful to exclude severe peptic ulcer disease or partial bowel obstruction. Endoscopic retrograde cholangiopancreatography (ERCP) delineates the anatomy of the pancreatic and biliary system. Stones in the common bile duct, stenoses of the pancreatic duct, and abnormalities of the union of the pancreatic and bile duct near the ampulla of Vater have been described in CF patients. ERCP is not usually performed after a single episode of pancreatitis because the risk of inducing pancreatitis with the examination is approximately 10%. Microlithiasis or crystals within bile may produce pancreatitis in normal individuals. Patients with CF have not been screened for this potential etiology.

Other causes of pancreatitis besides CF should be considered (Table 9).

Treatment of Pancreatitis

1. Give the patient nothing by mouth until pain remits. The elimination of intraluminal nutrients reduces pancreatic secretion, limiting flow of enzyme into inflamed tissue.

Table 9 Causes for Pancreatitis Other than Cystic Fibrosis

Abdominal trauma
Medications
    Azathioprine
    Thiazides
    Trimethoprim/sulfamethoxasole
    Azulfidine
    Corticosteroids
Infection
    Mumps
    Coxsackie virus
    Mycoplasma
    Ascariasis
Anatomical problems
    Gallstone obstruction
    Pancreas divisum
    Long common channel of pancreatic and bile duct
    Microlithiasis

2. Provide intravenous fluids and, possibly, parenteral nutrition.
3. Administer pain relief, usually with intravenous meperidine, in doses of approximately 1 mg/kg every 3–6 hours. If larger doses are needed, another opiate should be used to avoid inducing a seizure by metabolites of meperidine. Theoretically, morphine may cause spasm of the sphincter of Oddi and exacerbate pancreatitis. In practice, evidence of an adverse effect on the course of illness is slim.
4. Monitor the patient for complications. Systemic complications of acute pancreatitis appear to be uncommon in patients with CF. Systemic problems in patients without CF include shock, hemorrhage, hypocalcemia, ascites, pleural effusion, and adult respiratory distress syndrome.
5. Serial measurement of amylase and lipase is often performed but does not direct therapy. Enteral nutrition can resume when pain remits and before serum amylase and lipase are normal. Enzyme measurements can help determine whether pain is related to an exacerbation of pancreatitis because enzyme levels usually increase with increasing inflammation. As pancreatitis resolves, serum amylase concentration decreases more rapidly than serum lipase.
6. Many other therapies have been attempted to hasten the resolution or reduce the severity of an attack of acute pancreatitis; however, none of these therapies (e.g., nasogastric suction, somatostatin infusion, and ingestion of exogenous pancreatic enzymes) has been proven effective.

Course of Pancreatitis

Usually, pain remits in 2–5 days. Resolution of elevated serum amylase or lipase may take longer, but elevated enzyme levels should not preclude reintroduction of oral intake.

Local complications of pancreatic pseudocyst or abscess appear to be unusual. Serial imaging studies are not necessary if the patient is asymptomatic. Even if a pseudocyst is identified, watchful waiting would be the anticipated course. Many pseudocysts resolve without intervention within the first 6 weeks of the acute episode of pancreatitis.

Recurrence of Pancreatitis

Recurrent episodes of acute pancreatitis are common. If acute pancreatitis recurs, ERCP is often performed once the acute attack resolves. A correctable lesion such retained gallstone or pancreatic duct stricture is occasionally identified. Endoscopic interventional therapy (e.g., gallstone extraction, stricture dilation, sphincterotomy) may then prove beneficial to prevent further episodes of pancreatitis.

Supplemental pancreatic enzymes offer a theoretical benefit to prevent recurrent attacks of pancreatitis and to reduce abdominal pain. Unbound trypsin within the lumen of the duodenum may provide negative feedback inhibition of pancreatic secretion. Ingestion of uncoated or enteric-coated enzymes may supply sufficient trypsin to initiate this feedback, reducing stimulation of the pancreas. Adults with chronic pancreatitis not related to CF appear to receive some benefit from this therapy. The risk is minimal.

Patients who suffer recurrent pancreatitis are at risk of development of narcotic dependence. Abdominal pain may be the only symptom or sign of recurrent pancreatitis. Continuing pain and narcotic tolerance can gradually escalate medication requirements. Absence of elevation of serum amylase and lipase should prompt careful review of the diagnosis of pancreatitis, thoughtful consideration of alternative sources of abdominal discomfort, and hesitation in escalating doses of narcotics. If no new diagnosis is evident, alternative pain relief measures such as tricyclic antidepressants, transdermal electronic nerve stimulation (TENS), and behavioral therapy may deserve consideration.

IV. Liver

Several hepatobiliary tract disorders may occur in cystic fibrosis (Table 10).

A. Asymptomatic Elevation of Serum Transaminases or Alkaline Phosphatase

The most common abnormality is asymptomatic elevation of serum transaminases. Up to 30% of patients with CF may have elevated aspartate transaminase (AST) or alanine transaminase (ALT). Most of these patients have no other signs of liver dysfunction. Elevation of serum alkaline phosphatase may occur

Table 10 Hepatobiliary Disorders in Cystic Fibrosis

Common problems
    Asymptomatic elevation of serum transaminases
    Asymptomatic elevation of serum alkaline phosphatase
    Hepatic steatosis
    Multifocal biliary fibrosis
Uncommon problems
    Neonatal cholestasis
    Multilobular biliary cirrhosis, often with portal hypertension
    Gallstones
    Biliary tract obstruction

in 15%–30% of patients (44). Although the elevated serum alkaline phosphatase suggests biliary tract disease, symptomatic liver disease never develops in many patients. Longitudinal studies with long-term follow-up of patients with abnormal serum enzyme levels may allow determination of factors that predispose them to more severe hepatic disease.

B. Hepatic Enlargement

Apparent hepatic enlargement (liver edge palpated 3 or more centimeters below the right costal margin) is often attributable to pulmonary overinflation. True hepatic enlargement (increase in liver span) is frequently due to hepatic steatosis. In untreated cases in undernourished patients, steatosis may be generalized and prominent. In treated cases, the fat accumulation may be focal but is not clearly zonal. A clear-cut relationship between hepatic steatosis and progressive liver disease or cirrhosis has not been established. Autopsy examinations documented focal biliary fibrosis in up to 25% of CF patients, the frequency increasing with age. Most of these patients, however, had no clinical symptoms or signs of liver disease during life (45, 46).

C. Neonatal Cholestasis

Neonatal cholestasis occurs in approximately 5% of infants with CF. In one study, from one-fourth to one-half of these infants had meconium ileus in the newborn period, and many required surgery (47). Inspissated eosinophilic material in small and large bile ducts may produce local or generalized obstruction to bile flow within the liver, leading to intrahepatic cholestasis and jaundice. The location of CFTR within bile duct epithelium suggests that water and electrolyte secretion into bile may be abnormal, leading to thickened secretions that produce this obstruction. Hypoxemia, hypotension, bacterial or viral infection, and medications may accompany neonatal illness and surgery. In any newborn, transient cholestasis can follow these systemic problems. Infants with CF and meconium ileus are more likely to experience problems that predispose them to neonatal cholestasis and thus cholestasis is more likely to develop in these infants than in infants with CF but without neonatal illness. Neonatal cholestasis can persist for as long as 2 months, but usually does not progress to long-term or chronic liver disease (48).

D. Cirrhosis

Macronodular, multilobular cirrhosis and portal hypertension develop in from 2%–5% of patients with CF (45, 49). The degree of elevation of serum transaminases or alkaline phosphatase or the duration of elevation does not correspond with the risk of or presence of cirrhosis. Cirrhosis and portal hyper-

Table 11 Diagnosing Non-CF Liver Disease in CF Patients

Disorder	Screening laboratory tests
Chronic hepatitis B or C	Hepatitis B and C serologies (HbsAg, HbcAg, hepatitis C antibody, hepatitis C pcr)
Hepatitis E–G	Serologic assays being developed
Alpha$_1$-antitrypsin deficiency	Serum α_1-antitrypsin phenotype
Wilson's disease	Serum copper and ceruloplasmin, 24-hour urinary copper
Hemochromatosis	Serum ferritin, iron, and total iron-binding capacity
Autoimmune hepatitis	Antinuclear antibody, anti-DNA antibody, anti-LKM antibody, anti–smooth muscle antibody
Drug-induced hepatic dysfunction	Toxicological screens

tension develop silently and insidiously. A hard-edged, irregular liver and splenic enlargement are often first detected by careful physical examination. Superficial veins of the abdominal wall may be dilated and prominent. Digital clubbing and oxygen desaturation may occur with cirrhosis even without significant parenchymal pulmonary disease (50). Serum transaminases and alkaline phosphatase are mildly elevated or normal. Liver function, evaluated by measuring serum bilirubin, serum albumin, and coagulation studies, is initially normal. Increasing splenomegaly and diminution in liver size indicate progressive cirrhosis and portal hypertension, again usually without overt symptoms. Abdominal examination may reveal an asymmetric liver with shrinkage of the right lobe but prominence of the left lobe (51,52).

Patients with CF-related liver disease could suffer a coincident non-CF hepatic disorder (Table 11). A thorough search for these other conditions seems warranted because some have specific treatment. Both literature and personal experience suggest, however, that this search will not usually reveal additional problems. Liver biopsy is generally not necessary in the CF patient with cirrhosis but no indication of a second liver disorder. If one of these disorders is suspected by results of studies, liver biopsy may be essential to confirm histology or chemical analysis.

The complications of portal hypertension (e.g., ascites or hemorrhage from esophageal, gastric, duodenal, or colonic varices) rather than liver synthetic failure threaten the health of the CF patient (49,51–53). Portosystemic encephalopathy is uncommon. Splenomegaly, sometimes with pain and with the danger of rupture, results in thrombocytopenia and leukopenia from hypersplenism, but these do not usually contribute to clinical problems. Poor weight gain, slow growth, and delayed puberty may accompany cirrhosis and portal hypertension, but the mechanism is unclear.

Table 12 Diuretics for Treating Ascites

Drug	Dose
Spironolactone	2–3 mg/kg/day (given in 1–2 doses) by mouth
Aldactazide (Aldactone and hydrochlorothiazide)	1–2 mg/kg/day by mouth
Furosemide	0.5–2.0 mg/kg/day (1–2 doses) by mouth or intravenously

Ascites

Ascites requires treatment if the amount of fluid and abdominal distention are burdensome for the patient. The treatment of ascites in CF-related portal hypertension does not differ from that in other causes of portal hypertension and includes mild salt restriction and cautious use of diuretics (Table 12). Hypokalemic, hypochloremic metabolic alkalosis may necessitate potassium chloride supplementation. Hyponatremia with serum sodium concentration of approximately 130 mEq/L is common during diuretic therapy.

Refractory ascites can be reduced by periodic paracentesis with replacement of protein by infusion of 25% albumin (54). In adults, a liter or more of ascitic fluid is removed at each paracentesis, and the procedure is continued until the ascites resolves. The protein removed in the ascitic fluid is replaced gram for gram with intravenous albumin. In some series, this treatment produced fewer complications of fluid and electrolyte imbalance than the use of diuretics. No series of pediatric patients has been reported.

Spontaneous Bacterial Peritonitis

Spontaneous bacterial peritonitis is a serious complication of cirrhosis (55,56). Fever, abdominal pain, increasing ascites, diarrhea, and vomiting may herald the onset of bacterial infection. Diagnostic paracentesis demonstrates an absolute neutrophil count of more than 250 neutrophils per milliliter. In the 20–30 mL of ascitic fluid that is sent for bacterial culture, the density of organisms may be quite low. In cirrhotic patients, gram-negative bacteria, usually *Escherichia coli*, cause peritonitis. Patients with CF would appear to be at risk of *Pseudomonas* infection, but no series of patients has been reported to document this concern. The usual case of cirrhosis is treated with intravenous ampicillin and cefotaxime; replacement of cefotaxime with ceftazidime appears reasonable for the CF patient with peritonitis. Culture and sensitivity data along with clinical reponse guide specific antibiotic choices. Appropriate parenteral antibiotic therapy often reduces fever and abdominal tenderness within 24 hours. The neutrophil count in ascitic fluid also declines quickly. If coagulopathy or other clinical conditions interfere with paracentesis, then empirical antibiotic therapy is warranted. Intravenous antibiotic therapy is usually continued for 5–7 days. Oral antibiotics that match bacterial susceptibility profiles may extend therapy for another 7 days.

Bacterial peritonitis often recurs. Prophylactic therapy with oral norfloxacin appears effective in adults to prevent recurrent peritonitis. No trials have been performed in children.

Gastrointestinal Hemorrhage

To prevent gastrointestinal hemorrhage, avoid ingestion of aspirin and nonsteroidal antiinflammatory agents. These medications may produce esophageal, gastric, or duodenal mucosal injury and impair platelet function.

Hematemesis is most often due to bleeding from esophageal or gastric varices. Melena follows but may not appear for up to 24 hours. Hematochezia may indicate colonic variceal bleeding or rapid passage of blood from the upper gastrointestinal tract.

Are urgent endoscopic procedures necessary or helpful for the CF patient with gastrointestinal bleeding and portal hypertension? The data used to answer this question are extrapolated from series of adults with alcoholic cirrhosis. Pediatric experience is limited to various series of patients undergoing intervention; no controlled trials of the benefits of endoscopy, sclerotherapy, and variceal banding have been completed in children or adolescents (57–60). Most variceal hemorrhages in young patients are self-limited. Because spontaneous cessation represents the natural history of variceal bleeding, therapeutic manuevers appear successful. Cirrhotic adults often have complicating conditions such as chronic renal disease, arteriosclerotic heart disease, or severe pulmonary disease that predispose vital organs to dysfunction, adding significantly to morbidity and mortality. Uncompensated liver synthetic dysfunction and a propensity to portosystemic encephalopathy further complicate gastrointestinal hemorrhage in adults. Pediatric and adolescent patients suffer these complications less commonly. The decision to proceed with urgent endoscopy or therapeutic manuevers to prevent additional hemorrhages is complex and influenced by many factors. Sclerotherapy requires multiple endoscopies and has multiple potential morbidities (57–64). Endoscopic ligation necessitates fewer treatments and has a lower rate of rebleeding and complications (64). Availability in pediatric centers may be limited. The number of bleeding episodes, the degree of pulmonary disease, the potential candidacy for liver transplantation, the experience of the treating physicians, and the wishes of the patient and family represent some of the potential considerations guiding therapy.

Treatment focuses on maintenance of euvolemia. Close monitoring of pulse rate and perfusion is essential. Hypotension is a late and menacing sign of volume depletion in children and adolescents, indicating critical hypovolemia.

Two large-gauge intravenous lines are needed to provide sufficient crystalloid and packed red blood cell transfusion. A nasogastric tube may provide information about the volume of bleeding, but is not always required, particularly if the rate of bleeding appears to be slow. Coagulopathy is not often a complicating factor, but parenteral vitamin K (2–5 mg administered slowly intravenously and fresh frozen plasma (10–20 mL/kg) can be given, especially if the prothrombin time is more than 2 seconds above control values. Vitamin K can also be given intramuscularly because there is a small risk of anaphylaxis with intravenous administration. Intravenous H_2-receptor antagonists are often given to reduce gastric acid output, providing treatment for acid-related bleeding and, perhaps, reducing the frequency of stress-related bleeding.

Ascites often develops during or after the resolution of gastrointestinal bleeding in cirrhotic patients with portal hypertension. The mechanism is not clear, but the occurrence is so common that the patient and family should be advised of it. Gastrointestinal hemorrhage can be a presenting sign of bacterial peritonitis or bacteremia (65). After prompt evaluation with physical examination, culture of blood and urine, and possible paracentesis, broad-spectrum parenteral antibiotics are initiated until culture results are returned.

Progressive hepatocellular failure and complications of portal hypertension may prompt consideration of liver transplantation. Previously, various shunt procedures were recommended for recurrent gastrointestinal bleeding. Prophylactic shunts were considered to prevent bleeding episodes later in life when lung disease might be more severe. The use of therapeutic endoscopic procedures, transjugular intrahepatic portosystemic shunting (TIPS), and liver transplantation has replaced operative shunts for many patients. The TIPS may provide urgent decompression of the portal venous system and prevent further variceal hemorrhage. In a CF patient, TIPS provided a transient solution for gastrointestinal hemorrhage and refractory ascites (66).

Liver transplantation provides the dual benefits of replacing the diseased liver and decompressing the portal venous system. The risk of progressive liver disease with eventual failure of synthetic function and the risk of recurrent complications of portal hypertension can both be eliminated. Liver transplantation and the associated immunosuppression do not lead to rapidly progressive pulmonary disease. In one series, pulmonary function actually improved after liver transplantation (67). Short-term survival expectations for CF patients are similar to those of other patients undergoing liver transplantation. The decision to proceed with evaluation for transplantation, however, requires the careful consideration and participation of the entire health care team, including physicians, nurses, social workers, patient, and family, because the procedure is a major undertaking, requiring lifetime immunosuppression and considerable emotional and financial resources.

V. Biliary Tract

A. Cholelithiasis

Cholelithiasis occurs in 5%–15% of CF patients, the incidence increasing with age. In one review of 670 patients, 24 (3.6%) suffered symptomatic gallstone disease (68). The youngest symptomatic patient was 4 years old. Gallstones related to CF contain calcium bilirubinate and proteins (69). The exact conditions that predispose a person with CF to gallstone enucleation and enlargement are not known.

Symptoms from gallstones follow a characteristic pattern: pain is severe, colicky, and located in the right upper quadrant or epigastrium. Pain lasts a few to several hours and then remits spontaneously. Presumably, pain occurs when a stone impacts in the cystic or common bile duct, producing obstruction and proximal distention of the duct or gallbladder. Stones residing in the gallbladder are often asymptomatic. Jaundice occurs if the common bile duct is obstructed and the serum bilirubin increases above 3.0 mg%; lesser serum bilirubin elevation or transient mild elevation of serum alkaline phosphatase or serum transaminases may be present during or just after pain. Ultrasound reveals residual stones in the gallbladder or a stone within the cystic or common bile duct to confirm the diagnosis. In CF patients with characteristic pain and ultrasound findings, cholecystectomy is recommended because of the high risk of ascending cholangitis when stones are allowed to remain. Laparoscopic cholecystectomy produces less morbidity than laparotomy and is the preferred procedure. Residual stones within the common bile duct can be detected and removed by laparoscopic techniques or by ERCP.

B. Microgallbladder

A very small thick-walled gallbladder is a common finding on ultrasound or at autopsy in CF patients. A microgallbladder may not fill or empty normally, but it does not appear to cause particular symptoms (45,70).

C. Bile Duct Disorders

In 1981, Lambert et al. reported a single CF adult with intrapancreatic compression of the common bile duct, leading to obstructive jaundice (71). Gaskin et al. then described a group of 61 patients with liver disease and CF, two-thirds of whom had abnormal biliary tracts identified by radionucleotide scanning. Transhepatic cholangiography demonstrated intrapancreatic compression of the distal common bile duct with proximal dilatation in 14 patients. Many of these latter patients underwent surgical diversion of the common bile duct. This paper is unique in reporting such a high frequency of symptomatic bile duct abnormalities (72,73). The frequency of this finding in other CF populations is not

Table 13 Abdominal Pain in Patients with CF

Epigastric pain
    Common diagnoses
        Gastritis, duodenitis, ulcer disease, nonulcer dyspepsia, gastroesophageal reflux disease
    Less common diagnoses
        Pancreatitis, gallbladder or biliary tract disease, distal intestinal obstruction syndrome (DIOS)
    Usual approach
        Trial of H_2-receptor antagonist to treat acid peptic disease. Upper GI series small bowel follow through or upper GI endoscopy if empirical therapy is unsuccessful
Right upper quadrant pain
    Common diagnoses
        Gallstones or biliary tract disease
    Usual approach
        Hepatobiliary ultrasound
Right lower quadrant pain
    Common diagnosis
        DIOS
    Less common diagnoses
        Right colon fibrosis or stricture, appendiceal disease, intussusception, partial small bowel obstruction from adhesions from previous abdominal surgery, irritable bowel syndrome, ovarian cyst, renal colic
    Usual approach
        Evaluate and treat for DIOS; if no response to DIOS treatment, contrast fluoroscopy may be needed
Periumbilical or diffuse abdominal pain
    Common diagnosis
        Incorrect use of supplemental pancreatic enzymes
    Less common diagnoses
        Recurrent abdominal pain of childhood, partial small bowel obstruction, distal intestinal obstruction syndrome, irritable bowel syndrome, lactose intolerance, aerophagia, abdominal wall muscle pain (perhaps related to cough)
    Usual approach
        Investigate enzyme use; other evaluation as indicated if this does not reveal the problem.

known. Potentially affected CF patients have right upper quadrant pain with biochemical evidence of liver disease. If hepatobiliary ultrasound identifies dilatation of the extrahepatic or intrahepatic biliary tract, then invasive studies such as ERCP or transhepatic cholangiography delineate the exact biliary anatomy and site of presumed obstruction.

D. Abdominal Pain

Abdominal pain in a CF patient may relate to an intraabdominal complication of CF or may be the result of an unrelated disorder. Clinicians may be reluctant to subject a CF patient to a multitude of studies aimed at diagnosing a non-CF problem. Nonetheless, clinicians can approach abdominal pain of unknown cause as they would in the non-CF patient (Tables 13 and 14).

VI. Intestine

A. Neonatal Meconium Ileus

Approximately 10%–15% of CF patients experience neonatal meconium ileus or its complications (74,75). Viscous inspissated meconium blocks the small bowel lumen. Characteristically, abdominal distention and bilious vomiting develop within the first several hours of life. The infant does not pass meconium. Plain radiographs show air–fluid levels in the small bowel and a paucity or absence of gas in the colon. Small bowel ischemia and perforation may have occurred antenatally, producing intraabdominal calcifications, meconium cyst, or ileal atresia. In some infants, the intrauterine perforation seals with restoration of intestinal continuity. The clinical picture of distal small bowel obstruction necessitates the following measures:

1. Establish an intravenous line for restoration or maintenance of intravascular volume and electrolyte balance.
2. Place a number 10 French Replogle nasogastric tube to intermittent low suction.
3. Obtain surgical consultation.
4. Perform contrast enema, usually with Gastrografin water-soluble contrast material (76). This study is often diagnostic and therapeutic.

With meconium ileus, an unused "microcolon" or colon of normal shape with small caliber is delineated. If contrast refluxes into the distal small bowel, the contrast outlines filling defects of inspissated meconium. Caution is necessary because perforation may already be present or may occur with high-pressure filling of dilated or previously ischemic small bowel. Wagget recommends 60–90 mL of contrast to fill the colon without undue pressure (76). Ideally, contrast should flow back into the ileum until dilated small bowel proximal to the meconium obstruction is visualized. Gastrografin and similar radiocontrast materials are useful in this setting because the radiocontrast allows delineation of the anatomical structures, and the high osmolality pulls water into the lumen to liquify the obstructing meconium. More than one procedure may be necessary to achieve this goal. Several hours should elapse between attempts to allow for the hypertonic contrast material to draw fluid into the intestinal lumen and dilute the inspissated feces. This dilution facilitates passage of meconium to relieve the distal small bowel obstruction. The infant is carefully monitored for possible fluid and electrolyte imbalance that may occur with fluid secretion into the obstructed proximal bowel or into the colon. In 50%–75% of infants with

Table 14 Distinguishing Features of Abdominal Pain

Disease	Onset	Location	Referral	Quality	Comments
Irritable bowel syndrome	Recurrent	Right lower quadrant or left lower quadrant	None	Dull, crampy, intermittent, 2-h duration	Stress, variable diarrhea, constipation, tenesmus
Esophageal reflux disease	Recurrent, 1 h after meals, at night	Substernal	Chest	Burning	Acid brash, water brash, relieved by antacids
Duodenal ulcer	Recurrent, between meals, at night	Epigastric	Back	Severe burning; gnawing	Relieved by food, milk, antacids
Pancreatitis	Acute	Epigastric, left upper quadrant	Back	Constant, sharp, boring	Nausea, emesis, tenderness
Intestinal obstruction	Acute or gradual	Periumbilical, lower abdomen	Back	Alternating cramping (colic) and painless periods	Distention, obstipation, bilious emesis, increased bowel sounds
Appendicitis	Acute	Periumbilical, localized to right lower quadrant	Back or pelvis if retrocecal	Sharp, steady	Nausea, emesis, local tenderness, fever
Meckel diverticulum	Recurrent	Periumbilical, lower abdomen	None	Sharp	Hematochezia
Inflammatory bowel disease	Recurrent	Lower abdomen	Back	Dull cramping, tenesmus	Fever, weight loss, hematochezia
Intussusception	Acute	Periumbilical, lower abdomen	None	Cramping, with painless periods	Hematochezia, knees in pulled up position
Lactose intolerance	Recurrent with milk products	Lower abdomen	None	Cramping	Distention, bloating, diarrhea
Urolithiasis	Acute, sudden	Back	Groin	Sharp, intermittent, cramping	Hematuria
Urinary tract infection	Acute, sudden	Back	Bladder	Dull to sharp	Fever, costochondral tenderness, dysuria, urinary frequency
Recurrent abdominal pain	Recurrent	Periumbilical	None	Dull	Nausea, pallor, diaphoresis, begins at age 6 years

Source: Adapted from Behrman RE, Kliegman RM. Nelson Essentials of Pediatrics. Philadelphia: WB Saunders, 1990.

uncomplicated meconium ileus, the small bowel obstruction may be relieved with this treatment, eliminating the need for laparotomy.

If the meconium ileus is complicated by intestinal perforation, fixed obstruction by atresia, meconium cyst, or progressive illness due to persistent obstruction, laparotomy will be necessary (77). The exact procedure depends on the type of complication encountered (see Chapter 10). Before the advent of contrast enema therapy, parenteral nutrition, and special neonatal surgical and anesthesia techniques, the perioperative mortality rate of meconium ileus was approximately 50% (78,79). With current management, the mortality rate is approximately 5%.

Not all infants with meconium obstruction syndromes will have CF. Olsen et al. reviewed a series of infants with meconium plug syndrome, meconium ileus, and meconium peritonitis (77). Meconium plug syndrome differs from meconium ileus. In meconium plug syndrome, the initial symptoms and signs are similar but the obstruction is in the colon, caused by a mucous plug or plugs. The colon appears normal on contrast enema. The contrast enema generally mobilizes the inspissated plugs with subsequent passage and relief of obstruction. In the Olsen series, six of the 25 infants with meconium plug syndrome had CF; one infant had Hirschsprung's disease. The others appeared to be free of underlying disease. Of the 15 infants with meconium ileus, 12 had CF. Eight infants had meconium peritonitis. Four of them had CF. Thus, meconium obstructive disease is not always indicative of CF, but this finding should prompt a sweat test as soon as possible, despite the widely held misconception that sweat testing is not possible or not accurate in the newborn (see Chapter 1) (80). Most infants with meconium ileus will be shown to have pancreatic insufficiency.

In the uncommon situation when a sweat test cannot be accomplished and genetic testing is not available or is not diagnostic, strong consideration should be given to treating the infant as if CF is present rather than waiting for the development of poor weight gain or other nutritional problems. Many parents accept that the special nutritional therapies are reasonable and safe for the infant with the understanding that a definitive diagnosis requires more time and testing. With this approach, infants do not go untreated if lost to follow-up for a period of time and do not suffer nutritional compromise.

Complications of Meconium Ileus

The complications of ileal atresia, intestinal perforation, and meconium cyst all require laparotomy and probable intestinal resection and ileostomy. Usually, only a short section of ileum needs to be resected and sufficient small bowel remains for normal digestion and absorption. Rarely, longer sections of small bowel are resected, and short bowel syndrome may result. Prolonged parenteral nutrition and specialized formulas or feeding techniques may be necessary until small bowel function improves.

If an ileostomy is necessary, the infant will require salt supplementation when on complete enteral intake. Ileal effluent contains up to 100 mEq/L of sodium with variable amounts of chloride and bicarbonate as the anion. Usual infant stool contains approximately 20 mEq/L of sodium. Thus, fecal losses of sodium are high in the ileostomate. Most formulas contain only 15–20 mEq/L of sodium, enough to meet maintenance requirements in a normal infant, but insufficient for the infant with extra losses. Sodium depletion with poor appetite and slow weight gain is a common occurrence unless extra sodium supplements are provided. Serum sodium concentration remains normal unless depletion is severe. Urine sodium concentration does, however, decrease to less than 10 mEq/L on a random spot urine specimen, indicating the renal conservation of all available filtered sodium. Provision of oral sodium chloride supplements of 6–8 mEq/kg/day of sodium prevents sodium depletion (81). Sodium ionotrate contains 2.5 mEq of sodium chloride per milliliter and is a convenient form for administration. Mixing of salt solutions from table salt (approximately 100 mEq of NaCl per teaspoon) is problematic because there is potential for errors in measurement. Salt supplementation should be continued as long as the ileostomy is present.

Many infants who undergo surgery require a period of parenteral nutritional support. Total parenteral nutrition (TPN) requirements of CF infants do not differ from those of other neonates in the postoperative period. Most CF infants who do not have extensive intestinal resection quickly adapt to enteral feedings. Often, such infants feed with Pregestimil® or Alimentum®. These formulas contain hydrolyzed casein and a 50–50 mixture of long-chain and medium-chain triglycerides (MCT). Supplemental enzymes are still necessary to digest corn syrup solids and the long-chain triglycerides. Enzymes also optimize absorption of medium-chain triglycerides (82). Interruption of the enterohepatic circulation of bile acids due to ideal resection or dysfunction may have less effect on fat digestion, because intraluminal depletion of bile acids has no effect on MCT absorption.

B. Distal Intestinal Obstruction Syndrome

In the late 1960s, literature reports accumulated describing older CF patients who suffered distal small bowel obstruction due to inspissated intestinal contents in the terminal ileum (83). Originally, this clinical problem was labeled meconium ileus equivalent; presently, it is called distal intestinal obstruction syndrome (DIOS).

Etiology of DIOS

In the initial descriptions of DIOS, clinicians proposed that the condition occurred when CF patients failed to take adequate enzyme supplementation.

Subsequent experience suggests that most patients with DIOS are actually taking their enzymes in appropriate dosages. The CF patients with DIOS may have more severe residual steatorrhea, even with pancreatic enzyme treatment. Persistent steatorrhea may slow intestinal transit because neurotensin, a GI hormone that delays motility, is secreted from the distal ileum when unabsorbed fat reaches that location. Distal intestinal obstruction syndrome may result from inherently slow intestinal motility or from abnormal intraluminal secretions that occur as a basic part of CF (i.e., it is directly related to abnormal CFTR protein in crypt cells) (84, 85).

Slow intestinal motility in the postoperative period or in relation to narcotic analgesics may increase the risk of DIOS. Such patients should be closely monitored for the development of abdominal pain, distention, or fecal retention. Early intervention may prevent the development of small bowel obstruction and simplify the overall course.

Clinical Picture of DIOS

Distal intestinal obstruction syndrome may occur with acute or chronic symptoms. The cardinal features include crampy abdominal pain, often in the right lower quadrant or lower abdomen, a palpable mass in the right lower quadrant, and decreased frequency of defecation. The acute presentation may include abdominal distention and bilious vomiting, two signs of actual or impending complete small bowel obstruction. Approximately 10% of CF patients suffer this form of DIOS (86). In the chronic form of DIOS, the colicky abdominal pain may be provoked by meals, resulting in anorexia as a method of avoiding pain. The attacks of pain may remit for weeks or months, but return associated with right lower quadrant mass and relative constipation. In DIOS, physical examination reveals a mass or fullness in the right lower quadrant. The rectal examination is normal. Partial small bowel obstruction may produce diffuse abdominal distention and abdominal tenderness. Signs of dehydration and intravascular volume depletion are seen, not due to fluid losses from vomiting or reduced intake, but due to fluid and electrolyte secretion from the intestinal vasculature into the lumen of obstructed small bowel. Although abdominal plain films (flat plate and upright films) show bubbly fecal material in the right lower quadrant, this is a nonspecific finding and should not be overinterpreted. With acute obstruction, air–fluid levels appear in dilated proximal small bowel loops. If these "classic" physical and radiological findings are not present, then alternative causes of the abdominal pain or obstruction must be considered (Table 15). Often, DIOS is incorrectly implicated as a cause of abdominal pain in a CF patient. This error might delay the diagnosis of appendicitis, partial bowel obstruction due to adhesions, irritable bowel syndrome, and right colon fibrosis and may lead to inappropriate therapy.

Table 15 Causes of Colicky Abdominal Pain and Apparent Ileus in CF

Distal intestinal obstruction syndrome
Small bowel obstruction from adhesions from previous laparotomy
Appendicitis
Intussusception
Right colon fibrosis or stricture with partial bowel obstruction
Volvulus

Treatment of DIOS

Treatment of DIOS is directed at nonoperative relief of the small bowel obstruction.

Gastrografin Enema Procedure

As in infants with distal small bowel obstruction, Gastrografin enema confirms the diagnosis and may dislodge inspissated material from the distal ileum. In DIOS, the enema shows a nondilated colon and filling defects outlined in the distal ileum. Contrast material should reflux into the more proximal dilated small bowel. The hypertonic solution draws fluid into the small bowel lumen allowing for washout of the thick fecal material into the colon.

Advantages of Gastrografin enema are that exact diagnosis is established by direct visualization (other diagnoses such as distal bowel obstruction by adhesion or intussusception may also be evident) and that postevacuation films can document the success or failure of the contrast enema.

Disadvantages of Gastrografin enema are that intraluminal fluid shifts result in intravascular volume depletion or electrolyte imbalance, there is discomfort with the procedure, and the patient is exposed to x-rays.

The following are warnings about Gastrografin enema procedure:

1. An intravenous line is required in case there are fluid shifts.
2. A nasogastric tube may be needed if vomiting occurs frequently.
3. An experienced radiologist and, in some cases, a CF clinician may be required for optimal study. The procedure may produce marked abdominal distention and severe discomfort. The CF patient with significant lung disease and tachypnea may become dyspneic or even hypoxemic. While the radiologist monitors the progress of the radiographic examination, the CF clinician monitors the overall status of the patient, providing supplemental oxygen, pain relief, and reassurance.
4. Reflux into the terminal ileum or into dilated bowel may be difficult or impossible to achieve on the initial examination. Repeat enema may be needed in several hours if severe obstruction remains. Naso-

gastric tube suction is necessary if vomiting persists or if there is progressive dilation of proximal small bowel.

5. The procedure often causes such discomfort that most patients feel dramatically better at its conclusion, leading both patient and physician to conclude it has been therapeutic. The clinician must insist on objective evidence of improvement over a period of hours, or days, and be willing to entertain other possible diagnoses.

Lavage Treatment of DIOS

If the course of DIOS is chronic or if there is not evidence of complete small bowel obstruction, intestinal lavage treatment provides an alternative therapy to mobilize inspissated intestinal contents. Lavage treatment provides a large volume of isotonic fluid flowing from the stomach to the distal small bowel to dilute the impacted material. Older CF patients may take sufficient lavage solution by mouth; younger patients often require an infusion through a nasogastric tube (87). Details of the lavage procedure are listed in Table 16.

Benefits of lavage treatment (compared with Gastrografin enema) are that it is less uncomfortable than enemas, there is less x-ray exposure, it is less expensive, the procedure is easily repeated, and it can be done at home.

The disadvantages of lavage treatment are that it is contraindicated with complete bowel obstruction, there is exacerbation of intraluminal fluid accumulation, there may be vomiting and fluid or electrolyte imbalance, there is no delineation of exact diagnosis, and the relatively large volume required may not be tolerated, especially by the younger child.

If symptoms or findings worsen during lavage treatment, reevaluation is essential. Repeat physical examination and plain abdominal films are necessary.

Table 16 Lavage Procedure for Treating DIOS

1. The lavage solution is GoLYTELY® or similar isotonic solution. It can be mixed with flavoring such as Kool-Aid.
2. Rate of administration is 500–1000 mL/hour.
3. Often, an antiemetic such as metoclopramide (0.1 mg/kg intravenously up to 10 mg) must be given to prevent vomiting.
4. Volume administered varies from 4–6 L. The treatment is continued until the rectal effluent is almost clear. Abdominal masses should disappear; repeat abdominal films show disappearance of bubbly material from the right lower quadrant.
5. Intravascular volume status should be monitored by noninvasive techniques (e.g., peripheral perfusion, vital signs, urine output).
6. Serum electrolytes may be followed, but electrolyte disturbances have been uncommon.

Gastrografin enema may be helpful to confirm the diagnosis of DIOS and may help with relief of obstruction. Surgery consultation may be required.

Recurrences of DIOS

Recurrences of DIOS are fairly common. Increased fluid intake or bulk or lubricant laxatives have been offerred as prophylactic therapies, but have not been shown unequivocally to be effective. A therapy agent proven effective by careful clinical trial is cisapride, a prokinetic motility drug. Patients with CF treated with a continual course of cisapride had fewer recurrences of DIOS that required intestinal lavage treatment than CF patients given placebo (88). Cisapride treatment did not, however, abolish all recurrences of DIOS. An alternative therapy with anecdotal support is periodic intake of intestinal lavage solution in amounts less than that used in aggressive lavage treatments. Patients ingest lavage solution in amounts similar to that used as preparation for colonoscopy whenever they begin to have crampy abdominal pain or on a regularly defined schedule. No controlled study of this therapy is available.

An Essential Caveat

Not all crampy abdominal pain in CF patients is due to DIOS. If the CF patient's history, examination, radiographic findings, and response to therapy do not conform to the above description, DIOS may not be the correct explanation, and other diagnoses should be considered.

Intussusception

Ileocolic intussusception occurs in CF patients, reportedly at increased frequency and at an older age than in the general population. Idiopathic (non-CF) intussusception generally afflicts children aged 9 months to 2 years. In CF, the patient is usually older (89). The symptoms and signs can mimic the findings in DIOS. Early in the course, intussusception causes severe colicky pain, but without radiological signs of obstruction. Obstructive signs appear after the accumulation of bowel wall edema with ischemia. Gastrografin enema can be diagnostic and may prove therapeutic for the intussusception. Abdominal ultrasound may be useful to identify intussusception, demonstrating the "target sign" at the lead point of intussusception. Reduction is usually accomplished by a diagnostic contrast enema. Occasionally, repeat enemas are necessary. In rare cases, surgery, which may include cecectomy, is required.

Appendicitis

Acute appendicitis can also mimic the presenting signs of the acute form of DIOS. Fever and leukocytosis may be present. In one series, the appendix was often perforated by the time the diagnosis was made, but the perforation had been contained by surrounding structures. The frequent use of broad-spectrum antibiotics in CF patients may prevent severe complications of appendiceal perforation, blunting the clinical presentation. Contrast enema often shows deformity of the cecum with mass effect and not the findings expected in DIOS. Abdominal CT scan readily defines intraabdominal abscess or fluid collection near the cecum (90). In normal individuals, nonfilling of the appendix during contrast enema may indicate the presence of appendicitis. In a retrospective review of contrast enemas in series of CF patients, nonfilling of the appendix did not appear to be a reliable sign for the presence of appendicitis. Histological studies showed that nonfilling may be due to mucous plugging of the appendiceal lumen (91). Possibly, this mucous plugging could produce symptoms, even in the absence of inflammation, and require treatment with appendectomy. Percutaneous drainage of appendiceal abscesses by interventional radiologists and laparoscopic appendectomy permit avoidance of the morbidity of laparotomy.

VII. Colon

A. Colon Fibrosis

Several CF centers recently reported the occurrence of right colon fibrosis and stricture in CF patients who had been treated with very high dose pancreatic enzyme supplements (35, 39). Most of the patients were young children with symptoms and signs of partial distal bowel obstruction: crampy abdominal pain, decreased stool frequency, vomiting, and abdominal distention. Some had bloody diarrhea. Patients were often treated initially for possible DIOS; however, contrast enemas revealed narrowing and lack of distensibility of the cecum or right colon. Partial colon resection has been the usual therapy, but medical therapy with enzyme restriction and nutritional support may be effective (39a). Resected specimens show denudation of the surface epithelium, intermittent disruption of the muscularis mucosae, and inflammation with fibrosis in the submucosa. These pathological changes may represent postischmic repair, but the exact mechanism of injury is not known. The association with intake of high doses of pancreatic enzymes was strong enough, however, to initiate the removal of high-potency pancreatic enzyme supplements from the commercial market. This complication should be considered in patients who are taking very large doses of pancreatic enzymes, and who develop symptoms and signs that resemble DIOS but who do not have inspissated material evident on plain abdominal films or who respond poorly to lavage treatment for DIOS. Prevention of this complication appears possible if enzyme doses are not increased into very high ranges (>6000 units of lipase per kilogram of body weight per meal).

B. *Clostridium difficile* infection

Although CF patients receive multiple and prolonged courses of oral or parenteral antibiotics, the frequency of symptomatic infection with *C. difficile* appears to be low. In one series, 22% of CF patients had cytotoxin producing *C.*

difficile isolated from random stool specimens, but only three of 15 had any abdominal symptoms. No patient had the characteristic clinical picture of *C. difficile* colitis with fever and bloody diarrhea or the more uncommon presentation of chronic watery diarrhea (92). Thus, the finding of *C. difficile* or *C. difficile* toxin in the stools of CF patients is not usually associated with clinical illness. Treatment in asymptomatic patients would not, therefore, be required.

C. Rectal Prolapse

Rectal prolapse is often listed as a presenting feature of CF. Why rectal prolapse occurs in CF is not clear. Rectal prolapse can occur in any individual with frequent diarrhea, whether the cause is infection or malabsorption. With improvement in the diarrhea, the episodes of prolapse disappear. Rectal prolapse in the untreated CF patient usually resolves within a few months of institution of pancreatic enzyme therapy as stools decrease in amount and frequency. Rarely, more invasive measures such as submucosal injections of sclerosant or surgery are necessary to eliminate recurrent prolapse.

If rectal prolapse is occurring in the treated CF patient, then the differential diagnosis for possible causes must be expanded. Potential problems include giardiasis, excessive straining at stool due to a sensation of incomplete evacuation, the presence of a rectal polyp serving as a lead point, and anal intercourse or sexual abuse. Proctoscopy or flexible sigmoidoscopy can identify mucosal inflammation or a polyp. Anal cultures are useful to detect sexually transmitted infection. Stool specimens are used to identify giardia cysts or antigen.

VIII. Cancers

Cancer of any kind is uncommon in CF, but a few studies have suggested that there may be a slightly (but statistically significant) increased incidence of cancers of the GI tract in these patients.

IX. Summary

Because the cellular defect in cystic fibrosis alters fluid and electrolyte secretion in epithelia throughout the hepatobiliary, pancreatic, and gastrointestinal systems, the clinical symptoms and signs of CF can involve any or all of these systems. This chapter reviews the most common problems encountered in CF patients and the usual management of those problems. CF patients may, however, have gastrointestinal, pancreatic, and hepatobiliary problems that also occur in normal individuals. Thus, the differential diagnosis of abdominal complaints in CF patients must include a variety of CF-related and unrelated problems.

References

1. Coletti R, Christie D, Orenstein S. Indications for pediatric esophageal pH monitoring. J Pediatr Gastroenterol Nutr 1995; 21:253–262.
2. Stein H, Barlow A, DeMeester T, Hinder R. Complications of gastroesophageal reflux disease. Ann Surg 1991; 216(1):35–43.
3. Orenstein S, Orenstein D. Gastroesophageal reflux and respiratory disease in children. J Pediatr 1988; 112(6):847–858.
4. Bendig D, Seilheimer D, Wagner M, Ferry G, Harrison G. Complications of gastroesophageal reflux in patients with cystic fibrosis. J Pediatr 1982; 100(4):536–540.
5. Scott R, O'Loughlin E, Gall D. Gastroesophageal reflux in patients with cystic fibrosis. J Pediatr 1985; 106(2):223–227.
6. Feigelson J, Girault F, Pecan Y. Gastro-oesophageal reflux and esophagitis in cystic fibrosis. Acta Paediatr Scand 1987; 76:989–990.
7. Katz P. Pathogenesis and management of gastroesophageal reflux disease. J Clin Gastroenterol 1991; 13(suppl 2):S6–S15.
8. Ferreira C, Lohoues M, Bensoussan A, Yazbeck S, Brochu P, Roy C. Prolonged pH monitoring is of limited usefulness for gastroesophageal reflux. AJDC 1993; 147:662–664.
9. Low D, Mercer C, James E, Hill L. Post nissen syndrome. Surg Gynecol Obstet 1988; 167(1):1–5.
10. Negre J. Post-fundoplication symptoms. Ann Surg 1983; Dec:697–700, 1983.
11. Jolley S, Tunell W, Leonard J, Hoelzer D, Smith E. Gastric emptying in children with gastroesophageal reflux. The relationship to retching symptoms following antireflux surgery. J Pediatr Surg 1987; 22(10):927–930.
12. Amendola M, Spera T. Doxycycline-induced esophagitis. JAMA 1985; 253(7):1009–1011.
13. Haulk A, Sugar A. Candida esophagitis. Adv Intern Med 1991; 36:307–318.
14. Ashenburg C, Rothstein F, Dahms B. Herpes esophagitis in the immunocompetent child. J Pediatr 1986; 108(4):584–587.
15. Lubani M, al-Saleh Q, Teebi A, Moosa A, Kalaoui M. Cystic fibrosis and *Helicobacter pylori* gastritis, megaloblastic anaemia, subnormal mentality and minor anomalies in two siblings: a new syndrome? Eur J Pediatr 1991; 150(4):253–255.
16. Roth S, Bennett R. Nonsteroidal anti-inflammatory drug gastropathy. Arch Intern Med 1987; 147:2093–2100.
17. Bjarnason I, Zanelli G, Smith T, Prouse p, Williams P, Smethurst P, Delacey G, Gumpel M, Levi A. Nonsteroidal antiinflammatory drug-induced intestinal inflammation in humans. Gastroenterolosy 1987; 93:480–489.
18. Hermaszewski R, Hayllar J, Woo P. Gastro-duodenal damage due to non-steroidal anti-inflammatory drugs in children. Br J Rheumatol 1993; 32(1):69–72.
19. Gazarian M, Berkovitch M, Koren G, Silverman E, Laxer R. Experience with misoprostol therapy for NSAID gastropathy in children. Ann Rheumatol Dis 1995; 54(4):277–280.
20. Kendall M, Gibson R, Walt R. Co-administration of misoprostol or ranitidine with indomethacin: effects on pharmacokinetics, abdominal symptoms and bowel habit. Aliment Pharmacol Ther 1992; 6(4):437–446.

21. Konstan M, Byard P, Hoppel C, Davis P. Effect of high-dose ibuprofen in patients with cystic fibrosis. N Engl J Med 1995; 332(13):848–854.

22. Couper R, Corey M, Durie P, Forstner G, Moore D. J Pediatr 1995; 127(3):408–413.

23. Bronstein M, Sokol R, Abman S, Chatfield B, Hammond K, Hambidge K, Stall C, Accurso F. Pancreatic insufficiency, growth, and nutrition in infants identified by newborn screening as having cystic fibrosis. J Pediatr 1992; 120(4 Pt 1):533–540.

24. Couper R, Durie P. Pancreatic function tests. In: Pediatric Gastrointestinal Disease. Vol. 1. Toronto: BC Decker, 1991:1341.

25. Fleisher D, DiGeorge A, Barness L, Cornfeld D. Hypoproteinemia and edema in infants with cystic fibrosis of the pancreas. J Pediatr 1964; 64(3):341–348.

26. Mischler E, Parrell S, Farrell P, Odell G. Comparison of effectiveness of pancreatic enzyme preparations in cystic fibrosis. Am J Dis Child 1982; 136:1060–1063.

27. Dutta S, Hubbard V, Appler M. Critical examination of therapeutic efficacy of a pH-sensitive enteric-coated pancreatic enzyme preparation in treatment of exocrine pancreatic insufficiency secondary to cystic fibrosis. Dig Dis Sci 1988; 33(10):1237–1244.

28. Beverly D, Kelleher J, Macdonald A, Littlewood J, Robinson T, Walters M. Comparison of four pancreatic extracts in cystic fibrosis. Arch Dis Child 1987; 62:564–568.

29. Hendeles L, Dorf A, Stecenko A, Weinberger M. Treatment failure after substitution of generic pancrelipase capsules. JAMA 1990; 263:2459–2461.

30. Layer P, Groger G. Fate of pancreatic enzymes in the human intestinal lumen in health and pancreatic insufficiency. Digestion 1993; 54(2):10.

31. Constantini D, Padoan R, Curcio L, Giunta A. The management of enzymatic therapy in cystic fibrosis patients by an individualized approach. J Pediatr Gastroenterol Nutr 1988; 7(1):536–539.

32. Robinson P, Sly P. High dose pancreatic enzymes in cystic fibrosis. Arch Dis Child 1990; 65:311–312.

33. Carroccio A, Pardo F, Montalto G, et al. Use of famotidine in severe exocrine pancreatic insufficiency with persistent maldigestion on enzymatic replacement therapy. Dig Dis Sci 1992; 37:1441.

34. Zentler-Munro P, Fine D, Batter J, et al. Effect of cimetidine on enzyme inactivation, bile acid precipitation, and lipid solubilization in pancreatic steatorrhea due to cystic fibrosis. Gut 1985; 26:892.

35. Borowitz D, Grand R, Durie P, Consensus Committee. Use of pancreatic enzyme supplements for patients with cystic fibrosis in the context of fibrosing colonopathy. J Pediatr 1995; 127:681–684.

36. Brady M, Rickard K, Yu P, Eigen H. Effectiveness and safety of small vs. large doses of enteric coated pancreatic enzymes in reducing steatorrhea in children with cystic fibrosis: a prospective randomized study. Pediatr Pulmonol 1991; 10:79–85.

37. Beker L, Fink R, Shamsa F, Chaney H, Kluft J, Evans E, Schidlow D. Comparison of weight-based dosages of enteric-coated microtablet enzyme preparations in patients with cystic fibrosis. J Pediatr Gastroenterol Nutr 1994; 19:191–197.

38. Kraisinger M, Hochhaus G, Stecenko A, et al. Clinical pharmacology of pancreatic enzymes in patients with cystic fibrosis and in vitro performance of microencapsulated formulations. J Clin Pharmacol 1994; 34:158.

39. Smyth R, van Velzen D, Smyth A, Lloyd D, Heaf D. Strictures of ascending colon in cystic fibrosis and high-strength pancreatic enzymes. Lancet 1994; 343:85–86.
39a. Schwarzenberg SJ, Wielinski CL, Shamich I, Carpenter BL, Jessuwn J, Weisdorf SA, Warwick WJ, Sharp HJ. Cystic fibrosis associated colitis and fibrosing colonopathy. J Pediat 1995; 127(4):565–570.
40. Robb T, Lewindon P, Davidson G, et al. The natural history of entericcoated microsphere (pancrelipase) usage in a CF clinic. Pediatr Pulmonol Suppl 1992; 8:313.
41. Atlas A, Orenstein S, Orenstein D. Pancreatitis in young children with cystic fibrosis. J Pediatr 1992; 120(5):756–759.
42. Shwachman H, Lebenthal E, Khaw K. Recurrent acute pancreatitis in patients with cystic fibrosis with normal pancreatic enzymes. Pediatrics 1975; 55(1):86–95.
43. Tetrault G. Lipase activity in serum measured with ektachem is often increased in nonpancreatic disorders. Clin Chem 1991; 37(3):447–451.
44. Lloyd-Still J. Textbook of cystic fibrosis. Boston: John Wright, PSG, 1983.
45. Roy C, Weber A, Morin C, Lepage G, Brisson G, Yousef I, Lasalle R. Hepatobiliary disease in cystic fibrosis: a survey of current issues and concepts. J Pediatr Gastroenterol Nutr 1982; 1:469–478.
46. Hultcrantz R, Mengarelli S, Strandvik B. Morphological findings in the liver of children with cystic fibrosis: a light and electron microscopical study. Hepatology 1986; 6(5):881–889.
47. Maurage C, Lenaerts C, Weber A, Brochu P, Yousef I, Roy C. Meconium ileus and its equivalent as a risk factor for the development of cirrhosis: an autopsy study in cystic fibrosis. J Pediatr Gastroenterol Nutr 1989; 9:17–20.
48. Valman H, France N, Wallis P. Prolonged neonatal jaundice in cystic fibrosis. Arch Dis Child 1971; 46:805–809.
49. Psacharopoulos H, Howard E, Portmann B, Mowat A, Williams R. Hepatic complications of cystic fibrosis. Lancet 1981; July:78–80.
50. Barbe T, Losay J, Grimon G, Devictor D, Sardet A, Gauthier F, Houssin D, Bernard O. Pulmonary arteriovenous shunting in children with liver disease. J Pediatr 1995; 126(4):571–579.
51. Stern R, Stevens D, Boat T, Doershuk C, Izant R, Matthews L. Symptomatic hepatic disease in cystic fibrosis: incidence, course, and outcome of portal systemic shunting. Gastroenterology 1976; 70(5):645–649.
52. Tyson K, Schuster S, Shwachman H. Portal hypertension in cystic fibrosis. J Pediatr Surg 1968; 3(2):271–277.
53. Schuster S, Shwachman H, Toyama W, Rubino A, Taik-Khaw K. The management of portal hypertension in cystic fibrosis. J Pediatr Surg 1977; 12(2):201–206.
54. Quintero E, Arroyo V, Bory F, Viver J, Gines P, Rimola A, Planas R, Cabrera J, Rodes J. Paracentesis versus diuretics in the treatment of cirrhotics with tense ascities. Lancet, 1985; March:611–612.
55. Doershuk C, Stern R. Spontaneous bacterial peritonitis in cystic fibrosis. Gut 1994; 35(5):709–711.
56. Runyon B. Spontaneous bacterial peritonitis: an explosion of information. Hepatology 1988; 8(1):171–175.
57. Fox V, Carr-Locke D, Connors P, Leichtner A. Endoscopic ligation of esophageal varies in children. J Pediatr Gastroenterol Nutr 1995; 20(2):202–208.

58. Paquet K, Lazar A. Current therapeutic strategy in bleeding esophageal varices in babies and children and long-term results of endoscopic paravariceal sclerotherapy over twenty years. Eur J Pediatr Surg 1994; 4(3)165–172.

59. Goenka A, Dasilva M, Cleghorn G, Patrick M, Shepherd R. Therapeutic upper gastrointestinal endoscopy in children: an audit of 443 procedures and literature review. J Gastroenterol Hepatol 1993; 8(1):44–51.

60. Hill I, Bowie M. Endoscopic sclerotherapy for control of bleeding varies in children. Am J Gastroenterol 1991; 86(4):472–476.

61. Kochhar R, Goenka M, Mehta S. Esophageal strictures following endoscopic variceal sclerotherapy. Antecedents, clinical profile, and management. Dig Dis Sci 1992; 37(3):347–352.

62. Zeller F, Cannan C, Prakash U. Thoracic manifestations after esophageal variceal sclerotherapy. Mayo Clin Proc 1991; 66(7):727–732.

63. Rolando N, Gimson A, Philpott-Howard J, Sahathevan M, Casewell M, Fagan E, Westaby D, Williams R. Infectious sequelae after endoscopic sclerotherapy of oesophageal varices: role of antibiotic prophylaxis. J Hepatol 1993; 18(3):290–294.

64. Laine L, Cook D. Endoscopic ligation compared with sclerotherapy for treatment of esophageal variceal bleeding. Ann Intern Med 1995; 123(4):280–287.

65. Glass M, Berezin S, Boyle J. Bacterial peritonitis and sepsis presenting as acute gastrointestinal bleeding in patients with portal hypertension. Pediatr Emerg Care 1993; 9(1):19–22.

66. Kerns S, Hawkins I. Transjugular intrahepatic portosystemic shunt in a child with cystic fibrosis. AJR Am J Roentgen 1992; 159(6):1277–1278.

67. Noble-Jamieson G, Valente J, Barnes N, Friend P, Jamieson N, Rasmussen A, Calne R. Liver transplantation for hepatic cirrhosis in cystic fibrosis. Arch Dis Child 1994; 71(4)349–352.

68. Stern R. Rothstein F, Doershuk C. Treatment and prognosis of symptomatic gallbladder disease in patients with cystic fibrosis. J Pediatr Gastroenterol Nutr 1986; 5(1):35–40.

69. Angelico M, Gandin C, Canuzzi P, Bertasi S, Cantafora A, De Santis A, Quattrucci S, Antonelli M. Gallstones in cystic fibrosis: a critical reappraisal. Hepatology 1991; 14(5):768–775.

70. Quillin S, Siegel M, Rothbaum R. Hepatobiliary sonography in cystic fibrosis. Pediatr Radiol 1993; 23:1–3.

71. Lambert J, Cole M, Crosier D, Connon J. Intrapancreatic common bile duct compression causing jaundice in an adult with cystic fibrosis. Gastroenterology 1981; 80(1):169–172.

72. Gaskin K, Waters D, Howman-Giles R, DeSilva M, Earl J, Martin H, Kan A, Brown J, Dorney S. Liver disease and common-bile-duct stenosis in cystic fibrosis. N Engl J Med 1988; 318(6):340–346.

73. O'Brien S, Keogan M, Casey M, Duffy G, McErlean D, Fitzgerald M, Hegarty J. Biliary complications of cystic fibrosis. Gut 1992; 33(3):387–391.

74. Rescorla F, Grosfeld J, West K, Vane D. Changing patterns of treatment and survival in neonates with meconium ileus. Arch Surg 1989; 124(7):837–840.

75. Caniano D, Beaver B. Meconium ileus: a fifteen-year experience with forty-two neonates. Surgery 1987; 102(4):699–703.

76. Wagget J, Bishop H, Koop C. Experience with gastrografin enema in the treatment of meconium ileus. J Pediatr Surg 1970; 5(6):649–654.

77. Olsen M, Luck S, Lloyd-Still J, Raffensperger J. The spectrum of meconium disease in infancy. J Pediatr Surg 1982; 17(5):479–481.
78. Gross K, Desanto A, Grosfeld J, West K, Eigen H. Intra-abdominal complications of cystic fibrosis. J Pediatr Surg 1985; 20(4):431–435.
79. Donnison A, Shwachman H, Gross R. A review of 164 children with meconium ileus seen at the Children's Hospital Medical Center, Boston. Pediatrics 1966; 37(5):833–850.
80. Elian E, Shwachman H, Hendren W. Intestinal obstruction of the newborn infant. N Engl J Med 1961; 264(1):13–16.
81. Schwarz K, Ternberg J, Bell M, Keating J. Sodium needs of infants and children with ileostomy. J Pediatr 1983; 102(4):509–513.
82. Durie P, Newth C, Forstner G, Gall D. Malabsorption of medium-chain triglycerides in infants with cystic fibrosis: correction with pancreatic enzyme supplements. J Pediatr 1980; 96(5):862–864.
83. Lillibridge C, Docter J, Eidelman S. Oral administration of N-acetyl cysteine in the prophylaxis of "meconium ileus equivalent." J Pediatr 1967; 71(6):887–889.
84. Strong T, Boehn K, Collins F. Localization of cystic fibrosis transmembrane conductance regulator mRNA in the human gastrointestinal tract by in situ hybridization. J Clin Invest 1994; 93:347–354.
85. Dalzell A, Heaf D. Oro-caecal transit time and intra-luminal pH in cystic fibrosis patients with distal intestinal obstruction syndrome. Acta Univ Carol Med 1990; 36(1–4):159–160.
86. Matseshe J, Go V, DiMagno E. Meconium ileus equivalent complicating cystic fibrosis in postneonatal children and young adults. Gastroenterology 1977; 72(4):732–736.
87. Koletzko S, Stringer D, Cleghorn G, Durie P. Lavage treatment of distal intestinal obstruction syndrome in children with cystic fibrosis.
88. Koletzko S, Corey M, Ellis L, Spino M, Stringer D, Durie P. Effects of cisapride in patients with cystic fibrosis and distal intestinal obstruction syndrome. J Pediatr 1990; 117(5):815–822.
89. Holmes M, Murphy V, Taylor M, Denham B. Intussusception in cystic fibrosis. Arch Dis Child 1991; 66(6):726–727.
90. McCarthy V, Mischler E, Hubbard V, Chernick M, di Sant'Agnese P. Appendiceal abscess in cystic fibrosis. A diagnostic challenge. Gastroenterology 1984; 86(3):564–568.
91. Fletcher B, Abramowsky C. Contrast enemas in cystic fibrosis: implications of appendiceal nonfilling. AJR Am J Roentgen 1981; 137(2):323–326.
92. Welkon C, Long S, Thompson M, Gilligan P. *Clostridium difficile* in patients with cystic fibrosis. AJDC 1985; 139:805–808.

6

Nutrition and Electrolytes

DRUCY BOROWITZ

State University of New York at Buffalo
and The Children's Hospital of Buffalo
Buffalo, New York

CHRISTINE COBURN-MILLER

Cystic Fibrosis Center
The Children's Hospital of Buffalo
Buffalo, New York

I. Introduction

The nutrition of patients with cystic fibrosis (CF) has a direct impact on the length of their hospital stay. In general, patients who are well nourished have a shorter and less complicated stay than those who are malnourished. The more long-standing the malnutrition is, the harder it is to reverse and the more difficult it is for the patient to cope with the stress of a pulmonary exacerbation or other intercurrent problem. Management of inpatients depends largely on two factors: the severity of the energy deficit and the severity of the pulmonary disease.

II. Failure to Thrive

Malnutrition can be graded by determining the patient's percent ideal body weight for height (%IBW/ht). The patient's ideal weight for height is the weight on the same centile for the patient's height, age, and gender. For example, if a 1-year-old girl's height is at the 25 percentile, the ideal weight for height would be that found at the 25 percentile for a 1-year-old girl. For infants, the same

175

Example for a 1-year-old girl:
Actual height = 72 cm (25th percentile)
Actual weight = 7.2 kg (<5th percentile)
Ideal body weight = 8.8 kg (25th percentile)
Percent ideal body weight for height = 82% = (7.2/8.8 × 100)

Figure 1 Visual calculation of percent ideal body weight for height

approach can be used, substituting heel-to-crown length for height. The patient's actual weight is then divided by the ideal weight for height, and that number is multiplied by 100 (Fig. 1). Underweight is defined as patients who are 85%–89% IBW/ht. Those who are less than 85% IBW/ht are considered malnourished (1).

A. Previously Undiagnosed Infants and Toddlers Who Are Underweight (85%–89%IBW/ht)

Approximately 35% of patients newly diagnosed with CF present with failure to thrive according to the 1992 CF Registry statistics (2). Conversely, CF accounts for an important subset of infants with failure to thrive.

Insufficient pancreatic enzymes cause failure to thrive as a result of maldigestion and malabsorption. In many instances, weight gain can be achieved by providing pancreatic enzyme supplements along with a normal diet (see Chapter 4). Children who are admitted to the hospital because of failure to thrive and who subsequently are given the diagnosis of CF should be observed in the hospital for as many days as necessary to document control of steatorrhea and stabilization of weight. By the time of the patient's discharge, all caregivers should be comfortable giving pancreatic enzymes.

Human Milk and Formulas for Infants with CF

Mothers who strongly favor breast feeding should be encouraged to do so (3). Hyponatremic metabolic alkalosis can develop in both human milk–fed and formula-fed babies (4). Both groups should receive salt supplementation during hot weather (starting dose: 2–4 mmol Na/kg/day; this may be given as NaCl solution, which comes as 2.5 mmol/mL, or as table salt, which contains 87 mmol Na per teaspoon). Hypoproteinemia has been reported in the older literature in infants fed human milk, soy formula, and cow's milk–based formula. It is difficult to interpret these older reports because many babies are diagnosed at an earlier age and currently available enzyme preparations are more efficacious. Although protein intake is less in human milk–fed infants, growth, blood urea nitrogen, and albumin levels were well maintained in one small group of infants (5).

Predigested formulas containing medium chain triglycerides (MCT) are unnecessary, and routine cow's milk protein formulas should be used if a baby is not being breast-fed (6). If formulas containing MCT are used, pancreatic enzymes should be given (7). Soy-based formulas have been associated with poor growth in infants with untreated CF (8). Cow's milk–based formula has been shown to support good growth in infants with CF and is the preferred formula for non–breast-fed infants (3). Steatorrhea does not usually cause the transient lactose intolerance seen with infantile viral gastroenteritis; lactose-free formulas are rarely needed. Pancreatic enzymes (2000–4000 units of lipase per 4 ounces of formula or breast milk feeding) should be given before each feeding in patients who are pancreatic insufficient.

Foods for Toddlers

Toddlers should be allowed to eat foods appropriate for age. If cow's milk is used, it should be whole milk (4% fat). Pancreatic enzymes must be given before all fat- or protein-containing foods (including milk). Planning three meals and two or three snacks a day enables the child and caregiver to get used to the rule of enzymes before all foods. Primary care nursing should be encouraged so that mealtime routines are consistent. On occasion, feeding-related behavioral difficulties may require specialty consultation, and hospitalization may be prolonged. Follow-up with a CF center nutritionist after discharge from the hospital is important, because toddlers may have behavioral feeding problems that can only be resolved if there is persistent reinforcement of the prescribed intervention.

Vitamins

Vitamin supplementation should be started. A standard dose of an age-appropriate multivitamin preparation should be given each day (2). The content of children's vitamins is tightly regulated by the Food and Drug Administration, so generic formulations can be used (9). Eventually, pancreatic insufficient patients need fat-soluble vitamin (A, D, E, and K) supplementation beyond what is available in most multivitamins. Twenty-one percent of infants with CF diagnosed in the first 1 to 2 months of life by newborn screening were found to be vitamin A deficient and 35% had vitamin D deficiency; these values normalized after pancreatic enzyme supplements and multivitamins were begun (10). Vitamin E deficiency, found in 35% of these infants, was corrected in almost all infants after treatment with 5–10 IU/kg/day of a water miscible form of vitamin E. No infant was found to have vitamin K deficiency. A consensus statement sponsored by the CF Foundation recommends routine supplementation with water miscible vitamin E (Table 1) (2). An alternative strategy is to begin multi-

Table 1 Vitamin Supplementation in CF

Multiple vitamin supplementation	Vitamin E supplementation[a]	Vitamin K supplementation—if receiving intravenous antibiotics or if cholestatic liver disease is present:
Infants to 2 years: 1 mL/day Polyvisol or similar liquid multivitamin 2–8 years: standard pediatric multivitamin providing 400 IU vitamin D, 5000 IU vitamin A >8 years: standard adult multivitamin 1–2 tablets/day	0–6 months: 25 IU/day 6–12 months: 50 IU/day 1–4 years: 100 IU/day 4–10 years: 100–200 IU/day >10 years: 200–400 IU/day	0–12 months: 2–5 mg twice weekly >1 year: 5.0 mg twice weekly

[a]Dosages are for water-miscible vitamin E. Larger doses of fat-soluble vitamin E have been shown to be equivalent in children and adults (91). Excessive doses of vitamin E (>1000 IU/day) may exacerbate vitamin K deficiency coagulopathy.
Source: Ref. 1.

vitamins and check serum vitamin E levels 3 to 6 months after the start of therapy. Vitamin E supplements are then given to the patients who remain vitamin E deficient.

B. Previously Undiagnosed Infants with Mild Malnutrition (80%–85% IBW/ht)

Some infants with failure to thrive have mild malnutrition (80%–84% IBW/ht). These infants also benefit from pancreatic enzyme and vitamin supplementation, but need additional calories beyond the usual infant's intake. Often, hospitalization must be prolonged as a result of the patient's energy deficit.

When mild malnutrition is present (80%–84% IBW/ht) in an infant with a good appetite, formulas with increased calorie content may be used along with vitamin supplementation. Table 2 indicates methods for concentrating the calories in standard infant formula. Infants who are breast-fed may need supplemental feedings with high-calorie formula if observation of nursing technique does not reveal problems. If the mother's milk supply is inadequate, a nursing supplement device such as a LactAid (Fig. 2) can help ensure that the baby is getting adequate calories while allowing the baby to suckle. This helps the mother's milk volume to increase. The intervention for breast-fed infants depends on the degree of malnutrition present as well as a variety of psychosocial factors. The caloric content of breast milk cannot be altered by changing the

Table 2 Increasing Calories in Formula

To make 24 calorie/ounce formula:
    Mix one 13-oz can of concentrated formula with 9 ounces of water
    OR
    Mix 3 scoops[a] of powdered formula with 5 ounces of water
To make 27 calorie/ounce formula:
    Mix one 13-ounce can of concentrated formula with 9 ounces of water and add 3
        tablespoons of Polycose powder
    OR
    Mix 3 scoops[a] of powdered formula with 5 ounces of water[b] and add 2 teaspoons of
        Polycose powder

[a]The scoop included in a can of powdered formula is 8.7 g or 1 tablespoon.
[b]Add 1 ounce of water to the bottle, then the powder, fill to the 5-ounce line, then add Polycose.

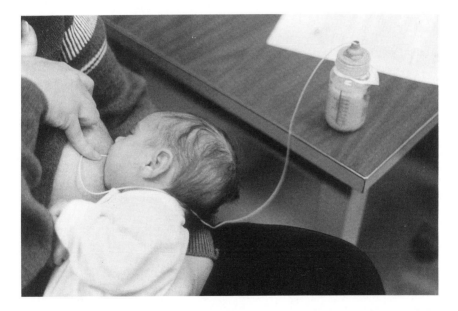

Figure 2 Use of a breast-feeding supplement device. To use an improvised lactation aid, cut the tab off one number 5 French, 36-inch feeding tube, and cut the top off a standard nipple. Place the cut end of tube through the nipple into the top of a 4-ounce bottle (glass is less likely to tip over). Position the bottle at the level of the baby's head or slightly above. Allow the baby to latch onto the mother's breast. Slip the other end of the feeding tube through the corner of the baby's mouth (as straight as possible), over the top of the tongue, but not extending beyond the mother's nipple. A manufactured lactation aid (e.g., LactAid) may be easier to use if long-term supplementation is needed.

Table 3 High Calorie Foods

Amount	Food	Added Calories	Suggested Uses
1 Teaspoon	Butter, margarine	34	Vegetables, breads, potatoes, hot cereal, soup
1 Tablespoon	Sour cream	26	Vegetables, dips, salads
1 Tablespoon	Mayonnaise	100	Salads, dips, deviled eggs, sandwiches, vegetables
1 Tablespoon	Half & half	20	Hot cereal, hot chocolate, shakes, pudding
1 Tablespoon	Evaporated whole milk	21	Hot cereal, hot chocolate, water in cooking
1 Tablespoon	Powdered milk	23	Whole milk, shakes, mashed potatoes, scrambled eggs, meatloaf
1	Hard-cooked egg	80	Casseroles, meatloaf, sandwiches
1 Tablespoon	Peanut butter	100	Vegetables, crackers, casseroles, meats, sandwiches, pasta, dips, soups, pizza
1 Teaspoon	Cream cheese	50	Toast, crackers, raw vegetables, eggs, gelatin molds
1 Tablespoon	Chopped nuts (not recommended for children younger than 4 years old)	49	Puddings, ice cream, salads, casseroles, cereal, fruit

mother's diet. If the child is eating solid foods, glucose polymer powder (Polycose; 23 calories/tablespoon) can be added to each feeding, starting at 1 tablespoon mixed with food at each meal and increasing to 2 tablespoons per meal.

Toddlers with mild malnutrition and a good appetite can be given a high-calorie formula in place of milk. Proprietary formulas such as Pediasure or Kindercal contain 30 calories per ounce, whereas whole milk (4% fat) has 20 calories per ounce. Calories should be added to each meal as high-fat foods (Table 3). Sugar can also be added, but 1 g of fat has 9 kcal, compared with 4 kcal/g of sugar or protein, so fat is the most calorie-rich food type.

Infants or toddlers who are 80%–84% IBW/ht should remain in the hospital until consistent weight gain is demonstrated. Psychosocial, educational, and financial factors that may interfere with adherence to the prescribed nutrition regimen should be addressed before discharge of the patient. The patient's nutrition status should be checked approximately 1 week after discharge. If traveling distance makes this difficult, the child should be weighed by the local physician within 1 to 2 days of discharge, so that a reliable comparison can be made 1 week later.

If addition of calories does not result in weight gain after 5 to 7 days of inpatient care, other factors should be considered (see discussion on persistent malnutrition). In some instances, purely nutritional factors account for inadequate weight gain. For example, the child may have a poor appetite or be a slow eater without a medical basis for this symptom. However, before beginning aggressive nutritional intervention (e.g., nocturnal enteral feedings), other possible causes for the inadequate weight gain should be considered. (Some of these possible causes include pulmonary disease, gastroesophageal reflux, and ongoing malabsorption.)

C. Moderate to Severe Malnutrition (<80% IBW/ht) in the Newly Diagnosed Infant or Persistent Malnutrition in Infants and Toddlers

Malnutrition may be moderate to severe (<80% IBW/ht) in newly diagnosed infants or may be persistent in those who have already been diagnosed. Other (non-CF) factors may also contribute to the child's failure to thrive. Thus, malnutrition can either prolong a hospitalization or by itself justify hospitalization in the patient with CF.

Many interdependent contributors can cause growth failure in a child with CF (11). The approach to the child with persistent malnutrition should be similar to that to any child who fails to thrive, taking into account certain factors that occur more frequently in children with CF (12). As with most children who fail to thrive, the history and physical examination usually point to the diagnosis.

Pulmonary Disease

The history should focus especially on pulmonary and gastrointestinal signs and symptoms. Weight loss is one of the signs seen during pulmonary exacerbations of CF. In older children and adults, worsening pulmonary disease is associated with increased oxygen consumption and energy expenditure at rest (13,14). Although it may be an oversimplification to say that "if you take care of the lungs, the nutrition will take care of itself," there is an important nugget of truth in this old saying among CF specialists. Use of intravenous antibiotics, chest physiotherapy, and bronchodilators or antiinflammatory medications may contribute to a more positive energy balance by decreasing the energy cost of breathing and coughing or the resting metabolic rate. If bronchodilators do not help the pulmonary situation, however, they should not be used, because there is some evidence that these drugs may increase energy expenditure in patients with CF (15).

Gastroesophageal Reflux

Cough can be a symptom of gastroesophageal reflux (GER), a problem that is common in malnourished children and in children with CF (16). It should be considered even in the absence of "spitting up," and especially if cough and poor weight gain persist despite nutritional and pulmonary treatments. A variety of diagnostic tests may be used, including upper gastrointestinal (UGI) series, scintigraphy, prolonged pH monitoring, and esophageal biopsy. Standard nutritional therapy for GER in infants involves thickening of formula with rice cereal, starting at 1 teaspoon of dry cereal per ounce of formula and increasing to 1 tablespoon per ounce. Although this intervention has the advantage of adding calories to formula (1 teaspoon of rice cereal = 5 calories), it may be detrimental to those infants in whom cough (as opposed to regurgitation) is a primary symptom (17). Although high-fat diets are associated with delayed gastric emptying (which can contribute to GER), the need for extra calories in infants with CF, failure to thrive, and GER outweighs this consideration, and a low-fat diet should not be prescribed. Prokinetic agents, such as metoclopramide or cisapride, can be useful in infants with CF who need to be on high-fat diets. Histamine blockers such as ranitidine are indicated when esophagitis is present (18). Treatment of GER in malnourished patients with CF is associated with weight gain (19).

Ongoing Malabsorption

The physician should inquire about flatulence, abdominal pain, and frequent loose stools. Patients with malabsorption often have protuberant, tympanitic abdomens with hyperactive bowel sounds. A 3-day fecal fat collection can help quantify the degree of steatorrhea. Patients with CF continue to have abnormally high amounts of fecal fat even when they are receiving pancreatic enzyme supplements, are asymptomatic, and appear to be growing well (20). Symptomatic steatorrhea may be the result of inadequate pancreatic enzyme supplementation; however, there are other possible explanations. Pancreatic lipase is irreversibly inactivated in an acid environment. For this reason, most pancreatic enzyme preparations come as capsules that contain enteric coated microtablets or microspheres. (These should not be crushed or the lipase will be released in the stomach and inactivated.) Because the patient with CF and pancreatic insufficiency does not produce the high-volume, bicarbonate-rich pancreatic secretion that neutralizes gastric acid, the duodenum and jejunum remain acidic. This can cause a delay in the dissolution of enteric coating until the microtablets or microspheres containing enzymes are far along in the small bowel, having passed a significant portion of the absorptive surface. Drugs that reduce gastric acidity (e.g., histamine blockers, antacids, protein pump inibitors) may help resolve this problem (21,22).

Overt liver disease is rare in infants and toddlers, but the decreased bile salt pool seen in patients with CF may lead to inadequate formation of micelles within the upper small intestine. Furthermore, bile salts can precipitate if the duodenum is acidic. These factors can contribute to steatorrhea despite adequate amounts of lipase.

On occasion, mucosal factors can contribute to malabsorption. Lactose malabsorption may occur in infants and children with CF (23). There have been case reports of severe giardiasis in individuals with CF, and one prevalence study found that older patients with CF harbored giardia significantly more than control subjects (24). Toxigenic *Clostridium difficile* have been recovered more frequently from the stools of patients with CF than controls, although most patients in this study were asymptomatic (25). Patients with poor growth who have positive *C. difficile* toxin titers or cultures should receive treatment because the small intestine, as well as the colon, can be inflamed, and this may contribute to poor growth. Crohn's disease (26) and celiac disease (27,28) have been reported in children with CF. Finally, there have been recent reports of colonic strictures associated with use of high doses of pancreatic lipase (29,30). Bacterial overgrowth of the small intestine can lead to severe nutritional problems and should be considered as well.

Poor Appetite

Infants and toddlers with CF may be poor eaters. It is essential to be sure that the patient does not have hyponatremic metabolic alkalosis. Sinusitis, nasal polyps, or both can cause poor appetite in children without CF by diminishing the ability to smell and taste, and by bloating caused by the constant swallowing of mucus. Almost all children with CF have sinuses filled with mucus: the clinician must decide whether sinusitis is contributing to failure to thrive. Constipation (a process that begins in the rectosigmoid and extends proximally) or the distal intestinal obstruction syndrome (a process that begins in the ileocecal area and extends distally) may contribute to a poor appetite. Neither should be treated by decreasing the pancreatic enzyme dose. A variety of behavioral issues can lead to poor intake and a thorough behavioral evaluation should be considered, especially in a toddler with willful food refusal.

Other Factors

Cystic fibrosis does not protect a child from other diseases that can contribute to malnutrition, and the concurrent diagnoses suggested above are not intended to be all inclusive.

Nutrition Intervention

Aggressive nutrition intervention should not be delayed until the diagnostic evaluation is completed. Although specific medical diagnoses may need

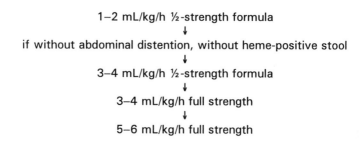

Figure 3 Tube feeding for infants

specific medical interventions, energy deficit is the final common denominator
and must be treated with calorie supplements. Nocturnal enteral feedings should
be started. Infants with moderate malnutrition are good candidates for
nasogastric (NG) feedings because nutritional repletion may be accomplished
within a relatively short time (weeks to a few months). A soft Silastic feeding
tube can be left in place during the day as the infant takes ad lib feedings and
then can be used at night for supplemental calories. Semielemental formulas
appropriate for infants, concentrated to 24–27 calories per ounce, can be used
for tube feedings (Fig. 3). Pancreatic enzymes can be given orally starting at
2000–4000 lipase units per 120 mL of full-strength formula. Infants with severe
malnutrition and toddlers with moderate to severe malnutrition may need
permanently implanted enteral access devices. Gastrostomies and jejunostomies
are discussed in subsequent paragraphs. Parenteral nutrition many be indicated
for the acute treatment of severe respiratory involvement.

A bulging anterior fontanel and rapid head growth may develop in infants
with CF following initiation of treatment (31,32). This phenomenon is probably
related to rapid brain growth as a result of the patient's improved nutrition. The
symptom may persist up to several months and does not require intervention.

D. Infants with the Syndrome of Anemia, Hypoproteinemia, and Edema

Some infants with previously unrecognized CF have the symptom complex of
edema, hypoproteinemia, and anemia (7). One review of 48 cases revealed that
27% of these infants had been fed cow's milk–based formula, 27% had been fed
breast milk, and 46% had been fed soy formula (33). The edema and hypoproteinemia are thought to be due to inadequate protein intake and absorption,
which can be corrected with pancreatic enzyme supplements (8). It is unclear
why some infants have this dramatic presentation while others do not. This
symptom complex is associated with high morbidity and mortality rates. In one

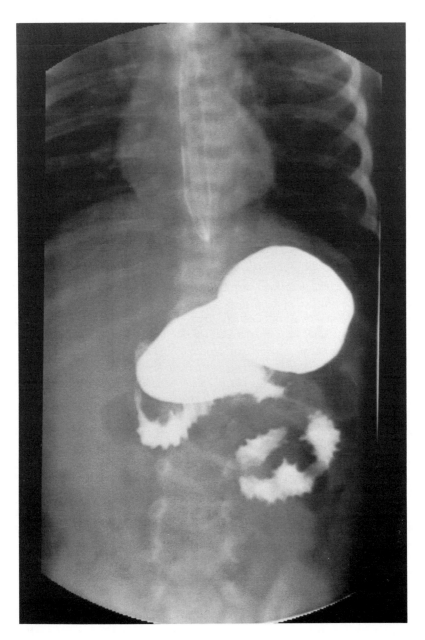

Figure 4 Bowel wall edema in an infant with hypoproteinemia and anemia. Thumbprinting is seen in the wall of the jejunum, which is indicative of mucosal edema.

recent study, five of nine affected infants required mechanical ventilation for respiratory failure, and three died (34). The average length of hospital stay for the survivors was 72 days (range 21–150).

These patients require aggressive treatment. Pulmonary symptoms should be treated with bronchial hygiene, antibiotics, bronchodilators, antiinflammatory medication, or a combination of these as indicated (see Chapter 4). Anemia may need to be treated with transfusions of packed red cells if it is severe or if the infant is hypoxemic. On occasion, albumin transfusions are needed to treat severe edema.

Decisions concerning nutritional intervention depend on the severity of the infant's medical status. Infants with severe respiratory distress may need total parenteral nutrition (TPN) because they are unable to suck and breathe adequately. Even nasogastric feeds may be difficult for them to tolerate because gastric distention may compromise respiration. Standard amounts of protein should be used in the TPN solution. Liver function tests should be obtained and followed routinely. Guidelines for use of TPN are given in Table 4.

Patients with less severe respiratory distress may be fed with continuous nasogastric feedings of elemental or semielemental formulas. In all likelihood, these infants have bowel wall edema and need a slow steady approach to enteral feeding (Fig. 4). Stool should be tested for the presence of blood before initiating tube feedings because many hypoproteinemic infants with CF have evidence of GI blood loss (7), although no systematic examination of the intestinal mucosal status of these patients has been published. Formulas should be given as half-strength and increased to three-fourths and then full strength as tolerated over the course of a few days (see Fig. 3). Hyperosmolar elemental formulas should not be given. Volume can be increased once the child is on full-strength formula. Pancreatic enzymes need to be given if the infant is receiving semielemental formula containing fat, even if the majority of the fat is medium chain triglycerides (7). Patients can be given enzymes orally starting at 2000–4000 lipase units per 120 mL full-strength formula.

Patients with less severe respiratory symptoms and mild malnutrition may be fed orally with high-calorie formula preceded by pancreatic enzyme supplements.

III. Meconium Ileus

Approximately 16% of infants with CF are born with meconium ileus (1). Neonates have a distended abdomen, bilious emesis, and failure to pass stool during the first 24 hours. The classic radiological picture by contrast enema is that of dilated small bowel loops and an unused, airless microcolon, with abrupt termination of the contrast stream in the right lower quadrant. Meconium ileus may be simple, or it may be complicated by intestinal volvulus, atresia, necrosis,

Table 4 Parenteral Nutrition Guidelines

Age	Fluid σ(/kg)	Calories (Cal/kg)	Protein (g/kg)	Initiation of therapy Dextrose (%)	Initiation of therapy Protein (g/kg)	Initiation of therapy Fat (g/kg)	Advance by - daily Dextrose (%)	Advance by - daily Protein (g/kg)	Advance by - daily Fat (g/kg)	Maximum daily amount Dextrose (%)	Maximum daily amount Protein (g/kg)	Maximum daily amount Fat (g/kg)
Preemle	80–150	110–130	2.5–3.0	5–10	0.5	0.5–1	1–2.5	0.5	0.5	35/g/kg	3–3.5	3
0–5 mo	100–150	110–120	2–2.5	10	1.0	0.5–1	2.5	1	0.5	24/mg/kg/min	3.0	4
6–12 mo	100–130	100–110	2	10	1.0	0.5–1	2.5	1	0.5–1	24/mg/kg/min	3.0	4
1–3 yr	100–120	90–100	1.5–2	10–15	50% of goal	1	5	Goal/day/2	1	24/mg/kg/min		
3–6 yr	100	80–90	1.5	10–15	50% of goal	1	5	Goal/day/2	1	24/mg/kg/min	20%	50%
6–9 yr	85	70–80	1–1.5	10–15	50% of goal	1	5	Goal/day/2	1	24/mg/kg/min	of	of
9–12/yr	75	60–70	1–1.5	10–15	50% of goal	1	5	Goal/day/2	1	24/mg/kg/min	total	total
12–15/yr	65	50–60	1.0	10–15	50% of goal	1	5	Goal/day/2	1	24/mg/kg/min	Calories	Calories
15–16/yr	50	10–50	0.5	10–15	50% of goal	1	5	Goal/day/2	1	24/mg/kg/min		
Adult	60	35	0.5	10–15	50% of goal	1	5	Goal/day/2	1	24/mg/kg/min		

Daily Mineral Requirements[a]

Age	Ha (mEq)	Cl (mEq)	K (mEq)	Phosphate (mH)	Calcium gluconate (mg)	Hg (mEq)
Neonates	3–5/kg	3–7/kg	2–4/kg	1.5–2/kg	400–950/kg	0.25–0.5/kg
Children	2–5/kg	2–4/kg	2–3/kg	1–2	100–500/kg	0.25–0.5/kg
Maximum	60–100	60–100	80–120	30–45	2000–3000	6–8

Source	kcal/g
Dextrose	3.4
Protein	4
Fat	9
	(101–1.1 kcal/mL)[b]
	(201–2 kcal/mL)[b]

$$\text{Flow rate of cycled TPN} = \frac{\text{vol TPH (ml)}}{(\text{total infusion time (hr)}) - 1/(0.375)} = \text{ml/hr}$$

[a] Miscellaneous: Trace Elements, 0.1/ml/kg, Max. 3/ml; HVI-pediatric, 2.0/ml/kg, Max. 5/ml; Calcium gluconate, 200/mg − 1 mEq. Ca; Potassium phosphate, 1/mH − 1.5/mEq; Sodium phosphate, 1/mH − 1.3/mEq; Maximum dextrose concentration; peripheral line, 12.5%; central line, 35%.

[b] Per manufacturer.

Source: Dickensen CJ, Reed MD, et al, Pediatr Res 1988; 23:390

perforation, meconium peritonitis, or meconium cyst. Simple meconium ileus may be treated with Gastrografin enemas. However, many infants (25%–50% of those with uncomplicated meconium ileus and most of those with complicated meconium ileus; see Chapters 5 and 9) require surgical intervention. The nutritional management of these infants varies with the complexity of the individual case.

There has been a remarkable increase in survival of patients with meconium ileus. In the 1960s, the long-term survival was approximately 20% (35). As a result of better perioperative management and the use of total parenteral nutrition, short-term infant survival has increased dramatically, to 90%–95% (36,37). The long-term survival rate has also improved. Although pulmonary function at age 8 and 13 years was the same in one study of CF patients with and without meconium ileus, weights and heights were lower in those with meconium ileus (38). This difference in long-term nutritional outcome may be a result of the early neonatal nutritional insult, or of some unidentified propensity for malnutrition in patients with meconium ileus.

There is a higher incidence of meconium ileus in patients whose genotype is homozygous for the ΔF508 mutation, or have the ΔF508/G542X mutation, although most patients with these genotypes do not have meconium ileus. Therefore, nongenetic factors must also contribute to the development of meconium ileus. Pathophysiological factors include pancreatic insufficiency (most infants with meconium ileus have pancreatic insufficiency), abnormal gut motility, dehydration of intraluminal contents, and increased gelling of intraluminal contents (39).

Infants with uncomplicated meconium ileus may be fed regular infant formula, enzymes, and vitamins. Those with a complicated surgical course may require either continuous enteral feedings or total parenteral nutrition. We recommend predigested infant formula (e.g., Pregestimil, Alimentum) for those who are fed enterally. Prestenotic dilatation of the small bowel, caused by the obstructing meconium, theoretically could lead to mucosal damage and thus contribute to malabsorption. Patients who have had serious complications of meconium ileus or sizable bowel resection may tolerate continuous feedings better than bolus feedings. These can be given by nasogastric tube if a gastrostomy tube was not placed at the time of the initial surgery. Feedings are begun with diluted formula, usually half strength, at low volume. If this is well tolerated, the strength and then volume may be increased (see Fig. 4). Pancreatic enzymes can be given orally starting at 2000–4000 lipase units per 120 mL of full-strength formula. Pancreatic enzymes should be given, even with MCT-oil containing formulas.

Infants who have had a major bowel resection may be left with the short gut syndrome and may be difficult to manage, especially if the ileocecal valve has been removed. An ileostomy may lead to excessive loss of water and electrolytes. These infants almost always need TPN. Guidelines for TPN differ from institution to institution; however, general suggestions are listed in Table 4. Gastric acid hypersecretion is commonly seen in patients with the short bowel syndrome (40). An acid pH inactivates pancreatic enzymes and impairs micelle formation and lipolysis. H_2 blockers should be used as an adjunct to pancreatic enzyme therapy in patients who have had major bowel resections. Urine sodium should be measured in infants with ileostomies who fail to grow, even if the serum sodium is normal. Those with urine sodium of less than 10 mEq/L need sodium (and possibly bicarbonate) supplementation (41).

Infants with meconium ileus who are managed with TPN are at increased risk for liver complications. One autopsy study found that a history of meconium ileus was recorded more frequently in persons with hepatic cirrhosis (42). Prolonged neonatal jaundice is sometimes seen in infants with CF (43). Cholestatic liver disease is a complication of TPN, which is seen especially in infants who have had bowel resections (44). Liver function should be monitored carefully in these infants.

IV. Nutrition Support in Children, Adolescents, and Adults with CF

A. Rationale

The major goal of nutritional care of the older hospitalized patient with CF is to provide adequate calories to help maintain immunocompetence, to promote optimal growth and development, and to prevent specific deficiencies (45).

The majority of hospitalizations for patients with CF are for treatment of pulmonary exacerbations. An increase in pulmonary infection and inflammation leads to an increase in energy expenditure. Loss of appetite also contributes to the unfavorable energy balance, which can compromise the ability to fight infection (11). As with infants, the patient's percent of ideal body weight for height should be calculated to determine whether patients are normally nourished, underweight, or malnourished.

B. Routine Diet for Patients Admitted for Treatment of a Pulmonary Exacerbation

While hospitalized, the patient with CF should be given an age-appropriate well-balanced diet with an emphasis on increased calories and protein. The increased calories are necessary because of the increased expenditure secondary to infection, work of breathing, and any energy loss via the stool (46). The best way to achieve a high-calorie diet is with unrestricted fat intake. Fat provides many calories in small volumes, which may be better tolerated in the patient admitted because of respiratory symptoms. Fat also improves that palatability of meals and provides necessary essential fatty acids. Some suggestions for ways to add fat to the diet are listed in Table 3. As fat is increased in the diet, the amount of enzymes needed may need to be adjusted. Most patients know that high-fat foods such as fried food or pizza call for more enzymes. Fat should make up 35%–40% of total caloric intake. This total intake should be divided into 5–6 meals per day, conveniently thought of as three regular meals, with two large snacks.

Low-fat diets should not be used. A study that compared patients with CF in Toronto and Boston found that the patients in Toronto, who received a high-fat diet with pancreatic enzyme replacement, had better heights and weights as well as improved survival, compared with those in Boston, where, in previous years, low-fat diets have been recommended. Most other aspects of care seemed comparable between centers (47).

Protein requirements are also increased in the patient with CF. Increased catabolism associated with infection and possible losses secondary to malabsorption can result in depletion of lean body mass. The diet should include foods high in protein (e.g., meat, eggs, dairy products, fish, poultry) and at least 15% 20% of the total calories should be from protein-rich foods (45).

C. Assessment of Caloric Needs in Malnourished Patients Admitted for Treatment of Pulmonary Exacerbations

Patients with CF have elevated energy expenditure (48,49). As pulmonary disease worsens, resting energy expenditure increases (14). However, caloric intake of patients with CF may be only 80%–90% of the recommended daily allowance (RDA). Those who maintain their weight consume calories in excess of the RDA (50). To determine actual intakes, an accurate 3- to 5-day food record is needed. Patients lose weight when energy intake is not adequate for energy requirements.

Table 5 presents one method of calculating caloric requirements in the CF patient. The method shown uses the RDA for patients aged 18 years and younger, and the Harris-Benedict equation for older patients.

If it becomes difficult to meet caloric needs with oral intake alone, or if the patient is less than 89% IBW/ht, then oral supplementation with proprietary formulas should be considered. A wide variety of calorically dense products are available (Table 6).

D. Aggressive Intervention for Malnourished Patients

If a patient with CF can no longer tolerate the taste of oral supplements or if weight slips to less than 85% IBW/ht, more aggressive nutritional intervention must be considered. Patients who receive nocturnal enteral feedings can achieve weight and height gains, along with an improved sense of well being, increased strength, improved body image, stabilization of pulmonary function, and

Table 5 Estimating Caloric Requirements

1–18 years:	RDA for age[a] X	1.2 mild CF
		1.3 moderate CF
		1.5 severe CF
18+ years:	Resting energy expenditure (REE) X	1.5 mild CF
		1.75 moderate CF, recent weight loss, infection
		2.0 severe CF, wasting

Harris–Benedict Equation

Males

$$REE = 66.5 + [13.8 \text{ wt (kg)}] + [5.0 \text{ ht (cm)}] - [6.8 \text{ A (yrs)}]$$

Females

$$REE = 655 + [9.6 \text{ wt (kg)}] + [1.7 \text{ ht (cm)}] - [4.7 \text{ A (yrs)}]$$

[a]RDAs for energy for age

	Age (yr)	kcal/kg
Infants	0–0.5	108
	0.5–1.0	98
Children	1–3	102
	4–6	90
	7–10	70
Male adolescents	11–14	55
	15–18	45
Female adolescents	11–14	47
	15–18	40

reduced weight loss during pulmonary exacerbations (51–54). These benefits can be realized even in patients with severe lung disease (55). The advantage of nocturnal enteral feedings is that the patient can carry on normal activity during the day and continue to eat regular meals, although patients thus fed have a diminished appetite, particularly in the morning. Most patients are reluctant to undertake this therapy (unless they have known another patient who has used such treatment successfully), and the idea often takes some adjusting to. There are no generally accepted criteria for when enteral tube feedings should be initiated. At our center, we consider 3 to 6 months with no catch-up growth despite aggressive oral calorie supplementation to be a fair trial and will initiate tube feeds then. Not every family can manage the logistics and the commitment that enteral tube feedings require. Families who have been habitually nonadherent to other aspects of prescribed CF care are not likely to benefit from tube feeds.

Nasogastric Tube Feedings

Nocturnal nasogastric tube feedings can be useful in a variety of settings. They are ideal when a short-term intervention is anticipated. Adolescents may prefer this route because it does not involve creation of an ostomy, which may worsen

Table 6 Proprietary Oral Supplements

Products for oral use	Cal/mL	g Fat	Type of fat	Comments
Ensure	1.06	37.2/L	Corn oil	Complete balanced nutrition
Ensure Plus	1.5	53.3/L	Corn oil	High calorie
Sustical	1.01	23/L	Partially hydrogenated soy oil	Complete balanced nutrition
Sustical Plus	1.52	58/L	Corn oil	High calorie
Resource	1.06	37/L	Corn oil	Lactose free
Resource Plus	1.5	53/L	Corn oil	Lactose free
Nutren 1.0	1.0	38/L	MCT and canola oil, lecithin	Complete balanced nutrition
Nutren 1.5	1.5	67.6/L	MCT, canola and corn oil, lecithin	High calorie
Scandishake	2.0	30 g/10 oz	Butter fat	Powder, mix with whole milk
Calories Plus	2.34	31 g/8 oz	Butter fat	Powder, mix with whole milk
Pediasure	1.0	49.7/L	High-oleic safflower oil, soy oil, MCT oil	Nutritionally complete formula for children 1–10 years of age
Carnation Instant Breakfast	1.17	8 g/8 oz	Butter fat	In grocery stores, inexpensive

the patient's body image. Even though a nasogastric tube may interfere with cough, nasogastric tube feedings may be indicated for some patients with severe lung disease who are unable to tolerate the anesthesia or sedation needed for placement of a gastrostomy or jejunostomy.

This method can be taught during the hospitalization once the patient's respiratory status stabilizes. If the patient and family are comfortable with the method, increases in the volume of tube feedings can be accomplished at home. The patient and family need to be highly motivated because a tube must be passed through the nose every night. Contact with another patient who has been successful with nasogastric tube feedings may help patients choose this method of nutritional intervention. An educational video is also helpful (56). Some patients may choose to leave a small nasogastric tube in place for a several-week intervention rather than undergo surgery or remove and replace the tube daily.

The initial goals should be to achieve greater than 120% of the RDA for energy needs by a combination of nasogastric tube feedings and oral intake (54). The volume and caloric content can be increased in the hospital or after discharge if this estimate does not result in weight gain. A variety of products can be infused overnight, but high-calorie formulas are recommended (Table 7). Tube feedings can be started at a rate of 30 mL (1 ounce) per hour over 8 hours (i.e., one 8-ounce can per night). Volume can be increased by 1/2 to 1 ounce per hour (i.e., one-half to one can per night) as tolerated until the goal is achieved. In our experience, four cans per night for children and six cans per night for adults of 1.5–2 calorie/mL of formula are tolerated and provide adequate calories for catch-up growth.

Pancreatic enzymes are needed with nasogastric tube feedings unless an elemental product is used. A wide variety of enzyme replacement strategies has been used for patients receiving tube feedings (57). Enzymes can be taken at bedtime in the amount usually taken with a meal (52). Some patients may need to take enzymes in the middle of the night. Powdered (non-enteric-coated) enzymes can be mixed with the formula. We have used Viokase, 1/2 teaspoon per 8-ounce can of formula, mixed before pouring the formula into the bag. (Because the nutrients are digested by the enzymes, the formula separates.) If patients have a large, loose stool each morning, the enzyme dose needs to be adjusted. It is best to have the nasogastric tube feedings finish a few hours before receiving chest physiotherapy in the morning because some patients vomit after coughing (58). Prokinetic agents are helpful if morning bloating is a problem.

Gastrostomies

Patients who require long-term nutritional support or who tire of passing a nasogastric tube nightly may choose to have a gastrostomy tube or button

Table 7 Tube Feeding Formulas

Products for tube feeding	Cal/ mL	g Fat/L	Type of fat	Osmolality, mOsm/ kg H$_2$O	Cost (range)[a]	Provider	Comments
Deliver 2.0	2.0	102	Soy oil, MCT oil	640	$.60–$.87 per 8 oz	Mead Johnson	High calorie and nitrogen
Magnacal	2.0	80	Soy oil	590	$.75–$.81 per 250 mL	Sherwood	High calorie, lactose free
Pulmocare	1.5	93.3	Canola oil, MCT and corn oil, high-oleic safflower oil, soy lecithin	475	$1.01–$1.19 per 8 oz	Ross	Lactose free, high fat, low carbohydrate, specialized for pulmonary patients
Lipisorb	1.35	57	MCT oil, soy oil	630	$2.63–$2.86 per 8 oz	Mead Johnson	High MCT (86%), lactose free
Reabilan HN	1.33	52	MCT oil, soy oil, venthera blennis oil	490	$11.32–$12.15 per 12.5 oz	Clintec	Semielemental/high nitrogen Note: each can contains 12.5 oz
Vital HN	1.0	10.8	Safflower oil, MCT oil	500	$2.65–$2.84 per 300-mL packet	Ross	Elemental product
TwoCal HN	2.0	90.9	Corn oil, MCT oil	690	$.91–$1.04 per 8 oz	Ross	High calorie, high nitrogen
Nutren 2.0	2.0	106	MCT oil, canola oil, lecithin	710	$.78–$.87 per 250 mL	Clintec	High MCT oil (73%)
Tolerex	1.0	1.5	Safflower oil	550	$4.38–$4.73 per 300-mL packet	Sandoz	Elemental product
Criticare HN	1.06	5.3	Safflower oil	650	$4.10–$4.56 per 8 oz	Mead Johnson	High nitrogen, elemental product
Vivonex Pediatric	0.8	23.5	MCT oil, soybean oil	360	$3.22–$3.85 per 250-ml pack	Sandoz	Elemental formula for children

[a]Prices as of June 1995; Coram Healthcare

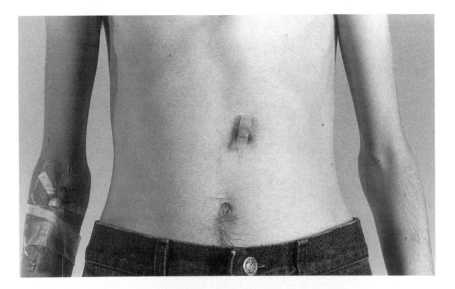

Figure 5 Gastrostomy button in situ.

placed. Tube placement can be done endoscopically, surgically, or by interventional radiologists. At our institution, local or epidural anesthesia with propofol sedation has been used during placement of gastrostomy buttons when general anesthesia is considered too risky. Patients should have stable pulmonary status before undergoing gastrostomy placement. Gastrostomy buttons are more aesthetically pleasing to patients than gastrostomy tubes (Fig. 5). There have been no instances of buttons dislodging during coughing spasms in our 10-year experience with these buttons.

Formula is delivered overnight while the patient sleeps, using the same guidelines as for nasogastric tube feedings. As with nasogastric tube feedings, pancreatic enzymes need to be given with the formula. Bloating and GER may be a problem with either method of tube feeding (59). The use of prokinetic agents, such as metoclopramide or cisapride, given at bedtime can alleviate this problem. A second dose may be given in the morning if needed.

Jejunostomy Feedings

Jejunostomy feedings are used at some centers when long-term nutritional support is needed. The advantage of this type of feeding is that delivery of formula distal to the ligament of Treitz makes gastroesophageal reflux unlikely. Jejunostomies may be placed by a variety of methods. The Witzel technique creates a serosal-lined conduit between the jejunum and the abdominal wall. A wide-bore catheter is then inserted into the jejunum. The tube may be replaced in the outpatient clinic if it is not fixed internally (60). Another technique involves threading a narrow catheter into the jejunum via a large needle. Only elemental formulas can be used with a needle catheter jejunostomy. With larger bore catheters, less expensive, nonelemental formulas can be used.

As with the other tube feeding modalities, jejunostomy feedings are usually and most conveniently delivered overnight. When nonelemental formulas are used, powdered pancreatic enzymes may be added to the formula (53) or pancreatic enzyme supplements can be given before the tube feeding. Likewise, the patient's pulmonary status should be stable before undergoing jejunostomy placement.

When a permanently implanted enterostomy is indicated, the choice of gastrostomy versus jejunostomy should be based on the clinical experience of the surgeons, gastroenterologists, radiologists, and CF clinic staff. Either method can be effective.

Parenteral Nutrition

Total parenteral nutrition or supplemental parenteral nutrition support may be indicated for patients with CF on a short-term basis for such problems as pancreatitis, short gut syndrome, or postoperative management (2). Total parenteral nutrition may also be used after lung transplantation. Weight gain can be achieved in the short term, and use of intravenous lipids can correct fatty acid deficiency (61,62). Guidelines for parenteral nutrition are listed in Table 4.

Long-term use of TPN is expensive, and complications occur more commonly with parenteral than with enteral supplementation (63). If long-term nutritional support will be needed after the patient is discharged, the enteral route should be used if possible.

E. Nutrition for Patients with Pancreatitis (see Chapter 5)

Patients with CF and pancreatitis should not eat while they have pain. They therefore need to be supported with intravenous fluids, and, if the pain lasts more than a few days, they need intravenous calories as well in the form of TPN delivered through a central line. Most cases of CF pancreatitis resolve without requiring TPN. Enteral feeds can be restarted when the pain remits, even if serum amylase and lipase levels remain elevated, as they often do. When food is reintroduced, it seems prudent to make it a gradual process, starting with a low-fat (40–50 g/day for adults) and relatively low-protein diet. The oft-used progression of "clear fluids" to "soft" diet to full diet makes no sense for someone with pancreatitis and teeth. In most dietary departments, for example, chicken soup (which has a very high fat content) is considered a clear fluid. Despite centuries of evidence supporting the curative powers of chicken soup, it would seem more rational in this setting to begin with a low-fat food to minimize pancreatic stimulation. A potato, for example, even a relatively hard one, should be better tolerated than a fatty broth. If the low-fat, low-protein diet is tolerated, with no recurrence of abdominal pain for a week or so, gradual liberalization of the diet can be undertaken. Teenagers and adults should be counseled to avoid alcohol.

F. Nutrition for Patients After Surgery (see Chapter 5)

There are only a few considerations for postoperative nutrition that are specific to CF. The first is the need for pancreatic enzyme supplementation in most patients. Countless episodes of distal intestinal obstruction syndrome (see Chapters 3 and 5) have occurred in CF patients because the postoperative team has overlooked the routine enzymes. Some of the considerations listed above for pancreatitis patients also apply, namely, the need to think of the physiology involved before automatically ordering a diet progression of clear fluids to soft foods.

G. Nutrition Support for End-Stage Patients

Aggressive nutritional intervention cannot reverse lung disease, although it may help prevent deterioration. Unfortunately, many patients delay initiation of these interventions until their lung disease has become so severe that they are then "willing to do anything." Because of the intrusiveness and expense of these interventions, it can be argued that nutritional intervention is not warranted in end-stage patients. Levy et al. developed a prognostic index to predict which patients were most likely to benefit from aggressive intervention (Table 8) (64). This index was developed before the advent of lung transplantation. Others have demonstrated good weight gain even in severely affected patients (55).

Although most patients who are evaluated for transplantation are severely malnourished (65), they can successfully gain weight using enteral feedings (66). Survival after transplant depends on many factors, and it is unclear whether patients with better weight before transplant have better survival. However, it has long been demonstrated that excessive postoperative morbidity and mortality can be predicted in general surgical patients who are malnourished (67). Based on these observations, aggressive pretransplant nutrition support is recommended (68).

Once a patient has been evaluated and accepted on the transplant list, enteral tube feedings should be initiated in those whose ideal weight for height is less than 85%. This group of patients may need slower infusions to prevent pulmonary compromise caused by abdominal distention. They may require diuretics to enable them to tolerate the fluid load in the face of cor pulmonale. Patients with CO_2 retention may benefit from high-fat formula, because less CO_2 is produced for each gram of fat metabolized as compared with carbohy-

Table 8 Prognostic Nutrition Index

P = 116.42 − 0.53 (average heart rate) − 12.98 (0 = absence,
1 = presence of *Burkholderia cepacia* in serum) − 0.95 ($Paco_2$) − 1.01 (age in years)
When P < 0, the likelihood of long-term survival after intervention is low.
When P > 0, prognosis for extended survival is good after nutritional intervention.

Source: Ref. 64.

drate. However, this effect is seen primarily in patients who are fed parenterally (69). Whatever the form of nutritional supplementation, indirect evidence suggests that an aggressive approach is useful after transplantation. In one recent series, patients who survived more than 1 year after lung transplantation differed from those who survived less than 1 year in that the survivors had gained weight between 1 and 3 months after transplant, whereas the group surviving less than 1 year did not gain weight between 1 and 2 months after transplant (70).

H. Cystic Fibrosis–Related Diabetes Mellitus (see Chapter 7)

Carbohydrate intolerance is common in patients with CF (71), and overt diabetes appears with increasing frequency in older patients. Cystic fibrosis–related diabetes mellitus (CFRDM) differs from type I and type II diabetes. It has a slow onset, and, because of persistent insulin secretion, there may be episodes of hyperglycemia interspersed between long periods of euglycemia. The hyperglycemia is not associated with ketosis. Furthermore, the presence of some insulin reserves may prevent the overwhelming lipolysis and ketogenesis seen in diabetic ketoacidosis (DKA). Because DKA does not develop, hypoglycemia is a greater short-term risk to patients with CFRDM than hyperglycemia.

Hyperglycemia is the metabolic abnormality that is recognized, but it is not the only problem associated with CFRDM. Insulin is an anabolic hormone, and lack of insulin contributes to wasting of muscle mass. This, along with loss of calories in the urine due to glycosuria, complicates the patient's already tenuous nutritional status.

The CFRDM may not be diagnosed until the patient is hospitalized for treatment of pulmonary exacerbation, because its onset is insidious and is superimposed on a chronic disease that could account for nonspecific symptoms such as weakness or fatigue. It is not uncommon for infection and fever to cause transient elevations of blood glucose in patients with CF, because of their predisposition to carbohydrate intolerance. Glucocorticoids may also cause hyperglycemia. Persistent elevations of blood sugar may signal the onset of CFRDM. Intervention should be considered when multiple daily fasting blood sugar measurements are greater than 140 mg/dL or 2-hour postcibal values are greater than 180 mg/dL (72).

The prevalence of carbohydrate intolerance increases with increasing age (73). CFRDM has been reported to have either no effect (74) or a negative effect on prognosis (75). Microangiopathy has been described in patients with long-standing CFRDM (76).

Dietary Management

Cystic fibrosis–related diabetes mellitus complicates dietary management in patients with CF. We emphasize weight gain in patients with CFRDM, whereas patients without CF who have diabetes are encouraged to keep their body weight low. Patients with CFRDM should not be automatically placed on a low-calorie American Diabetes Association diet. We continue to encourage high-fat meals and snacks with a limited amount of concentrated sweets. If concentrated sweets are consumed, they should be eaten with a meal and not as an individual snack to minimize dramatic swings in postprandial blood sugar levels. Beverages such as fruit drinks or soft drinks should be free of sucrose and glucose. When a patient is taking insulin, the timing of meals and snacks needs to be consistent from day to day to prevent wide swings in blood sugar levels and rapidly changing insulin doses. Some centers have advocated no change in the patient's usual diet, with multiple insulin doses given titrated to the meal's carbohydrate load (77). Table 9 outlines the conflicts in dietary management.

Medical Management

Because the course of CFRDM is variable, medical management must be individualized. There are no studies on the role of oral hypoglycemic agents, but there have been anecdotal reports of success. One study of insulin responses in eight well-nourished patients with CF indicated that there may already be an upregulation of peripheral glucose receptors as a compensation for decreased endogenous insulin production (78). We have used glipizide, 5–15 mg by mouth

Table 9 Nutritional Advice

	CF-related diabetes	Non-CF-related diabetes
Energy intake	100%–200% of recommended daily allowance (RDA)	100% or less of RDA
Fat	30%–40% of calories	<30% of calories
Monosaccharides and disaccharides	No concentrated sweets	Limited or no intake
Salt	Encouraged, especially in hot weather	Low intake

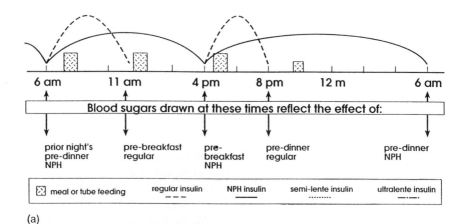

(a)

Figure 6 Insulin regimens for management of hypergylcemia in patients with CFRDM. (a) Routine CFRDM. (b) Tube feeding–induced hyperglycemia (i.e., daytime blood sugars only mildly elevated). (c) Tube feeding in patients with CFRDM.

every morning, along with dietary management to control moderate hyperglycemia (pretreatment blood sugar levels, 180–250 mg/dL) with some success. Some of these patients have ultimately been able to control their diabetes with diet alone, and others have intermittently required insulin. Patients who are started on an oral hypoglycemic agent should have fasting blood sugar levels monitored (on arising or before dinner) for hypoglycemic. Two-hour postprandial blood sugar levels reflect whether this therapeutic strategy is controlling hyperglycemia. There is a 24- to 48-hour lag between changing a dose of oral hypoglycemic medicine and its effect on blood sugars. On an outpatient basis, measurement of fasting blood sugar and glycosylated hemoglobin can be used to monitor therapy.

A variety of insulin preparations is available. In most instances, twice-daily injections of a combination of short- and intermediate-acting insulin are used. The amount of insulin needed to maintain euglycemia in patients with CFRDM is generally less than that needed for patients with type I diabetes. Starting doses of 0.3–0.5 units/kg/day are usually effective. Initially, two-thirds of the dose can be given before breakfast and one-third is given before dinner. Of this amount, two-thirds can be given as regular insulin and the remaining one-third as intermediate-acting insulin [neutral protamine Hagedorn (NPH) or lente]. Blood sugars are measured before each meal and before the evening snack. Insulin dose can then be adjusted based on these data (Fig. 6). If the first morning blood sugar measurement is consistently high, a 2 AM blood sugar level should be checked for evidence of the "Sovmogyi effect" (reactive hyperglycemia). In our experience, few patients actually fit this classic "two-thirds,

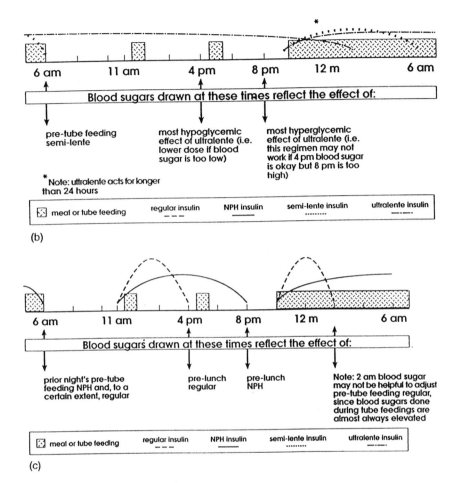

(b)

(c)

one-third" pattern, but it is still a reasonable starting point from which adjustments can be made.

Many factors can affect insulin dosing. Use of prednisone can cause transient hyperglycemia or may lead to a permanent insulin requirement (79). It can be exceedingly hard to regulate blood sugars in patients on high-dose prednisone. Frequent blood sugar measurements are the most useful therapeutic tool. Use of alternate-day steroids may not be logistically feasible in patients with CFRDM, because alternate-day insulin dosing is also needed. Adherence to this regimen is highly unlikely, except in the most motivated and well-educated patients.

Likewise, use of nocturnal enteral feedings may cause feeding-related hyperglycemia (i.e., daytime blood sugar levels are normal) or may unmask CFRDM (80). High-fat formulas may be better tolerated than high-carbohydrate formulas (see Table 7). If blood sugar levels are elevated only during the time of the infusion, a single injection of regular insulin plus NPH just before tube feedings may normalize blood sugars. In our experience, 4–6 units of insulin per 360 calories (i.e., 8-ounce can of 1.5 calorie/mL formula) can be given to start, with one-fourth of the dose as regular insulin. We do not usually check blood sugar levels during the time of the infusion. Absence of glycosuria in the first morning void and a blood sugar level of less than 180 one to two hours after the tube feeding has ended indicate reasonable metabolic control. Glycosylated hemoglobin measured every few months can give an indication of longer-term control.

If a patient on nocturnal enteral feedings has CFRDM, a combination of semilente and ultralente insulin given before the tube feeding may provide adequate glycemic control. If needed, additional insulin can be given before lunch (regular insulin plus NPH) or dinner (regular insulin), depending on the patient's eating habits and blood sugar levels (see Fig. 6b).

Patients who are given large amounts of insulin before tube feedings or those who use long-acting insulins can be given glucose-containing intravenous fluids while they are hospitalized if, for some reason, they are unable to tolerate their tube feedings or are unable to eat after being given insulin.

Patients may develop CFRDM while receiving total parenteral nutrition. Regular insulin can be added to the TPN solution, starting at 1 unit of regular insulin for each 4–8 g of carbohydrate infused.

V. Electrolyte Abnormalities

A. Abnormalities Caused by the Primary Genetic Defect

The observation that patients with CF have abnormal sweat electrolytes dates from 1948 when, during a heat wave in New York City, Kessler and Andersen identified heat exhaustion in five patients with CF (81). Serum chlorides were found to be low in the two patients in whom it was measured. di Sant' Agnese et al. collected and analyzed sweat from patients with CF and found the concentration of chloride and sodium greatly exceeded that of control subjects (82). More than 40 years later, it was recognized that the electrolyte abnormalities are directly due to the primary genetic defect.

Acute hyponatremic dehydration can be seen in infants with CF, especially during heat waves or during febrile illnesses. Typically, patients are anorectic, irritable, and then lethargic. Vomiting may be a prominent symptom, and patients are febrile. As a result of excessive salt loss, the effective circulating fluid volume is depleted, leading to increased antidiuretic hormone (ADH) secretion and renal reabsorption of sodium. Urine output decreases, along with serum sodium and osmolarity. Therapy is directed at controlling the cause of excess sweating and estimating and replacing the fluid and sodium chloride losses (Table 10.)

Table 10 Treatment of Hyponatremia

Serum sodium >120 mEq/L

Estimate fluid deficit (hyponatremic children may appear more depleted than they actually are).

Give 20 mL/kg fluid bolus of isonatremic (normal) saline or lactated Ringer's solution over 1–2 hours (faster if the patient is hypotensive).

Give 1/3 maintenance and 1/2 remaining estimated deficit plus ongoing losses as D5 1/2 normal saline plus 20–40 mEq/L of potassium[a] over 8 hours.

Give maintenance, remaining deficit, and replacement of ongoing losses with D5 1/2 normal saline plus 20–40 mEq/L of potassium over the remainder of the 24-hour period.

Continue maintenance and replacement of ongoing losses as indicated.

Serum sodium <120 mEq/L (in the absence of hyperglycemia)

Infuse hypertonic (3%) saline to bring serum sodium above 125 mEq/L (12 mL/Kg raises serum sodium approximately 10 mEq/L) added to initial bolus.

Some clinicians do not give hypertonic saline unless patients have symptoms such as malaise, confusion, stupor, coma, or seizures. Never give more than 4–5 mEq/kg in less than 90–120 minutes—pontine myelolysis can develop.

[a]Do not give potassium until urine output has been established.

Hyponatremia, hypochloremia, hypokalemia, and metabolic alkalosis can be seen in infants with CF who do not have apparent heat stress (83–85). They may have poor appetite and failure to thrive, and they do not appear to be dramatically dehydrated. An intercurrent illness, which, by itself, would not cause metabolic derangement, is superimposed on chronic salt loss in sweat, resulting in a pseudo-Bartter's syndrome (86). The syndrome has also been attributed to a low-salt diet (87). Before restoration of fluid and electrolyte balance, patients have elevated plasma renin and aldosterone. In individuals without CF, a low-salt diet results in hyperaldosteronism and diminution in sweat sodium and chloride. In patients with CF, a salt-free diet also causes hyperaldosteronism, but sweat sodium and chloride concentrations remain high (88). The hyperaldosteronism may contribute to hypokalemia by increasing sweat and urine potassium losses (89). Potassium can also be lost in the stool, as is seen in the hyperaldosteronism of patients with chronic renal failure.

Therapy is outlined in Table 10. These patients should be placed on chronic oral salt supplements during infancy to prevent further episodes of hypoelectrolytemia (2–4 mmol of Na/kg/day; this may be given as NaCl solution, which comes as 2.5 mmol/mL or as table salt, which contains 87 mmol of Na per teaspoon). Urine sodium concentrations of less than 10 mEq/L suggest inadequate replacement.

Older patients may also develop hypoelectrolytemia. Even mildly affected patients with CF lose significantly more sodium and chloride per square meter of body surface area compared with control subjects when they exercise in the heat (90). In one study, patients with CF drank less than control subjects when allowed to consume liquids ad lib during exercise (91).

B. Abnormalities Caused by Advanced Pulmonary Disease

Hypercapnia and Cor Pulmonale

As pulmonary disease advances, patients begin to retain carbon dioxide. The kidneys compensate for the resulting respiratory acidosis by retaining bicarbonate ions. There is a 3.5-mEq/L increase in bicarbonate ions for every 10-mm Hg increase in Pco_2. The extracellular pH returns toward normal. Hypoxemia usually precedes chronic hypercapnia, so most patients have pulmonary artery hypertension (as a result of hypoxemia) at this stage of their disease. When heart failure complicates cor pulmonale, there may be fluid transudation into the lungs. Diuretics are used to improve gas exchange, but they complicate the metabolic picture.

Loop diuretics such as furosemide and bumetanide cause large amounts of sodium, chloride, and calcium to be lost in the urine. Distal tubule and connecting segment diuretics such as thiazides, chlorthalidone, and metolazone also cause electrolyte loss, but to a lesser extent. Spironolactone, amiloride, and triamterene act in the cortical collecting tubule and cause weak natriuresis while preventing potassium depletion.

Patients with compensated respiratory acidosis who are taking diuretics often have hyponatremia, hypochloremia, and elevated serum bicarbonate. Chronic chloride depletion may lead to metabolic alkalosis, worsening the patient's hypoventilatory state. KCl, NH_4Cl, or arginine Cl supplements may be needed if patients are unable to tolerate sodium because of heart failure. Some antibiotics contain large amounts of sodium (Table 11), which can aggravate heart failure. Overzealous use of diuretics can lead to volume depletion and poor tissue perfusion, with acute metabolic (lactic) acidosis superimposed on the chronic respiratory acidosis.

Syndrome of Inappropriate ADH Secretion

In uncommon cases, end-stage patients with hyponatremia may have the syndrome of inappropriate ADH secretion (SIADH). These patients have decreased serum sodium and osmolarity in the face of inappropriately high urine sodium and osmolarity. However, urine electrolyte concentrations are not diagnostically useful in a patient who is taking diuretics. It is possible that ADH is released in response to the decreased left atrial filling pressure caused by cor pulmonale, not by intrinsic lung disease (92). The treatment is fluid restriction until serum electrolytes become normal. In severe cases, hypertonic saline along with intravenous furosemide may be needed. Two-thirds to three-fourths maintenance fluid is given, but the sodium requirements of the entire day should be given in this volume.

Table 11 Sodium Content of Selected Antibiotics

Antibiotic	Sodium content per gram
Ceftazidime	54.0 mg (2.3 mEq)
Imipenem-cilastin[a]	75.0 mg (3.2 mEq)
Piperacillin	42.5 mg (1.85 mEq)
Ticarcillin	119.6 mg (5.2 mEq) to 149.5 mg (6.5 mEq)
Timentin (ticarcillin-clavulanate)	109.0 mg (4.75 mEq)[b]

[a]Imipenem is usually diluted in 100 mL normal saline per dose.
[b]Theoretical.

Hypomagnesemia

Symptomatic hypomagnesemia may develop in patients with CF (93,94). Some have typical tetany, whereas others have nonspecific symptoms such as weakness, fatigue, or muscle cramps. Secondary hyperaldosteronism, due either to the sweat defect in CF or to aminoglycosides, causes increased excretion of magnesium in the urine. Aminoglycosides may also cause accumulation of magnesium in the proximal tubule leading to necrosis. Diuresis, either due to drugs or glycosuria from diabetes, can also increase magnesium excretion. Magnesium can also bind to fat in the stool and be lost secondary to steatorrhea. Treatment is with intravenous magnesium sulfate, 4–5 g, given over 4–5 hours, and repeated daily until the serum magnesium level is greater than 1.5 mEq/L (94).

Hyperkalemia

Hyperkalemia may result from a variety of causes. Renal failure alters urinary excretion of potassium. Patients with CF often have enormous lifetime exposure to aminoglycosides, a known nephrotoxic agent. In end-stage patients, hypoperfusion can lead to chronic renal insufficiency.

A variety of drugs can elevate serum potassium, including angiotensin-converting enzyme inhibitors such as captopril or enalapril, and the antirejection drugs cyclosporine and FK506. We have seen one instance of trimethoprimsulfamethoxazole–related hyperkalemia, which resolved when the drug was withdrawn, a complication reported in patients with acquired immunodeficiency syndrome (95). Potassium-sparing diuretics can cause hyperkalemia.

Treatment should be initiated only if the potassium level is increasing rapidly or if an electrocardiogram shows peaked T waves, widened QRS, or arrhythmias. Intravenous calcium should be given if a widened QRS is seen (10% calcium gluconate, 0.5–1.0 mL/kg as a rapid intravenous injection over 3–5 minutes). Intravenous insulin and glucose can shift potassium into cells (50%

glucose, 1 mL/kg over 30 minutes, accompanied by regular insulin, 1 unit per 3 g of glucose). Sodium bicarbonate should be used if metabolic acidosis is present (2 mEq/kg as a rapid intravenous injection over 3–5 minutes). Following this, Kayexalate may be given (0.5–1.0 g/kg by mouth or by rectum, repeated every 4–6 hours as needed).

VI. Conclusion

Nutritional intervention should be considered in every hospitalized patient with cystic fibrosis. Those who are well nourished need ongoing encouragement to continue to consume high-calorie foods. Those who are underweight or malnourished need special interventions. When CF physicians pay attention to nutrition, the health and quality of life for patients with CF is improved.

References

1. Ramsey B, Farrell PM, Pencharz P, et al. Nutritional assessment and management in cystic fibrosis: a consensus report. Am J Clin Nutr 1992; 55:108–116.
2. FitzSimmons SC. The changing epidemiology of cystic fibrosis. J Pediatr 1993; 122:1–9.
3. Holliday KE, Allen JR, Waters DL, Gruca MA, Thompson SM, Gaskin KJ. Growth of human milk-fed and formula-fed infants with cystic fibrosis. J Pediatr 1991; 118:77–79.
4. Laughlin JJ, Brady MS, Eigen H. Changing feeding trends as a cause of electrolyte depletion in infants with cystic fibrosis. Pediatrics 1981; 68:203–207.
5. Bronstein MN, Sokol RJ, Abman SH, et al. Pancreatic insufficiency, growth, and nutrition in infants identified by newborn screening as having cystic fibrosis. J Pediatr 1992; 120:533–540.
6. Brennan J, Ellis L, Kalnins D, et al. Do infants with cystic fibrosis and pancreatic insufficiency require a predigested formula? (abstr) Pediatr Pulmonol Suppl 1991; 6:295.
7. Durie P, Newth C, Forstner G, Gall D. Malabsorption of medium-chain triglycerides in infants with cystic fibrosis: correction with pancreatic enzyme supplements. J Pediatr 1980; 96(5):862–864.
8. Fleisher DS, DiGeorge AM, Barness LA, Cornfeld D. Hypoproteinemia and edema in infants with cystic fibrosis of the pancreas. J Pediatr 1964; 64:341–348.
9. Park YK, Kim I, Yetley EA. Characteristics of vitamin and mineral supplement products in the United States. Am J Clin Nutr 1991; 54:750–759.
10. Sokol RJ, Reardon MC, Accurso FJ, et al. Fat-soluble vitamins in infants identified by cystic fibrosis newborn screening. Pediatr Pulmonol Suppl 1991; 7:52–55.
11. Durie PR, Pencharz PB. A rational approach to the nutritional care of patients with cystic fibrosis. J R Sock Med 1989; 82:11–20.
12. Sills RH. Failure to thrive. The role of clinical and laboratory evaluation. Am J Dis Child 1978; 132:967–969.

13. Cropp GJA, Rosenberg PN. Energy costs of breathing in cystic fibrosis and their relation to severity of pulmonary disease. Monogr Paediatr (Karger, Basel) 1981; 14:91–94.
14. Fried MD, Durie PR, Tsui LC, Corey M, Levison H, Pencharz PB. The cystic fibrosis gene and resting energy expenditure. J Pediatr 1991; 119:913–916.
15. Vaisman N, Levy LD, Pencharz PB, Tan YK, Soldin SJ, Canny GJ, Hahn E. Effect of salbutamol on resting energy expenditure in patients with cystic fibrosis. J Pediatr 1987; 111:137–139.
16. Scott RB, O'Loughlin EV, Gall DG. Gastroesophageal reflux in patients with cystic fibrosis. J Pediatr 1985; 106:223–227.
17. Orenstein SR, Orenstein DM. Gastroesophageal reflux and respiratory disease in children. J Pediatr 1988; 112:847–858.
18. Cystic Fibrosis Foundation Consensus Conferences. Gastrointestinal problems in CF. Gastroesophageal reflux. Concepts in Care 1991; II (II):
19. Malfroot A, Dab I. New insights on gastro-oesophageal reflux in cystic fibrosis by longitudinal follow up. Arch Dis Child 1991; 66:1339–1345.
20. Murphy JL, Wootton SA, Bond SA, Jackson AA. Energy content of stools in normal healthy controls and patients with cystic fibrosis. Arch Dis Child 1991; 66:495–500.
21. Durie PR, Bell L, Linton W, Corey ML, Forstner GG. Effect of cimetidine and sodium bicarbonate on pancreatic replacement therapy in cystic fibrosis. Gut 1980; 21:778–786.
22. Boyle BJ, Long WB, Balistreri WF, Widzer SJ, Huang N. Effect of cimetidine and pancreatic enzymes on serum and fecal bile acids and fat absorption in cystic fibrosis. Gastroenterology 1980; 78:950–953.
23. Antonowicz I, Reddy V, Khaw KT, Schwachman H. Lactase deficiency in patients with cystic fibrosis. Pediatrics 1968; 42:492–500.
24. Roberts DM, Craft JC, Mather FJ, Davis SH, Wright JA. Prevalence of giardiasis in patients with cystic fibrosis. J Pediatr 1988; 112:555–559.
25. Welkon CJ, Long SS, Thompson CM, Gilligan PH. *Clostridium difficile* in patients with cystic fibrosis. Am J Dis Child 1985; 139:805–808.
26. Lloyd-Still JD. Crohn's disease and cystic fibrosis. Dig Dis Sci 1994; 39:880–885.
27. Goodchild MC, Nelson R, Anderson CM. Cystic fibrosis and coeliac disease: coexistence in two children. Arch Dis Child 1973; 48:684–691.
28. Taylor B, Sokol G. Cystic fibrosis and coeliac disease. Arch Dis Child 1973; 48:692–696.
29. Smyth RL, van Velsen D, Smyth AR, Lloyd DA, Heaf DP. Strictures of ascending colon in cystic fibrosis and high-strength pancreatic enzymes. Lancet 1994; 343:85–86.
30. Freiman JP, FitzSimmons SC. Colonic strictures in patients with cystic fibrosis: results of a survey of 114 CF care centers in the United States. Lancet. In press.
31. Bray PF, Herbst JJ. Pseudotumor cerebri as a sign of "catch-up" growth in cystic fibrosis. Am J Dis Child 1973; 126:78–79.
32. Roach ES, Sinal SH. Increased intracranial pressure following treatment of cystic fibrosis. Pediatrics 1980; 66:622–623.
33. Gunn T, Belmonte MM, Colle E, Dupont C. Edema as the presenting symptom of cystic fibrosis: difficulties in diagnosis. Am J Dis Child 1978; 132:317–318.

34. Abman SH, Accurso FJ, Bowman CM. Persistent morbidity and mortality of protein calorie malnutrition in young infants with CF. J Pediatr Gastroenterol Nutr 1986; 5:393–396.
35. McPartlin JF, Dickson JAS, Swain VAJ. Meconium ileus. Immediate and long-term survival. Arch Dis Child 1972; 47:207–210.
36. Rescorla FJ, Grosfeld JL, West KJ, Vane DW. Changing patterns of treatment and survival in neonates with meconium ileus. Arch Surg 1989; 142:837–840.
37. Del Pin CA, Czyrko C, Ziegler MM, Scanlin TF, Bishop HC. Management and survival of meconium ileus. A 30-year review. Ann Surg 1992; 215:179–185.
38. Kerem E. Corey M, Kerem B, Durie P. Tsiu LC, Levison H. Clinical and genetic comparisons of patients with cystic fibrosis, with or without meconium ileus. J Pediatr 1989; 114:767–773.
39. Wilcox DT, Borowitz DS, Stovroff MC, Glick PL. Chronic intestinal pseudo-obstruction with meconium ileus at onset. J Pediatr 1993; 123:751–752.
40. Hyman PE, Everett SL, Harada T. Gastric acid hypersecretion in short bowel syndrome in infants: association with extent of resection and enteral feeding. J Pediatr Gastroenterol Nutr 1986; 5:191–197.
41. Bower TR, Pringle KC, Soper RT. Sodium deficit causing decreasing weight gain and metabolic acidosis in infants with ileostomy. J Pediatr Surg 1988; 23:567–572.
42. Maurage C, Lenaerts C, Weber A, Brochu P, Yousef I, Roy CC. Meconium ileus and its equivalent as a risk factor for the development of cirrhosis: an autopsy study in cystic fibrosis. J Pediatr Gastroenterol Nutr 1989; 9:17–20.
43. Valman HB, France NE, Wallis PG. Prolonged neonatal jaundice in cystic fibrosis. Arch Dis Child 1971; 46:805–809.
44. Hodes JE, Grosfeld JL, Weber TR, Schreiner RL, Fitzgerald JF, Mirkin LD. Hepatic failure in infants on total parenteral nutrition (TPN): clinical and histopathologic observations. J Pediatr Surg 1982; 17:463–468.
45. Adams E. Nutrition care in cystic fibrosis. Nutr News 1988; 3:1–6.
46. Luder E. Nutritional care of patients with cystic fibrosis. Top Clin Nutr 1991; 6(2):39–50.
47. Corey M, McLaughlin FJ, Williams M, Levison H. A comparison of survival, growth, and pulmonary function in patients with cystic fibrosis in Boston and Toronto. J Clin Epidemiol 1988; 41:593–591.
48. Grunow JE, Azcue MP, Berall G, Pencharz PB. Energy expenditure in cystic fibrosis during activities of daily living. J Pediatr 1993; 122:243–246.
49. Tomezsko JL, Stallings VA, Kawchak DA, Goin JE, Diamond G, Scanlin TF. Energy expenditure and genotype of children with cystic fibrosis. Pediatr Res 1994; 35:451–460.
50. Tomezsko JL, Stallings, VA, Scanlin TF. Dietary intake of healthy children with cystic fibrosis compared with normal control children. Pediatrics 1992; 90:547–553.
51. Levy LD, Durie PR, Pencharz PB, Corey ML. Effects of long-term nutritional rehabilitation on body composition on clinical status in malnourished children and adolescents with cystic fibrosis. J Pediatr 1985; 107:225–230.
52. Shepherd RW, Holt TL, Thomas BJ, et al. Nutritional rehabilitation in cystic fibrosis: controlled studies of effects on nutritional growth retardation, body protein turnover, and course of pulmonary disease. J Pediatr 1986; 109:788–794.

53. Boland MP, Stoski DS, MacDonald NE, Soucy P, Patrick J. Chronic jejunostomy feeding with a non-elemental formula in undernourished patients with cystic fibrosis. Lancet 1986; 233–234.

54. O'Loughlin E, Forbes D, Parson H, Scott B, Cooper D, Gall G. Nutritional rehabilitation of malnourished patients with cystic fibrosis. Am J Clin Nutr 1986; 43:732–737.

55. Steinkamp G, von der Hardt G. Improvement of nutritional status and lung function after long-term nocturnal gastrostomy feedings in cystic fibrosis. J Pediatr 1994; 124:244–249.

56. Coburn-Miller C, Kontos M, Borowitz D. Does a video designed to educate and motivate patients impact on caregivers? Pediatr Pulmonol Suppl 1994; 10:293.

57. Holben D, Wilmott R. Enzyme replacement therapy and enteral tube feedings in cystic fibrosis (CF). Pediatr Pulmonol Suppl 1991; 6:295.

58. Bowser E. Evaluating enteral nutrition support in cystic fibrosis. Top Clin Nutr 1990; 5(3):55–61.

59. Scott RB, O'Loughlin EV, Gall DG. Gastroesophageal reflux in patients with cystic fibrosis. J Pediatr 1985; 106:223–7.

60. Boland MP, Patrick J, Stoski DS, Soucy P. Permanent enteral feeding in cystic fibrosis: advantages of a replaceable jejunostomy tube. J Pediatr Surg 1987; 22:843–847.

61. Mansell AL, Muttart CR, Loeff DS, Heird WC. Short-term pulmonary effects of total parenteral nutrition in children with cystic fibrosis. J Pediatr 1984; 104:700–705.

62. Lester LA, Rothberg RM, Dawson G, Lopez AL, Corpuz Z. Supplemental parenteral nutrition in cystic fibrosis. J Parenter Enter Nutr 1986; 10:289–295.

63. Allen ED, Mick AB, Nicol J, McCoy KS. Prolonged parenteral nutrition for cystic fibrosis patients. Nutr Clin Pract 1995; 10:73–79.

64. Levy L, Durie P, Pencharz P, Corey M. Prognostic factors associated with patient survival during nutritional rehabilitation in malnourished children and adolescents with cystic fibrosis. J Pediatr Gastroenterol Nutr 1986; 5:97–102.

65. Robbins MK, Paradowski L, Thompson J. Nutritional status of cystic fibrosis patients before and after lung transplantation. Pediatr Pulmonol Suppl 1993; 9:273.

66. Nagy R, Mallory G. Efficacy of nutritional supplementation via nocturnal gastrostomy tube feedings in children and adolescents with cystic fibrosis awaiting lung transplantation. Pediatr Pulmonol Suppl 1993; 9:283.

67. Buzby GP, Mullen JL, Matthews DC, Hobbs CL, Rosato EF. Prognostic nutritional index in gastrointestinal surgery. Am J Surg 1980; 139:160–167.

68. Tamm M, Higenbottam T. Heart-lung and lung transplantation for cystic fibrosis: world experience. Semin Respir Criti Care Medi 1994; 15:414–425.

69. Memsic L, Silberman AW, Silberman H. Respiratory failure and malnutrition: what to do. J Respir Dis 1990; 11:693–701.

70. Fulton JA, Orenstein DM, Koehler AN, Kurland G. Nutrition in the pediatric double lung transplant patient with cystic fibrosis. Nutr Clin Pract 1995; 10:67–72.

71. Handwerger S, Roth J, Gorden P, di Sant'Agnese P, Carpenter DF, Peter G. Glucose intolerance in cystic fibrosis. N Engl J Med 1969; 281:451–461.

72. Cystic Fibrosis Foundation Consensus Conferences. Consensus Conference on CF-Related Diabetes Mellitus. January 11–12, 1990; Vol 1, Sec IV.

73. Lanng S, Thorsteinsson B, Erichsen G, Nerup J, Koch C. Glucose tolerance in cystic fibrosis. Arch Dis Child 1991; 66:612–616.
74. Reisman J, Corey M, Canny G, Levison H. Diabetes mellitus in patients with cystic fibrosis: effect on survival. Pediatrics 1990; 80:374–377.
75. Finkelstein SM, Wielinski CL, Elliot GR, et al. Diabetes mellitus associated with cystic fibrosis. J Pediatr 1988; 112:373–377.
76. Sullivan MM, Denning CR. Diabetic microangiopathy in patients with cystic fibrosis. Pediatrics 1989; 84:642–647.
77. Sheehan JP, Ulchaker MM, Doershuk CF, Stern RC, Amini SB. Diet, cystic fibrosis, and diabetes: making friends with the perfect enemy. Lancet 1990; 336:501.
78. Wilmshurst EG, Soeldner JS, Holsclaw DS, et al. Endogenous and exogenous insulin responses in patients with cystic fibrosis. Pediatrics 1975; 55:75–82.
79. Rosenstein BJ, Eigen H. Risks of alternate-day prednisone in patients with cystic fibrosis. Pediatrics 1991; 87:245–246.
80. Kane RE, Black P. Glucose intolerance with low-, medium-, and high-carbohydrate formulas during nighttime enteral feedings in cystic fibrosis patients. J Pediatr Gastroenterol Nutr 1989; 8:321–326.
81. Kessler WR, Andersen DH. Heat prostration in fibrocystic disease of the pancreas and other conditions. Pediatrics 1951; 8:648–656.
82. di Sant'Agnese PA, Darling RC, Perera GA, Shea E. Abnormal electrolyte composition of sweat in cystic fibrosis of the pancreas. Pediatrics 1953; 12:549–563.
83. Nussbaum E, Boat TF, Wood RE, Doershuk CF. Cystic fibrosis with acute hypoelectrolytemia and metabolic alkalosis in infancy. Am J Dis Child 1979; 133:965–966.
84. di Sant'Agnese P. Salt depletion in cold weather in infants with cystic fibrosis of the pancreas. JAMA 1960; 172:2014–2021.
85. Beckerman RC, Taussig LM. Hypoelectrolytemia and metabolic alkalosis in infants with cystic fibrosis. Pediatrics 1979; 63:580–583.
86. Kennedy JD, Dinwiddie R, Daman-Willems, C. Dillon MJ, Matthew DJ. Psuedo-Bartter's syndrome in cystic fibrosis. Arch Dis Child 1990; 65:786–787.
87. Laughlin JJ, Brady MS, Eigen H. Changing feeding trends as a cause of electrolyte depletion in infants with cystic fibrosis. Pediatrics 1981; 68:203–207.
88. Siegenthaler P, DeHaller J, DeHaller R, Hampai A, Muller AF. Effect of experimental salt depletion and aldosterone load on sodium and chloride concentration in the sweat of patients with cystic fibrosis of the pancreas and of normal children. Arch Dis Child 1964; 39:61–65.
89   Rapaport R, Levine LS, Petrovic M, et al. The renin-aldosterone system in cystic fibrosis. J Pediatr 1981; 98:768–771.
90. Orenstein DM, Henke KG, Costill DL, Doershuk CF, Lemon PJ, Stern RC. Exercise and heat stress in cystic fibrosis patients. Pediatr Res 1983; 17:267–269.
91. Bar-Or O, Blimkie CJR, Hay JA, MacDougall JD, Ward DS, Wilson WM. Voluntary dehydration and heat intolerance in cystic fibrosis. Lancet 1992; 339:696–699.
92. Cohen LF, di Sant'Agnese P, Taylor A, Gill JR. The syndrome of inappropriate antidiuretic hormone secretion as a cause of hyponatremia in cystic fibrosis. J Pediatr 1977; 90:574–578.
93. Orenstein SR, Orenstein DM. Magnesium deficiency in cystic fibrosis. South Med J 1983; 76:1586.

94. Green CG, Doershuk CF, Stern RC. Symptomatic hypomagnesemia in cystic fibrosis. J Pediatr 1985; 107:425–428.
95 Choi MJ, Fernandez PC, Patnaik A, et al. Brief report: trimethoprim-induced hyperkalemia in a patient with AIDS. N Engl J Med 1993; 328:703–706.

7

Cystic Fibrosis–Related Diabetes Mellitus

WILLIAM B. ZIPF

The Ohio State University
and Children's Hospital
Columbus, Ohio

I. Introduction

Cystic fibrosis–related diabetes mellitus (CFRDM) differs considerably from the more common forms of diabetes types I and II in its clinical course, genetics, and biochemical features. This chapter reviews the history, clinical features, biochemical abnormalities, possible cause, and therapy, particularly inpatient therapy, for CFRDM.

II. Historical Perspective

The association between CF and diabetes mellitus was first thought to be uncommon. Although Andersen reported a decrease in the number of islets of Langerhans in the pancreases of individuals with CF in 1938 (1), the first report of a case of diabetes in a CF patient did not appear until 1949 (2). In 1969, Handwerger et al. (3) and Milner (4) made important observations: serum insulin responses to oral glucose were decreased in all glucose-intolerant CF subjects they studied but the response could be augmented with tolbutamide or glucagon. The family histories, clinical characteristics, and postmortem signs of diabetes mellitus were absent. Because glucagon and tolbutamide were both capable of augmenting insulin release (3,4) and because the histological evaluation of the pancreas of individuals who had died with both CF and diabetes did not show the paucity of beta cells observed in the pancreases of patients with classic juvenile onset diabetes (3,4), both groups of investigators concluded that the increased incidence of diabetes in CF was not an independent second disease, but a consequence of CF itself.

III. Complications of Combined Cystic Fibrosis and Diabetes Mellitus

Insulin-dependent diabetes occurs in approximately 10% of all CF patients (5) and in as many as 30% of patients older than 25 years compared with an incidence of type I diabetes in the normal population of approximately 0.01%. Furthermore, 50%–75% of patients with CF have decreased insulin secretory capacity and impaired glucose tolerance. Even young children with CF with no evidence of overt diabetes have subnormal insulin responses to meal stimulation tests (6).

Most (7,8), but not all (9), studies suggest that diabetes has negative effects on both morbidity and mortality in CF. In one large study, fewer than 25% of the patients with CFRDM survived beyond the age of 30 years, whereas 60% of those without diabetes survived until at least 30 years of age (7). In another study, CF patients with diabetes had worse weights, body mass indices, and pulmonary function than matched control CF patients without diabetes, even years before the diabetic patients required insulin therapy (8). Insulin therapy narrows or may even close the gap in pulmonary function and nutritional status between those with and without diabetes (8).

In non-CF diabetes, chronic or intermittent hyperglycemia is associated with a significant loss of calories and some essential vitamins and trace elements, increased risk for infection, and small vessel disease, particularly affecting the kidney and retina. It appears that patients with CF and diabetes may be at risk for some of these same complications. One recent study of patients with CFRDM (10) showed a 21% incidence of microangiopathy. In this study, longer than 10 years of glucose intolerance and poor compliance with the diabetic care program was associated with a strong probability of diabetic complications (10). These complications will probably be seen more frequently as CF patients live longer.

Insulin deficiency can also have negative effects on metabolism and growth even when glycosuria is minimal. Uncontrolled diabetes is characterized by muscle wasting, fatigue, and impaired ability to respond to infections. In part, these changes are due to the absence of actions of insulin beyond that of controlling glucose. Insulin is a potent anabolic hormone and may promote the secretion of other peptides and proteins necessary for normal growth (11–14). Insulin controls amino acid uptake and is a direct stimulator of other growth factors and growth factor receptors. It also influences cellular protein metabolism by its effects on the sodium–proton pump. Partial or complete loss of these anabolic effects is apparent in classic type I (insulin deficient or juvenile onset) diabetes mellitus. Children with diabetes also have less than expected linear growth even with adequate insulin therapy (15).

Cystic fibrosis is characterized by a poor adaptation to protein-energy metabolism (16,17). It is reasonable to assume that insulin deficiency presents further metabolic complications for the already nutritionally deprived CF patient, even when the classical symptoms of diabetes have not yet occurred. Even though there are no long-term studies evaluating the effect of correcting the chronic insulin-deficient state with long-term supplemental insulin or oral hypoglycemic agents on growth and health of children with CF, two reports have shown improved growth and lean body mass in children with CF treated with the oral hypoglycemic agent tolbutamide (18,19). In one of these studies, the subject was diabetic (18), whereas, in the other, the subjects were not (19), Thus, there is accumulating theoretical and empirical evidence that the individual with CF has a high probability for insulin insufficiency throughout life and a significant risk for the development of diabetes mellitus. The insulin-deficient state may impair growth during childhood and place both the child and adult at a metabolic disadvantage. Progression of the insulin-deficient state to clinical diabetes mellitus appears to be associated with increased nutritional and pulmonary morbidity and mortality.

Diabetes complicates the management of CF. Independently, both diabetes and CF are complex illnesses to treat. Together, the therapeutic programs can be a formidable challenge. The onset of diabetes therapy confounds an already complicated and demanding treatment program, has conflicting therapeutic demands that must be integrated into a single program, and is associated with additional financial costs. In addition to the complications to the patient and family, there are additional demands placed on the care team. The primary team managing the patient needs to become familiar with the management of diabetes or must involve another team of specialists. Although the latter option has obvious advantages, a team of very good diabetologists and their dieticians and nurses may not have sufficient understanding of CF to manage the diabetes without frequent interactions with the CF team. If health care teams managing the patient are inconsistent and prescribe different and possibly conflicting therapies, the patient is not likely to adhere to any program. Trade-offs with respect to treatment plans and therapeutic goals are likely needed.

IV. Characteristics of Diabetes in the Patient with Cystic Fibrosis

The usual clinical picture, manners of presentation, and biochemical abnormalities of CFRDM are well known. The presentation can be with classical polyuria, polydipsia, weight loss, and exercise intolerance. To this extent, CFRDM is similar to both type I and type II diabetes. However, even though CFRDM is associated with a young age of onset, as is juvenile onset diabetes (type I diabetes mellitus), it is almost always nonketotic, has a slow, insidious onset, and glucose control is often maintained easily with very low doses of insulin, frequently less than 0.5 units/kg/day (37,38). Furthermore, CFRDM does not show either the inheritance pattern, genetic markers, or autoimmune markers of type I diabetes mellitus (22–24).

Whereas CFRDM does not occur as classical type I diabetes mellitus, it is also different from type II diabetes mellitus. Patients with CFRDM are not obese and rarely show evidence of severe insulin resistance, and they do not have the inheritance pattern for type II diabetes (22).

Before the onset of insulin dependency, the CF patient often has abnormal glucose homeostasis if stressed with corticosteroids, intravenous or enteral feedings, surgery, or pregnancy. Hyperglycemia may be mild or severe, but is rarely accompanied by ketonuria. Once the stress is resolved, fasting and after-meal glucose values usually return to normal. This pattern can repeat itself many times before the development of persistent diabetes when either insulin deficiency has progressed to a point at which the residual beta cells can no longer maintain euglycemia or the chronic stress of the disease creates sufficient insulin resistance to cause clinical symptoms of diabetes mellitus even though insulin secretory capacity has not changed significantly.

Cystic fibrosis does not protect against the development of either type I or type II diabetes. Thus, CF patients in whom either one of these more classical forms of the disease develops may need further modification of therapy.

Insulin secretion in the small number of CF patients with exocrine pancreatic sufficiency appears to be normal (21,25). However, insulin secretion patterns in patients with CF and exocrine insufficiency generally show abnormalities even when there is no clinical evidence for diabetes or biochemical evidence for either diabetes or glucose intolerance. The almost universal finding is a marked blunting of the early insulin release pattern after an oral (15–20 minutes) or intravenous (2–5 minutes) glucose challenge (26–32). We have seen this abnormality in children as young as 2 years of age (6,33). Insulin secretory responses are generally approximately 50% of normal (26–32). The general pattern is then for a progressive decline in insulin secretion with time (34). For approximately 10%–20% of CF patients, this leads to diabetes by the third decade of life. In rare instances, and for unknown reasons, mild to moderate hyperinsulinemia rather than hypoinsulinemia has developed (35,36).

Even though insulin deficiency is the rule, patients with CF still have normal or only slightly impaired glucose levels. This observation suggests an increase in both peripheral and hepatic insulin sensitivity. Some studies have found an increased number of insulin receptors on monocytes (37–39) of patients with CF—possibly inducing increased sensitivity—and others have shown an increased insulin suppressability of hepatic glucose output. Thus, the decrease in insulin secretion may be partly compensated for by increased sensitivity to insulin.

In contrast to the consistency for insulin secretion in CF patients, glucagon secretion can be normal, increased, or decreased. In the patient with normal glucose and insulin, glucagon secretion is generally normal (21,40).

When insulin deficiency develops in the CF patient, glucagon deficiency generally also occurs (21,25). When insulin secretory capacity has further deteriorated and fasting hyperglycemia is present, glucagon responses are exaggerated, as is typically seen in the non-CF diabetic patient.

V. Etiology of Insulin Deficiency Associated with Cystic Fibrosis

Insulin deficiency in the CF patient has generally been thought to be secondary to the loss of beta cells from pancreatic destruction and loss of normal islet cell architecture (2,3). The pancreas of the CF patient shows either the classic fibrotic changes of the exocrine pancreas with disruption of the islet cell architecture or, less commonly, a fatty infiltration of the pancreas (3,4) with fragmentation and isolation of the islet cells. There is a strong relationship between pancreatic destruction and insulin deficiency in both patients with and without CF, but this single explanation does not seem to be sufficient. The onset of diabetes as a consequence of pancreatic destruction is difficult to reconcile with a number of other observations. Most importantly, insulin-dependent diabetes develops in only 15%–20% of patients with CF, despite the majority having comparable degrees of exocrine insufficiency. Histological studies have generally been unable to correlate degree of fibrosis with glucose intolerance (3,42). Abdul-Karim et al. (42) showed in seven adult CF patients with insulin dependent diabetes that there remained 16%–47% (mean, 28%) of normal beta cell number. Patients with classical type I diabetes mellitus generally do not show clinical evidence of diabetes until their beta cell population is reduced to less than 10% of normal number. Although there is not a strong correlation between genotype and phenotype with respect to the occurrence of CFRDM, this complication may be somewhat more common in patients with the ΔF508 genotype (43). Genetic studies to determine whether there is a genetic linkage between

CFRDM and type I or type II disease have not uncovered such a linkage (44). Other possible causes of diabetes may relate to other elements of the disease or even to current therapy. In non-CF settings, nutritional forms of diabetes have been well described (45). In some retrospective human studies (46) and in animal studies (47), it has been shown that protein–calorie malnutrition, even when transient, can predispose the subject to insulin deficiency. No study has been done to determine whether there is a relationship between the development of diabetes and the nutritional state of the individual during infancy and childhood. Other possible factors that might be involved in beta cell destruction or that could interfere with normal insulin release include acute and chronic deficiencies of essential fatty acids (48), potassium (49), and trace elements known to be important in insulin secretion such as zinc (50), magnesium, and manganese. Any one or a combination of these factors might partially determine in which patients CFRDM develops.

VI. Screening and Diagnosis

Patients with CF should be asked routinely whether they are experiencing symptoms of diabetes such as polyuria, polydipsia, nocturia, weight loss, and decreased exercise tolerance. However, because CFRDM can be slow in onset, these symptoms might appear so gradually that they are not recognized by the patient. The recommended screening guidelines as outlined by the Cystic Fibrosis Consensus Conference on CFRDM (51) include routine urinalysis two to three times a year and fasting and 2-hour postprandial glucose determinations once every 2 to 4 years during late childhood and at least every 2 years during and after adolescence.

It is also suggested that, during the patient's hospitalizations, fasting and 2-hour postprandial glucose checks be obtained as part of the initial evaluation. Many patients are hospitalized for intravenous antibiotic therapy, intensified pulmonary therapy, and intensified nutritional therapy one or more times a year. During those hospitalizations, the patient is under increased stress because of infections, corticosteroid therapy, increased enteral or parenteral feedings, or any combination of these factors. All may increase insulin requirements and thus unmask a patient with suboptimal insulin secretion or even overt diabetes mellitus. Fasting or postprandial hyperglycemia under these circumstances may be transient and require either only short-term therapy or no therapy at all. By the time of the patient's discharge, normal fasting and postprandial glucose concentrations may have been reestablished, even without low-sugar diets, oral hypoglycemics, or insulin. However, such patients still need to be identified as individuals at risk and should be followed at 6-month to 1-year intervals with more definitive glucose tolerance testing.

The use of glycosylated hemoglobin concentrations has not been found to be adequate for screening for either type I or type II diabetes mellitus, but is used by some clinicians to help rule out CFRDM (52–54). It does appear to be useful for following patients with CFRDM. However, the levels often accepted as reflecting reasonable control in the adolescent with diabetes mellitus (i.e., 8.0%–10.0%), which tend to be more liberal than the levels used in adults with diabetes mellitus (7.0%–9.0%), should not be used for the patient with CFRDM. The patient with CFRDM is not prone to ketoacidosis and is generally much more sensitive to insulin. The adolescent with CFRDM rarely experiences the marked swings in blood glucose that are common in the non-CF adolescent patient with diabetes mellitus. As a consequence of these differences between the adolescent with CFRDM and type I diabetes mellitus, the patient with CFRDM can achieve a glycosylated hemoglobin value in a range considered as evidence of acceptable control for the type I diabetes patient (7.0%–9.0%) with little effort and very small doses of insulin. In practice, additional effort and greater doses of insulin with corresponding increases in insulin anabolic effects and appetite-stimulating effects could easily be achieved and would be associated with normal or near-normal glycosylated hemoglobin values.

VII. Diagnosis of Diabetes in Patients with Cystic Fibrosis

The definition of diabetes in a patient with CF is not different from that in a non-CF individual, although confirming the diagnosis is not always as straightforward. The definitive diagnosis of diabetes is based on the National Diabetes Data Group criteria for the standard oral glucose tolerance test. This test includes the administration of 1.75 g of dextrose per kilogram of body weight (maximum dose, 75 g) as an oral challenge. The test is standardized to the non-diabetic, healthy individual who has been ambulatory, is adequately nourished, and has received at least 150 g of carbohydrate daily for the previous 3 days. In practice, however, the diagnosis is often made and treatment instituted on purely clinical grounds. If a glucose tolerance test is used, interpretation of the glucose response requires adjustment for age. These criteria are presented in Table 1.

In occasional patients with atypical clinical presentation or unexpected glucose tolerance test results, additional testing (e.g., islet cell antibody studies) may be needed. By chance alone, ketotic-prone type I diabetes mellitus or type II diabetes mellitus is expected to develop in some CF patients. Family history, documentation of ketosis, and the presence of elevated insulin levels or islet cell antibodies are of value in differentiating these types from CFRDM.

VIII. Treatment of the Patient with Cystic Fibrosis and Diabetes

The challenge to developing a therapeutic program for the CF patient in whom diabetes develops is that classical therapies for diabetes mellitus are at odds with many of the therapies for CF (Table 2).

Table 1 Serum Glucose Responses to Oral Glucose Tolerance Tests (mg/dL)

	Fasting	0.5 h	1.0 h	1.5 h	2.0 h	Urine ketones
Normal adult	<115	<200	<200	<200	<140	
Normal prepubertal child	<130				≤140	
Glucose intolerance	<140	≥200[a]	≥200[a]	≥200[a]	140–200	
Diabetes mellitus type II (nonketotic) adult[b]	≥140		≥200		≥200	Negative
Diabetes mellitus type I (ketotic) adult[c]	≥140	≥200	≥200	≥200	≥200	Positive
Diabetes mellitus type I (ketotic) prepubertal child[d]	≥140	≥200	≥200	≥200	≥200	Positive
Abnormal, but not diagnostic[e]	115–140	≥200	≥200	≥200	≤140	

[a]0.5 h, 1 h, or 1.5 h at this level
[b]Fasting levels as listed on at least two occasions and/or 1-h and 2-h values as listed
[c]Fasting levels as listed on at least two occasions and/or 0.5-h, 1-h, and 2-h values and urine as listed or fasting levels as listed and 2-h levels and urine as listed
[d]Fasting, 0.5 h, 1 h, or 1.5 h as listed or fasting, 2-h levels and urine as listed
[e]Fasting as listed; 0.5 h, 1 h, or 1.5 h as listed; 2 h as listed

In diabetes management, achieving weight loss or preventing excess weight gain is preferred, whereas, in CF management, weight gain is preferred. In diabetes, insulin is used for glucose control, whereas, in CF, insulin is used for glucose control and for its anabolic effects. Nutritional recommendations for diabetes emphasize a low-fat, simple-sugar diet, as opposed to the diet for CF, which often works toward increasing fat and allowing or encouraging ad lib

Table 2 Contrast of Treatment Goal for CF and Diabetes

	CF	Diabetes
Weight	Weight gain	Weight loss
Energy intake	100%–200% Recommended daily allowance (RDA)	≤RDA
Fat	30%–40% of Calories	<30% of Calories
Monosaccharides and disaccharides	Limited or no concentrated sweets	Limited or no intake
Meals	Frequent, when hungry	Tightly scheduled
Salt	Encouraged, especially in hot weather	Low intake
Insulin	Adequate control of blood sugar; push dose as tolerated to use anabolic effects	Tight control of blood sugar

simple sugars in the diet to promote weight gain. The diabetes diet encourages establishing a routine and tightly scheduled meal plan, whereas, in CF, patients are encouraged to "eat frequently, when you have time or are hungry." The approach to diabetes management over the last decade has been one of adding increasing complexity to day-to-day living schedules (frequent glucose testing, multiple insulin injections, strict meal planing, scheduled exercise) to reduce the potential for diabetes-related complications; however, the already complex lifestyle of the CF patient necessitates that every effort be made to simplify the elements of therapy.

The philosophy of diabetes management has been to "look ahead" and maintain strict glucose control to prevent long-term complications. There is some controversy as to whether to apply this principle to CF. Some clinicians feel that the more limited longevity of CF patients tends to suggest that, in respect to the nonfatal medical problems, attention to more immediate goals with correspondingly less concern for 20- to 30-year complications might be the better approach. This is particularly important if additional diabetes therapies decrease attention to pulmonary care. However, as the prognosis for patients with CF improves and the possibility of an outright cure becomes imaginable, other clinicians feel that the CFRDM patient should also be treated with a "look-ahead" approach. This may include multiple daily injections of regular insulin. Currently, there is relatively little known about the outcome of treatment of CFRDM to help guide choices.

As a consequence of the diametrically opposed therapeutic approaches to CF and diabetes, the CFRDM treatment program must have predefined goals based on a clear understanding of the patient's condition. The overall goals are to eliminate the diabetes symptoms, allow optimal growth, weight gain, and resistance to infection, and to accomplish this with a program acceptable to the patient.

Patients with CF may have many degrees of glucose homeostasis problems, from only an occasional elevated serum glucose to overt symptomatic diabetes. This variability is a consequence of the size of the individual's pancreatic beta cell population, adjunctive therapies, and metabolic stress factors that affect tissue insulin sensitivity and hepatic glucose output. The following discussion of treatment of the various CFRDM situations often applies to the inpatient setting.

A. Treating Transient Diabetes in the CF Patient

Most patients with CF have no metabolic difficulties in handling stress. Some patients without overt diabetes, however, have elevations in the serum glucose values at times of substantial illness or stress. Such stress-associated glucose intolerance could be due to any one or combination of factors including (1) a "sluggish pancreas" from chronic decreased caloric intake, (2) reduction in functional beta cell number or responsiveness, (3) insulin resistance from infection and stress, (4) corticosteroid therapy, (5) parenteral nutrition with high glucose concentrations, (6) enteral tube feedings, (7) pregnancy, or (8) surgery. Short-term insulin therapy should be considered for these patients if daily fasting glucose values are consistently more than 140 mg/dL or the 2-hour postprandial values are greater than 180 mg/dL. Short-term therapy, lasting a few days or weeks, is usually most easily implemented as multiple injections of short-acting regular insulin. The usual daily dose ranges from 0.1 to 0.3 units/kg/24 h given as three to four divided doses before meals and before bedtime. Elevated temperature, sepsis, or high-dose corticosteroid treatment necessitates greater doses (0.5–1.0 units/kg/day). For patients on alternate-day corticosteroids, an increase in the dose may be required on the dosing days, but if the doses are very high, there may be minimal difference in the insulin dose between days on and off. Corticosteroids should always be tapered and discontinued as rapidly as possible. Patients without prior glucose problems usually return to a euglycemic state after resolution of the stress, and the insulin can be discontinued. However, these individuals are at greater risk for development of diabetes at a later date and require close follow-up with repeated oral glucose tolerance test (OGTT) at 6-month to 1-year intervals.

B. Treating Persistent Diabetes Mellitus in the CF Patient

A greater reduction in functional beta cell number or responsiveness leads to persistent glucose intolerance or diabetes as defined by OGTT. Continuous, long-term therapy of diabetes should be started when the diagnosis of diabetes is made using standardized criteria, when the 2-hour postprandial glucose values are repeatedly more than 180 mg/dL while the patient is in a usual state of health, or when persistent impaired glucose tolerance is associated with weight loss or absent weight gain in the undernourished patient. Instituting the treatment program is best done in the hospital.

The onset of diabetes forces difficult decisions concerning management strategies. These difficulties arise because CFRDM is different from the two main types of diabetes mellitus. Furthermore, the treatment program for CF has requirements that appear to be contradictory to those of diabetes (see Table 2), and, finally, the addition of a second chronic illness can complicate the already stressed life of the patient. Nonetheless, a rational approach should lead to improved health and well being. As with other forms of diabetes, treatment for CFRDM includes (1) insulin injections (or, in rare cases, oral hypoglycemic agents), (2) dietary measures, and (3) routine monitoring of the response to these therapies. However, the differences between CFRDM and other forms of diabetes suggest modifications of the traditional approaches. The goal of therapy is to achieve optimal metabolic conditions for cellular function and normal growth while avoiding hypoglycemia and keeping the patient's overall medical regimen as simple as possible.

Insulin Therapy (and Oral Hypoglycemic Agents)

Insulin therapy generally includes twice-daily (before breakfast and before dinner) standard combinations of intermediate- and short-acting insulins. A typical starting dose schedule is presented in Table 3. However, nontraditional insulin dose types and schedules, such as regular insulin only before each meal or ultralente Humulin with regular insulin before each meal, may occasionally be useful. A few patients may be able to achieve adequate glucose control with a single injection of intermediate-acting insulin in the morning. However, this approach albeit convenient in its simplicity, is seldom appropriate because a single injection increases the risk of late afternoon hypoglycemia. Because hypoglycemia is uncomfortable, patients often decrease their dose to prevent these afternoon episodes, thereby receiving inadequate insulin the rest of the day. It should be understood that a regimen can be tried for a few months and discarded if the results are unsatisfactory.

Teaching patients to adjust their own insulin doses is a major goal of the education program. Adolescent and adult patients often adjust their insulin doses, whether they have been so instructed or not. If the patient does not understand self-management, dangerous dose errors may occur. These errors may not come to the physician's attention because of patient reluctance to share information on self-initiated treatment. Patients must also be competent in adjusting their insulin dose so they can accommodate prescribed use of diet supplements or more frequent and larger meals.

Home blood glucose monitoring is essential for rational adjustment of insulin doses. For most patients with CFRDM, a glucose check (fasting) in the morning and another 1 to 2 hours after a regular meal are needed for optimal

Table 3 Treatment of CF-Related Diabetes

Transient diabetes
    Short-acting regular insulin 0.1–0.3 units/kg/24 h, given in 3–4 divided doses (If the patient is taking daily steroids, 0.5–1.0 units/kg/24 h may be needed; if the patient is taking alternate-day steroids, a higher dose on steroid days may be needed.)
Persistent diabetes
    Combined short- and intermediate-acting insulins, total starting dose 0.3–0.5 units/kg/24 h in 2 doses: 2/3 of total before breakfast, 1/3 before dinner; 2/3 of each dose is regular insulin, 1/3 is intermediate-acting neutral protamine Hagedorn (NPH) or lente
    Sample starting dose for 50-kg patient
        Before breakfast: 7 units regular and 3 units NPH
        Before dinner: 3 units regular and 2 NPH

monitoring of glucose control. If the patient is stable and the test times are varied, only two tests need be obtained daily.

When the patient is given either enteral tube or intravenous feedings, additional insulin is needed to maintain euglycemia. For enteral feeding, multiple subcutaneous doses of regular insulin, intermediate-acting insulin, or long-acting insulin can be used. For parenteral feedings, insulin can be added to the solution just before its administration. The usual dose is 1 unit of insulin for each 4–8 g of carbohydrate, although this can vary among patients. This method has the potential safety advantage that, if the nutrient line is compromised, the patient does not receive the extra insulin, and it is more simple in that it does not require an added insulin infusion control pump. However, a separate insulin drip "piggy backed" into the hyperalimentation line can be used during the first few days to determine the insulin dose required for the rate of nutrient administration, or it can be continued for the entire course of therapy and is preferred in some centers because of the added level of glucose control that can be achieved.

The goals of treatment include weight gain, normal growth, elimination of symptoms of diabetes, and control of blood glucose levels. In diabetic CF patients, even those with a markedly abnormal glucose tolerance profile, fasting glucose values may be normal or near normal. Normal or near-normal glucose levels can be achieved with minimal doses of supplemental insulin, but achieving these levels should not be the only or even the main goal of control. Attempting to use minimal doses of insulin as a primary therapeutic goal deprives the patient of an important growth factor. As discussed, because the patient with CF is insulin deficient and insulin has significant anabolic effects, the dose of insulin should be increased to the amount that is comfortably tolerated without hypoglycemic symptoms. Most patients tolerate 0.5–1.0 units/kg/day. This dose is often 2–3 times greater than the insulin dose needed for what is usually considered adequate glucose control. However, as the insulin dose is increased, the patient and support team must be careful to monitor for potentially dangerous hypoglycemia. With a cooperative, well-prepared, and supported patient, control can often be titrated to achieve normal fasting glucose values, 2-hour postprandial glucose values of less than 140 mg/dL, rare episodes of mild to moderate hypoglycemia, and near-normal or normal glycosylated hemoglobin concentrations. Further support for the importance of insulin therapy, even if patients could "sqeak by" with normal or near-normal glucose levels, is found in a Danish study (55) that showed that insulin therapy closed the gaps between diabetic and nondiabetic CF patients with regard to anthropometrics and pulmonary function. Repeated evaluations on a regular basis, usually once every 3 to 4 months, must be maintained as part of the schedule so that trends in glucose control can be detected early and appropriate adjustments be made in the treatment program.

Table 4 Symptoms of Hypoglycemia

Shakiness
Sweating
Tachycardia
Hunger
Drowsiness

It is essential for any patient who is taking insulin to be taught to self-monitor for hypoglycemia by recognizing characteristic symptoms (Table 4). Confirmation of hypoglycemia should be made by blood glucose monitoring. Patients with CFRDM tend to be more prone to hypoglycemia because glucagon deficiency frequently accompanies the insulin deficiency and because of a tendency toward increased peripheral insulin sensitivity.

In the CF patient with impaired glucose tolerance of diabetes with glucose elevations that rarely exceed 250 mg/dL, a trial of an oral hypoglycemic agent may be reasonable. However, even if there is initial success, it is probable that subcutaneous insulin will be required during times of stress (Table 5). The patient should be informed at the onset of treatment that eventual drug failure is common with these agents.

Nutritional Management of the Patient with CFRDM

In rare well-nourished patients whose body weights are near or better than 100% ideal for age and height, CFRDM can be managed by diet alone. Even in these patients, insulin therapy is likely to be needed eventually.

Diet recommendations in CFRDM may need to be modified from the program usually implemented for type I or type II diabetes. An important goal of therapy in CFRDM, second only to alleviating the classical symptoms of diabetes, is promoting normal weight gain and prevention of weight loss. Tight glucose control is important, but not at the cost of weight loss or decreased weight gain because of a difficult meal schedule or decreased palatability of the

Table 5 Stresses that May Worsen Glucose Control in CF Patients

Severe pulmonary infection
Fever
Corticosteroid therapy
Enteral tube feedings
Pregnancy
Sepsis

diet. As a consequence, the diet program of the child or adult with CFRDM must be an amalgam of the traditional programs used separately for diabetes and CF.

The traditional goals for optimal nutritional management of non-CF diabetes mellitus include (1) avoidance of prolonged hyperglycemia (2) avoidance of hypoglycemia, (3) avoidance of hyperlipidemia, (4) maintenance of ideal body weight for height with avoidance of obesity, and (5) avoidance of possible long-term nephrotic complications of a high-protein diet. The diet plans used to achieve these goals generally (1) allow for no more than normal weight gain in the child and achievement of a normal weight in the adult (which most often requires a decrease in usual caloric intake) and (2) limit both simple sugars and fats to reduce long-term complications of diabetes.

In contrast, the dietary plan for the nondiabetic patient with CF often focuses on increasing energy stores by using highly palatable simple sugars and calorically dense fats. Thus, some compromises need to be made. In respect to total energy intake, the priority should be to maintain normal to slightly above normal stores and to meet the higher than usual energy requirement that occurs in the patient with CF. Thus, the guidelines for total caloric intake in CFRDM are not different from those for the typical CF patient, namely, 100% to 200% of the recommended daily allowance.

To achieve the high caloric intake needed for CF, the proportion of total fat is increased from the 30% or less recommended for diabetes to 30%–40%. To maintain palatability, simple sugars are not routinely excluded from the diet of the patient with CFRDM. To maintain glucose control, however, these are limited to meals at which their impact on blood sugar is mitigated by the digestion of other food items and are covered by premeal regular insulin. High-calorie snacks with high concentration of monosaccharides or disaccharides are avoided, and all snacks should include a mix of macronutrients and complex carbohydrates.

The meal plan for both diabetes mellitus and CF is similar in that both include three meals and three snacks. However, with CFRDM, it is critical that these be maintained on a tight schedule and that the quantity of the meal is constant to ensure that the caloric load is matched to the insulin absorption pattern.

As with insulin therapy, nutritional management must include detailed consideration of the patient, the manifestations of the CF, and the manifestations of the diabetes. Traditionally, the nutritional management of CF requires consideration of the pulmonary status, current nutritional deficit, and the need for exocrine enzyme replacement. The patient's glucose control status needs to be assessed in a similar fashion. This includes the characterization of glucose intolerance (transient or persistent), the type of therapy being used (single, multiple, combined insulin injections, or oral therapy), the severity of the hyperglycemia on glucose control treatment, and the frequency and severity of any hypoglycemia on glucose control therapy. For both conditions, each individual must be evaluated for adjunctive problems such as liver disease, bowel disease, need for steroids, and any complicating conditions such as acute infections or pregnancy.

Meal planning should continue to be based on the nutritional requirements and practice needed for optimal health of the child, adolescent, or adult with CF. Diet modifications for CFRDM include more regularly scheduled meals, more consistency in meal size and composition, and elimination of snacks with a high simple sugar content as the primary source of calories. Moderate amounts of such items could still be allowed into the regular meal as a dessert if given on a routine basis such that the caloric load could be offset by an appropriate adjustment in the insulin dose. Including the dessert in each meal should allow for sufficient consistency that the 1- and 2-hour postprandial glucose checks can be used to determine how well the insulin is matched to the calories. Including these simple sugar items at the end of the meal allows additional time for the regular portion of the insulin dose given 20 minutes before the meal to be absorbed and available to handle the glucose load.

Monitoring Glucose Control in CFRDM

Glucose control should be monitored in patients with CFRDM by symptoms and by objective measurement of glucose levels. Patients must be taught to recognize the signs and symptoms of hypoglycemia (see Table 4) and its treatment. They should also check blood glucose levels by finger stick blood samples and glucometer before meals and at bedtime.

The diagnosis of a second major chronic illness may create serious psychological problems that require attention from experienced support staff. Psychological and psychosocial support for these patients must be available. Anticipatory counseling and monitoring of the patient's psychological health is necessary to deal with depression or denial of the disease processes and possible alienation from the medical program.

Available data and experience are still insufficient to allow a clear understanding of the long-term implications of insulin deficiency and abnormal glucose homeostasis or the impact of aggressive treatment of these problems on the overall health of the CF patient. There is a need to evaluate the effects of these therapeutic recommendations and alternatives (e.g., oral hypoglycemic agents). Important variables to study include not only glucose control but also growth, adolescent development, progression of other elements of the CF disease complex, and complications of long-standing hyperglycemia and insulin deficiency as well as the effects of therapy on the general well being of the patient.

References

1. Anderson DH. Cystic fibrosis of the pancreas and its relation to celiac disease. Am J Dis Child 1938; 56:344–399.
2. Anfanger H, Bass M, Heavenrich R, Bookman JJ. Pancreatic achylia and glycosuria due to cystic fibrosis of the pancreas in a 9 year old child. J Pediatr 1949; 35:151–164.
3. Handwerger S, Roth J, Gorden P, di Sant'Agnese P, Carpenter DF, Peter G. Glucose intolerance in cystic fibrosis. N Engl J Med 1969; 281:451–460.
4. Milner AD. Blood glucose and serum insulin levels in children with cystic fibrosis. Arch Dis Child 1969; 44:351–355.
5. Lanng S, Thorsteinsson B, Erichsen G, Nerup J, Koch C. Glucose tolerance in cystic fibrosis. Arch Dis Child 1991; 66:612–616.
6. Zipf WB, McCoy K, O'Dorisio TM. Effects on glucose and insulin of GIP normalization by exocrine replacement in cystic fibrosis. Pediatr Res 1986; 337A.
7. Finkelstein SM, Wielinski CL, Elliott GR, Warwick JB, Wu S, Klein DJ. Diabetes mellitus associated with cystic fibrosis. J Pediatr 1988; 112:373–377.
8. Lanng S, Thorsteinsson B, Nerup J, Koch C. Influence of the development of diabetes mellitus on clinical status in patients with cystic fibrosis. Eur J Pediatr 1992; 151:684–687.
9. Reisman J, Corey M, Canny G, Levison H. Diabetes mellitus in patients with cystic fibrosis: effect on survival. Pediatrics 1990; 86:374–377.
10. Sullivan MM, Denning CR. Diabetic microangiopathy in patients with cystic fibrosis. Pediatrics 1989; 84:642–647.
11. Straus DS. Growth-stimulatory actions of insulin in vitro in vivo. Endocr Rev 1984; 5:356–69.
12. Heinze E, Beischer W, Teller WM. Insulin secretion in growth hormone deficient children and the effect of the sulfonyluria drug glibenclamide on linear growth. Eur J Pediatr 1978; 128:41–48.
13. Van Wyk JJ, Underwood LE, Hintz RL, Clemmans DR, Voina SJ, Weaver RP. The somatomedins: a family of insulin like hormones under growth hormone control. Recent Prog Horm Res 1974; 30:259–318.
14. Costin G, Kogurt MD, Philipps LS, Daughaday WH. Craniopharyngioma: the role of insulin in promoting postoperative growth. J Clin Endocrinol Metab 1976; 42:370–379.
15. Tattersol RB, Pyke DK. Growth of diabetic children: studies in identical twins. Lancet 1973; II:1105–1108.
16. Miller M, Ward LC, Thomas BJ, Cooksley WGE, Shephered RW. Altered body composition and muscle protein degradation in children with cystic fibrosis. Am J Clin Nutr 1982; 36:492–499.
17. Hubbard VS. Nutrient requirements of patients with cystic fibrosis. In: Sturgess JM, ed. Perspective in Cystic Fibrosis. Proceedings of the Eighth International Cystic Fibrosis Congress. Toronto: Canadian Cystic Fibrosis Foundation, 1980:149–160.
18. Peden VH, Powell KR, Rejent AJ. Glucose intolerance in a three year old child with cystic fibrosis. Clin Pediatr 1974; 13:10–15.
19. Zipf WB, Kien CL, Horswill CA, McCoy KS, O'Dorisio T, Pinyerd BL. Effects of tolbutamide on growth and body composition of nondiabetic children with cystic fibrosis. Pediatr Res 1991; 30:309–314.

20. Hayes FJ, O'Brian A, Obrien C, Fitzgerald MX, McKenna MJ. Diabetes mellitus in an adult cystic fibrosis population. Irish Med J 1995; 88:102–104.
21. Moran A, Pyzdrowski KL, Weinreb J, Kahn BB, Smith SA, Adams KS, Seaquist ER. Insulin sensitivity in cystic fibrosis. Diabetes 1994; 43:1020–1026.
22. Lanng S, Thorsteinsson B, Pociot F, Marshall MO, Madsen HO, Schwartz M, Nerup J, Loch C. Diabetes mellitus in cystic fibrosis: genetic and immunological markers. Acta Paediatr 1993; 82:150–154.
23. Stutchfield PR, O'Halloran SM, Smith CS, Woodrow JC, Bottazzo GF, Heaf D. HLA type, islet cell antibodies and glucose intolerance in cystic fibrosis. Arch Dis Child 1988; 63:1234–1239.
24. Cucinotta D, Nibali SC, Arrigo T, Di Benedetto A, Magazzu G, Di Cesare E, Costantino A, Pezzino V, De Luca F. Beta cell function, peripheral sensitivity to insulin and islet cell autoimmunity in cystic fibrosis patients with normal glucose tolerance. Horm Res 1990; 34:33–38.
25. Moran A, Diem P, Klein DJ, Levitt MD, Robertson RP. Pancreatic endocrine function in cystic fibrosis. J Pediatr 1991; 118:715–723.
26. Cucinotta JD, De Luca F, Arriago T, Di Benedetto A, Sferlazzas, C, Gigante A, Rigoli L, Magazzu G. First phase insulin response to intravenous glucose in cystic fibrosis patients with different degrees of glucose tolerance. J Pediatr Endocr 1994; 7:13–17.
27. Hamdi I, Green M, Shneerson JM, Palmer CR, Hales CN. Proinsulin, proinsulin intermediate and insulin in cystic fibrosis. Clin Endocrinol 1993; 38:21–6.
28. Mohan V, Alagappan V, Snehalatha C, Ramachandran A, Thiruvengadam KV, Viswanathan M. Insulin and C-peptide responses to glucose load in cystic fibrosis. Diabetes Metab 1985; 11:376–379.
29. Adrian TE, McKiernan J, Johnstone DI, Hiller EJ, Vyas H, Sarson DL, Bloom SR. Hormonal abnormalities of the pancreas and gut in cystic fibrosis. Gastroenterology 1980; 79:460–465.
30. Hinds A, Sheehan AG, Machida H, Parsons HG. Postprandial hyperglycemia and pancreatic function in cystic fibrosis patients. Diabetes Res 1991; 18:69–78.
31. De Schepper, J, Hachimi-Idrissi S, Smitz J, Dab I, Loeb M. First-phase insulin release in adult cystic fibrosis patients: correlation with clinical and biological parameters. Horn Res 1992; 38:260–263.
32. Holl RW, Heinze E, Wolf A, Rank M, Teller WM. Reduced pancreatic insulin release and reduced peripheral insulin sensitivity contribute to hyperglycaemia in cystic fibrosis. Eur J Pediatr 1995; 154:356–361.
33. Kjellman N-IM. Larsson Y. Insulin release in cystic fibrosis. Arch Dis Child 1975; 50:205–209.
34. Lanng S, Thorsteinsson, B, Erichsen G, Nerup J, Koch C. Glucose tolerance in cystic fibrosis. Arch Dis Child 1991; 66:612–616.
35. Lippe BM, Sperling MA, Dooley RR. Pancreatic alpha and beta cell function in cystic fibrosis. J Pediatr 1977; 90:751–755.
36. Geffner ME, Lippe BM, Kaplan SA, Itami RM, Gillard BK, Levin SR, Taylor IT. Carbohydrate tolerance in cystic fibrosis is closely linked to pancreatic exocrine function. Pediatr Res 1984; 18:1107–1111.
37. Cucinotta D, Nibali SC, Arrigo T, Di Benedetto A, Magazzu G, Di Cesare E, Costantino A, Pezzino V, De Luca F. Beta cell function, peripheral sensitivity to insulin and islet cell autoimmunity in cystic fibrosis patients with normal glucose tolerance. Horm Res 1990; 34:33–38.

38. Lippe BM, Kaplan SA, Neufeld ND, Smith A, Scott M. Insulin receptors in cystic fibrosis: increased receptor number and altered affinity. Pediatrics 1980; 65:1018 1022.

39. Andersen O, Garne S, Heilmann C, Perersen KE, Petersen W, Loch C. Glucose tolerance and insulin receptor binding to monocytes and erythrocytes in patients with cystic fibrosis. Acta Paediatr Scand 1988; 77:67–71.

40. Ahmad T, Nelson R, Taylor R. Insulin sensitivity and metabolic clearance rate of insulin in cystic fibrosis. Metabolism 1994; 43:163–167.

41. Lohr M, Goertchen, P, Nizze H, Gould NS, Oberholzer M, Heitz PU, Kloppel G. Cystic fibrosis associated islet changes may provide a basis for diabetes: an immunocytochemical and morphometrical study. Virchows Arch A Pathol Anat Histopathol 1989; 414:179–185.

42. Abdul-Karim FJW, Dahms BB, Velasco ME, Rodman HM. Islets of Langerhans in adolescents and adults with cystic fibrosis. Arch Pathol Lab Med 1986; 110:602.

43. Rosenecker J, Eichler I, Kuhn L, Harms HK, von der Hardt H. Genetic determination of diabetes mellitus in patients with cystic fibrosis. J. Pediatr 1995; 127:441–443.

44. Lanng, S, Schwartz M, Thorsteinsson B, Koch C. Endocrine and exocrine pancreatic function and the delta F508 mutation in cystic fibrosis. Clin Genet 1991; 40:345–348.

45. Rao RH. Diabetes in the undernourished: coincidence or consequence? Endocr Rev 1988; 9:67–87.

46. James WPT, Coore HG. Persistent impairment of insulin secretion and glucose tolerance after malnutrition. Am J Clin Nutr 1970; 23:382–394.

47. Dixit PK, Sorenson RL. Effect of protein malnutrition on insulin secretion. Indian J Med Res 1987; 86:663–670.

48. Opara EC, Burch W, Hubbard VS, Akwari OE. Enhancement of endocrine pancreatic secretions by essential fatty acids. J Surg Res 1990; 48:329–332.

49. Becker DJ, Mann MK, Weinkove E, Pimstone BL. Early insulin release and its response to potassium supplementation in protein calorie malnutrition. Diabetologia 1975; 11:237–242.

50. Anderson RA, Polansky MM, Bryden NA, Roginski EE, Mertz W, Glinsman W. Chromium supplementation of human subjects: effects on glucose, insulin and lipid variables. Metabolism 1983; 32:894–895.

51 Cystic Fibrosis Foundation Consensus Conference. Concepts in care: CF Related Diabetes Mellitus. Vol. I. Section IV. Bethesda, MD: Cystic Fibrosis Foundation, 1990.

52. Bistritzer T, Sack J, Eshkol A, Katznelson D. Hemoglobin A1 and pancreatic beta cell function in cystic fibrosis. Isr J Med Sci 1983; 19:600–603.

53. Mulherin D, Ward K, Coffey M, Keogan MT, FitzGerald M. Cystic fibrosis in adolescents and adults. Ir Med J 1991; 84:121–124.

54. DeLuca F, Arriago T, Conti Nibali S, Sferlazzas C, Gigante A, Di Cesare E, Cucinotta D. Insulin secretion, glycosylated haemoglobin and islet cell antibodies in cystic fibrosis children and adolescents with different degrees of glucose tolerance. Horm Metab Res 1991; 23:495–498.

55. Lanng S, Thorsteinsson B, Nerup J, Koch C. Diabetes mellitus in cystic fibrosis: effect of insulin therapy on lung function and infections. Acta Paediatrica 1994; 83:849–853.

8

Thoracic Surgery for Patients with Cystic Fibrosis

THOMAS M. EGAN

University of North Carolina School of Medicine
Chapel Hill, North Carolina

Indications for thoracic surgery for patients with cystic fibrosis (CF) can be regarded as surgical therapy for conditions unrelated to cystic fibrosis and surgical therapy for consequences of the disease. The incidence of congenital heart disease or other non-CF conditions requiring thoracic surgery is the same for patients with CF as it is for the general population, and the general principles for perioperative management suffice for these clinical situations. This chapter focuses on conditions arising from the diagnosis of CF for which thoracic surgery has a role in management. These clinical problems are summarized in Table 1.

I. Principles of Perioperative Management for Patients with CF

Certain aspects of perioperative management are common to all patients undergoing thoracic surgery, but there are items that should be specifically emphasized for patients with CF.

A. Preoperative Issues

Avoidance of accumulation of airway secretions should begin preoperatively, with planned chest physical therapy and postural drainage before elective

Table 1 Indications for Thoracic Surgery for Consequences of CF

Consequence of CF	Indications for surgery
Pleural processes	
Pneumothorax	First persistent pneumothorax
	Ipsilateral recurrent pneumothorax
Empyema	Persistent undrained pleural space collection with evidence of infection
Parenchymal lung disease	
Hemoptysis	Failure of bronchial artery embolization to control major hemoptysis
	Major hemoptysis from a lobe or segment that is essentially destroyed
	Major hemoptysis associated with cavitary lung disease
Bronchiectasis	Severe bronchiectasis limited largely to one lobe or segment, with evidence of ongoing symptoms (e.g., copious purulent secretions, recurrent infections) without other major areas of parenchymal disease

procedures. For patients in the midst of a pulmonary exacerbation, elective procedures should be postponed. For patients who are particularly debilitated, serious consideration should be given to participation in a preoperative rehabilitative program of aerobic exercise for 6–8 weeks. Although this is clearly impractical for urgent or emergent situations, it should be seriously considered when elective thoracic surgery is contemplated. In CF patients with end-stage lung disease awaiting lung transplantation, pretransplant aerobic exercise has been shown to increase exercise performance, even in patients with severe end-stage lung disease (1).

Extremely compromised pulmonary function [e.g. forced expiratory volume in 1 second (FEV_1) < 30% predicted] may preclude elective surgery.

Psychological preparation is important, particularly in young patients. In general, a well-informed patient is less anxious postoperatively.

B. Intraoperative Considerations

Most thoracic surgical procedures are facilitated by periods of one-lung ventilation. This necessitates a double lumen tube or, in smaller patients, appropriately placed bronchus-blocking balloons. To facilitate gas exchange during single-lung ventilation, it is imperative that airway secretions be evacuated. In patients with significant airway secretions, it has been our practice to intubate the CF patients with a large-bore endotracheal tube and pass a flexible bronchoscope for aspiration of secretions, followed by placement of a double lumen tube, usually in the left main stem bronchus. In younger patients, the use of a pediatric bronchoscope augmented by an endotracheal suction catheter may be a useful adjunct to anesthetic management.

Anesthetic technique should take into consideration the patient's liver function, which may influence the metabolism of narcotic agents or paralytics. Liver function also has an impact on coagulation factors. Clotting factors in the form of fresh-frozen plasma should be available for all CF patients undergoing thoracotomy. Prothrombin times may be normal, but, in our experience, blood loss in CF patients is usually accompanied by a coagulation defect, presumably because of slower replacement of coagulation factors in these patients.

C. Postoperative Issues

Particular attention must be paid to adequate clearance of airway secretions postoperatively. This necessitates excellent postoperative pain control, aggressive chest physical therapy and postural drainage, and early ambulation. Patients must have adequate analgesia to tolerate chest percussion after thoracotomy, yet they must be awake enough to cough and clear secretions. Strategies that may be useful in this regard include the use of thoracic epidural analgesia or augmentation of intravenous narcotic analgesia with intercostal nerve blocks using bupivacaine. The disadvantage of this approach is the necessity to repeat the intercostal blocks every 8 hours, but this can be an extremely effective method of pain control after thoracotomy and should be considered in patients who do not tolerate epidural analgesia or in whom epidural analgesia proves ineffective.

Although complete reversal of paralytic agents is always optimal before extubation after thoracic surgery, it is particularly important in patients with CF because of the requirement for early deep breathing and coughing for airway clearance. To facilitate effective cough, we use the nebulized beta-agonist albuterol (2.5 mg or 0.5 mL in 2.5 mL normal saline). For patients with thick, tenacious secretions, *N*-acetyl cysteine (2 mL of 20% solution diluted in 5 mL normal saline) may be a useful adjunct to the nebulizer with every other dose of inhaled bronchodilator. DNase is a potent mucolytic agent in vitro; its effectiveness after surgery in CF patients has not been studied, but it may be useful in this regard (see Chapter 4).

Early ambulation is particularly useful and facilitates airway clearance. We believe that postoperative exercise hastens recovery by promoting airway clearance, even for patients who have not participated in a preoperative exercise program. Patients who participated in a preoperative exercise program should be encouraged to resume this type of activity even before removal of pleural drainage tubes, and certainly before discharge. Early ambulation has many benefits, including reduced incidence of pulmonary embolism, earlier resumption of gut function, and improved appetite.

Particular attention must be paid to the gastrointestinal (GI) tract after thoracic surgery for CF patients. Intrathoracic vagal nerve injury may be the result of surgical mobilization of lungs, particularly in the presence of adhesions of the lung to the mediastinum. Intrathoracic vagal nerve injury has been a postulated cause of postoperative ileus after heart-lung transplant for patients with CF. The intestines of patients with CF are no more sensitive to narcotics than are the intestines of other patients. However, in CF patients, narcotics can precipitate distal intestinal obstruction syndrome (DIOS). The consequences of DIOS may be more devastating in a postoperative patient who is receiving narcotic analgesics because these tend to mask any peritoneal signs that may be developing.

Nutrition is an important consideration in all patients undergoing major surgical procedures, but is of particular concern in patients with CF, many of whom are already malnourished. Postoperative enteral or parenteral nutritional support is necessary in these patients if there is any delay in the resumption of oral intake. Although the enteral route is preferable, intravenous hyperalimentation can be useful, particularly in patients whose bowel function is unreliable. Nutritional support is particularly important for patients who require mechanical ventilation postoperatively. In our experience, it is difficult to wean catabolic patients from ventilatory support.

Full recovery from thoracic surgical procedures should occur by several months postoperatively. For patients who recover uneventfully, no external limitations need be placed on activity by 6 weeks. Pulmonary function tests (PFTs) can be obtained by the third postoperative morning.

II. Thoracic Surgical Procedures for Complications of CF

A. Pleural Procedures

Pleural Effusions and Empyema

Despite the frequency of pulmonary infections in CF patients, pleural effusions requiring drainage are distinctly unusual. As a general rule, however, parapneumonic effusions should be drained with thoracentesis or tube thoracostomy if fluid reaccumulates. Parapneumonic effusions can become colonized with bacteria and can lead to the development of an empyema.

Pus in the pleural space necessitates drainage. When an empyema becomes loculated, an open procedure may be necessary to deal with the chronically infected space. Surgical options for empyema include tube thoracostomy for a simple, uncomplicated empyema or the creation of a pleural window for protracted drainage of more chronic cavities. Thoracotomy with decortication of underlying lung and evacuation of infected, organized material from the pleural space is the preferred approach to a chronic empyema cavity, but it may be impractical in patients with advanced lung disease. When decortication is performed, we prefer to leave patients intubated and mechanically ventilated for approximately 24 hours to encourage obliteration of the pleural space by maintaining expansion of the lung.

Illustrative Case 1

An 18-year-old man with CF was referred for further management of a complex pleural fluid collection (Fig. 1A). Despite therapy at another institution with appropriate intravenous antibiotics for a pulmonary exacerbation, a right pleural effusion developed. Culture of aspirated fluid revealed *Pseudomonas aeruginosa*, and a chest tube was inserted. Despite adequate tube placement confirmed by computed tomography (CT) scan, the pleural collection persisted and appeared to become organized. With no further drainage, the chest tube was withdrawn after 1 week, and intravenous antibiotics continued, but the patient continued to have temperature spikes to 39.5°C daily and a persistent leukocytosis. A CT scan (see Fig. 1B) demonstrated loculated fluid in the right pleural space.

Spirometry performed 6 months earlier showed forced vital capacity (FVC), of 2.31 L (52% predicted) and forced expiratory volume in 1 second (FEV_1) of 0.87 L (23% predicted). Intravenous antibiotics were based on in vitro susceptibility studies, and the patient started a program of aerobic exercise (treadmill and bicycle ergometry) in preparation for thoracotomy. Four weeks later, a right posterolateral thoracotomy through the seventh interspace was performed, and the pleural space was debrided of loculated, infected debris (see Fig. 1C). Culture of pleural fluid retrieved at operation revealed *P. aeruginosa*. The patient was ventilated for 24 hours and then extubated. He had an uneventful recovery and participated in the aerobic exercise program until his discharge 3 weeks after surgery. His chest film 1 year after operation is shown in Fig. 1D. The patient's pulmonary function tests have improved. One year after thoracotomy, his FVC was 3.47 L (74% of predicted) and his FEV_1 was 1.52 L (37% of predicted). These have remained stable for another year.

Consideration was given to creation of a chronic pleural window, but it was thought that this might jeopardize a future opportunity for bilateral lung transplantation, whereas a thoracotomy and decortication would deal with the problem of chronic pleural sepsis and preserve his candidacy for transplantation. In our experience, prior thoracic surgical procedures have not had an adverse impact on survival after bilateral lung transplants for CF (2) using the clamshell incision and bilateral implantation techniques (3).

Pneumothorax

Participants in a consensus conference on the management of pulmonary complications of CF recently made recommendations for an approach to management of pneumothorax in CF (4). Pneumothorax can be either spontaneous,

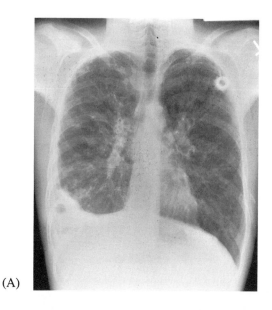

(A)

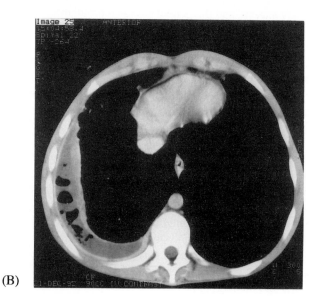

(B)

Figure 1 (A) Posteroanterior chest radiograph demonstrating a loculated fluid collection in the right pleural space. (B) Computed tomography scan demonstrating a complex right pleural fluid collection. (C) A portion of the resected decortication surgical specimen. (D) Posteroanterior chest radiograph 1 year after decortication, showing resolution of the right pleural process.

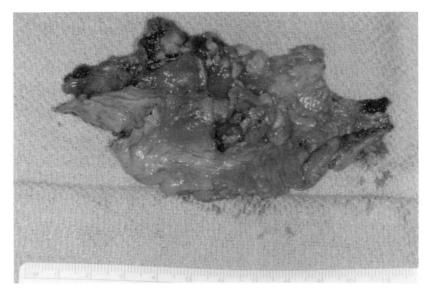

(C)

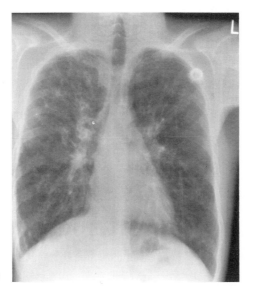

(D)

related to the rupture of subpleural blebs and egress of air into the pleural space, or iatrogenic, due to lung injury during procedures such as line placement. According to Cystic Fibrosis Foundation Registry data, 5%–8% of all patients with CF eventually experience a pneumothorax. The incidence increases with age, so that up to 20% of adults with CF experience a pneumothorax (4).

A small (less than 20% of the volume of the hemithorax) asymptomatic or minimally symptomatic pneumothorax in a CF patient can be managed with observation alone. A symptomatic pneumothorax or a pneumothorax occupying more than 20% of the volume of the hemithorax should be treated, initially with tube thoracostomy and application of negative pressure to the pleural space. The principle of tube thoracostomy is to evacuate all air from the pleural space, which should result in coaption of the visceral and parietal pleural surfaces. If the visceral and parietal pleural surfaces come into contact, then there is a possibility for resolution of the pneumothorax without any further intervention. In patients in whom tube thoracostomy does not result in resolution of the pneumothorax, serious consideration should be given to placing additional chest tubes until the lung is fully expanded and the pleural space is completely evacuated of air. If the air leak stops and the lung remains inflated after removal of the chest tubes, then the pneumothorax has resolved. For patients with recurrent pneumothorax on the same side or a persistent air leak, therapy to prevent future pneumothoraces is indicated in most patients. The consensus conference (4) defined a persistent air leak as one lasting more than 5 days, which is a reasonable time for resolution of air leak. Occasionally, the air leak persists even though the lung is adherent to the chest wall; accordingly, a trial of placing the chest tube to underwater seal or removing it may be reasonable before judging that the pneumothorax is persisting.

Both medical and surgical approaches to preventing recurrence of pneumothorax have usually entailed trying to initiate pleural inflammation to promote scarring of the pleural surface. This scarring is intended to prevent lung collapse even if there is a new leak.

Chemical sclerosing agents have been used to manage pneumothorax, with mixed results. Agents used include tetracycline, quinacrine, silver nitrate, and talc. Tetracycline and silver nitrate had a high recurrence rate in two small series (5,6). Quinacrine was more successful (6,7), but this agent is no longer available. Talc, instilled thoracoscopically (8,9), has a high success rate in preventing recurrence of pneumothorax, but some caution should be exercised in its application because of its tendency to initiate exuberant inflammation and fibrosis.

Talc administered thoracoscopically necessitates a general anesthetic and thoracoscopy. Talc may be the agent of choice in the management of malignant pleural effusions because it is so effective at inducing pleural scarification. The intensity of the inflammatory response frequently causes considerable discomfort and fever in the recipient. Granulomatous inflammation of the lung has been documented after instillation of talc. The dense adhesions produced make subsequent explantation particularly difficult and may increase the morbidity of lung transplantation. A theoretical concern is the calcification that can occur along the pleural surfaces and, in particular, along the diaphragm as a long-term consequence of talc poudrage, because this might seriously hamper diaphragmatic motion. Although instillation of talc is effective, a surgical approach to pneumothorax may be preferable.

Bleomycin is another agent that has been used extensively for the management of malignant pleural effusions. It is difficult to justify the use of such a potent antimetabolite in a patient with benign disease. Because of reduced contact of the sclerosing agent with the pleural surface in the face of an air–fluid interface, it is reasonable that, in general, chemical sclerosing agents are less likely to be successful in the management of pneumothorax than in the management of chronic pleural effusion.

A surgical approach to recurrent or persistent pneumothorax is associated with a very low recurrence rate. The surgical approach involves identifying actual leaks or potential leaks (blebs) and excising them. Most surgeons have also created pleural inflammation either by removing or abrading the parietal pleura. Spector and Stern reported a 95% success rate with thoracotomy and apical pleurectomy among 57 patients with pneumothorax (6). Using a similar approach, Schuster et al. reported 100% success in 20 patients (5). It is not clear whether pleurectomy is necessary or whether mechanical pleural abrasion coupled with removing the ruptured blebs would be sufficient. The latter approach is successful in the management of recurrent spontaneous pneumothorax, and I believe it affords the best opportunity for resolution of the pneumothorax while still allowing for subsequent pulmonary transplantation.

Interest has grown in recent years in the use of thoracoscopy in the management of recurring spontaneous pneumothorax, either as a method to eliminate bullae (10) or for insertion of Nd-YAG or CO_2 laser for pleurodesis (11). This technology may be more difficult to use in patients with CF because of the tendency of their lungs not to deflate fully with a pneumothorax due to inspissated airway secretions and fibrosis of the underlying lung. This tendency may seriously hamper visualization of the diseased area at the apex of the lung and the apex of the superior segment, the most common site of ruptured blebs.

A small transaxillary thoracotomy (12) provides excellent exposure of the apex of the lung and of the superior segment of the lower lobe for stapling ruptured blebs, and it affords good access to the pleural space for mechanical abrasion. This remains our first choice for management of recurrent or persistent pneumothorax in patients with CF. However, pneumothorax often occurs in patients whose disease is clearly advanced and for whom even a limited thoracotomy constitutes a substantial surgical risk. In general, patients awaiting lung transplantation pose a considerable dilemma if they develop a pneumothorax that does not resolve with tube thoracostomy.

Although less effective than surgery, chemical pleurodesis may have some utility in very ill patients in whom the risk of surgery and general anesthesia outweighs its benefits.

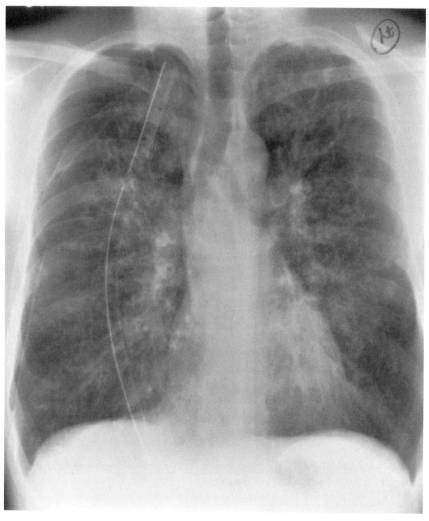

(A)

Figure 2 (A) Despite a right-sided chest tube, a large (approximately 30%) pneumo-thorax persists. (B) Placement of a second tube positioned at the apex of the right chest has resulted in resolution of the pneumothorax; however, the patient's air leak has persisted.

Illustrative Case 2

A 27-year-old man with CF diagnosed at age 16 years and multiple left-sided pneumothoraces was referred for treatment of a persistent right pneumothorax,

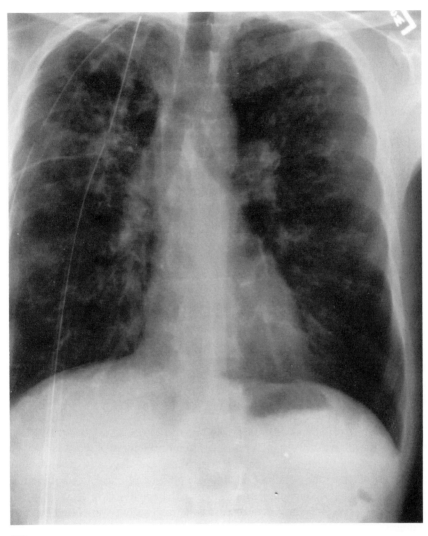

(B)

for which he had undergone placement of chest tubes four times in the preceding month. Before insertion of chest tubes, his most recent pulmonary function tests had documented an FEV_1 of 1.34 L (30% predicted). A chest radiograph showed a large right pneumothorax, despite the presence of a tube in the right pleural space (Fig. 2A). A second chest tube was placed to the apex of the chest, resulting in complete expansion of the right lung, but air leak persisted despite resolution of the pneumothorax. After 5 days, the tubes were placed to underwater seal and a small apical pneumothorax recurred, with evidence of ongoing air leak. At surgery, a right transaxillary incision revealed areas of blebs both in the apex of the upper lobe and along the posterior superior margin of the superior segment of the lower lobe. These were resected with surgical staples, and mechanical abrasion was undertaken. A small air leak resolved after 4 days. Chest tubes were removed, and the patient was discharged 6 days postoperatively. He remained well, with no recurrence of pneumothorax, and was seen again for evaluation of transplant candidacy 2 1/2 years later, when his FEV_1 was 1.22 L (28% predicted). By this time, his exercise capacity had begun to decline, and he had required embolization for hemoptysis (see Chapter 4). Both preoperatively and postoperatively, the patient was treated with chest physical therapy to aid in mobilizing secretions. There is no evidence that properly performed chest physical therapy interferes with resolution of pneumothorax, and this therapy should be continued postoperatively. The patient was also treated with intravenous antibiotics appropriate to the suscepti-bility of his *P. aeruginosa.*

B. Surgery for Parenchymal Disease

Hemoptysis

Blood streaking of sputum in patients with CF is a common occurrence. Major hemoptysis, often defined as 240 mL in a 24-hour period, is life threatening, primarily because of the risk of asphyxiation from airway obstruction; rarely, death from exsanguination may occur. Approximately 1% of CF patients have an episode of major bleeding each year, according to the Cystic Fibrosis Foun-dation, Patient Registry 1994 Annual Data Report, Bethesda, Maryland, August 1995. Most such patients are older than age 16. Major hemoptysis in patients with CF is almost always of systemic arterial origin (4). However, in CF patients in whom mycobacterial or fungal disease develops, consideration should be given to the possibility that a new episode of major hemoptysis may be related to cavitary lung disease. A CT scan may be useful in establishing the presence of severe cavitary lung disease. The distinction is important because therapy may be different.

Although pulmonary resection can be life saving in some individuals with CF and hemoptysis (13,14), most of these patients do not require dramatic inter-vention (see Chapter 4). In those whose bleeding persists despite observation and medical therapy, bronchial artery embolization has become the treatment of choice (15–17). Bronchial artery embolization is largely ineffective at control-ling hemoptysis from cavitary lung disease (15,18); therefore, patients with CF who have refractory bleeding from known cavitary lung disease should undergo resection if they are suitable candidates for thoracotomy.

Surgery may have a role in patients who continue to bleed after bronchial artery embolization or whose bleeding recurs despite embolization. In these circumstances, accurate preoperative localization of the bleeding site is essential. Angiography, CT scan, and bronchoscopy may be useful in this regard. If the lobe in question has been substantially destroyed, then resection may have benefits other than controlling hemoptysis, as explained in subsequent paragraphs. If the lobe appears to be intact but bleeding continues, it may be possible to salvage the lobe by surgically interrupting all systemic vessels that supply the bleeding lobe. This approach is likely to be difficult and tedious, and has never been reported, but may be reasonable, particularly in patients with minimal pulmonary reserve who fail bronchial artery embolization. It is based on the premise that hemoptysis from bronchiectasis always involves the systemic bronchial circulation. Presumably, failure of embolization to control hemoptysis is related to missing an aberrant bronchial artery or a collateral artery from the chest wall.

Many patients who have had bronchial artery embolization are subsequently found to have substantial pleural adhesions at the time of transplant. Neither embolization nor the pleural adhesions appear to affect bronchial healing after lung transplantation.

C. Resection Surgery for Cystic Fibrosis

In the 1960s and 1970s, some enthusiasm was seen for the role of pulmonary resection to control symptoms in patients with CF. Mearns et al. (19) reported on 23 patients with CF undergoing lobectomy or segmental resection. Half of these patients underwent resection of what was presumed to be a single gross airway lesion. One operative death occurred, and one patient had no benefit from surgery, whereas 21 of 23 patients were judged to have derived some benefit from the surgery. Marmon and associates (20) reported similar results in 10 patients with CF undergoing 11 pulmonary resections, but cautioned that pulmonary resection in patients with CF was safe and therapeutically rewarding only when resection was limited to the most diseased portion of the lung without sacrificing functional tissue. Smith et al. (21) cautioned that an FEV_1 less than 30% predicted was uniformly associated with a poor outcome after surgery in a series of 17 pulmonary resections for CF, which included some resections for hemoptysis.

With improvement in medical treatment of CF lung disease, the role of surgery has declined. Nevertheless, a subset of patients remains whose disease is largely localized to one lobe or segment and who may benefit from resection to reduce copious secretions and to prevent soiling of relatively uninvolved lung tissue.

Illustrative Case 3

A 36-year-old man with CF had an increasing need for hospitalizations and intravenous antibiotics. He had been expectorating 2 cups of purulent sputum daily for more than a year, and a chest film documented progressive volume loss

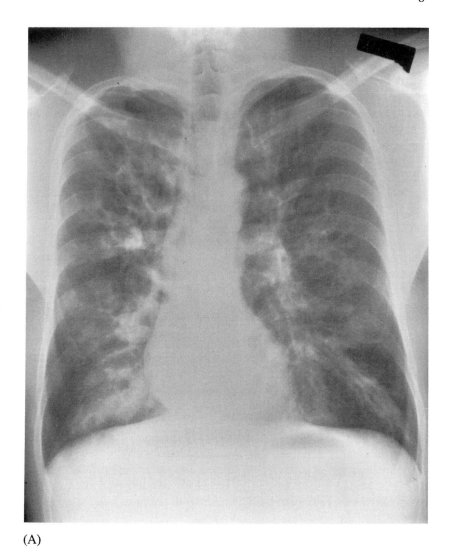

(A)

Figure 3 (A) Posteroanterior chest radiograph showing right-sided volume loss and right lower lobe consolidation. (B) Computed tomography scan demonstrating destruction of most of the right lower lobe with large cystic spaces filled with fluid. (C) Resected right lower lobe showing extensive parenchymal destruction and replacement by large cysts filled with pus.

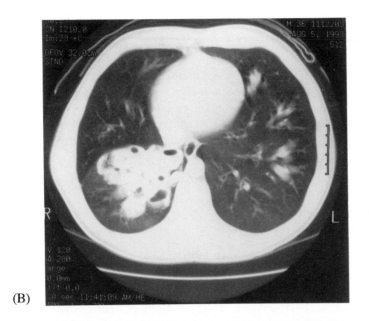

(B)

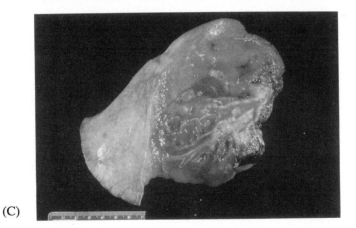

(C)

in the right hemithorax and consolidation of the right lower lobe (Fig 3A). A CT scan (see Fig. 3B) confirmed that much of the right lower lobe had been destroyed and replaced with cystic lesions. At bronchoscopy, a large amount of purulent material could be aspirated from the right lower lobe. Preoperative pulmonary function tests demonstrated an FVC of 3.2 L (70% predicted) and an FEV_1 of 1.78 L (47% predicted). The patient underwent a right posterolateral thoracotomy with right lower lobectomy, which was complicated by accumulation of right pleural fluid requiring drainage for infected fluid in the pleural space. The resected specimen, shown in Figure 3C, confirmed that much of the lobe had been destroyed. These complications extended his hospital stay for a total of 34 days. However, there was a dramatic reduction in sputum production and in the necessity for hospital admissions. Three months postoperatively, the FVC was 60% predicted and the FEV_1 was 41% predicted. These pulmonary function tests remained essentially unchanged at 1 year postoperatively. The patient has not required further hospital admissions in the ensuing 18 months.

III. Summary

Patients with CF who require thoracic surgery pose substantial challenges to the thoracic surgeon and the surgical unit. Meticulous attention to perioperative clearance of airway secretions is mandatory. Indications for thoracic surgery related to complications of CF include the management of recurrent or persistent pneumothorax, the management of some pleural space infections, the emergency management of massive hemoptysis, and the occasional resection of isolated bronchiectatic segments or lobes. Although contraindications to lung transplantation differ from center to center, prior thoracotomy does not preclude successful lung transplantation.

Because of the severity of adhesions after talc poudrage or surgical pleurectomy, the preferred management of spontaneous or recurrent pneumothorax is a surgical approach to the leaking lung with bleb-stapling and mechanical pleural abrasion.

Assessment of perioperative risk is important in determining which patients should be surgical candidates for the thoracic complications of CF. Vigorous preoperative and postoperative physical therapy, pain control, nutritional support, intravenous antibiotics if appropriate, and early ambulation all contribute to a successful thoracic surgical outcome in these challenging patients.

References

1. Arnold CD, Westerman JH, Downs AM, Egan TM. Benefits of an aerobic exercise program in CF patients waiting for double lung transplantation (abstr). Pediatr Pulmonol 1991; 6(suppl):287.
2. Egan TM, Detterbeck FC, Mill MR, Paradowski LJ, Lackner RP, Ogden WD, et al. Improved results of lung transplantation for cystic fibrosis. J Thorac Cardiovasc Surg 1995; 109:224–235.
3. Egan TM, Detterbeck FC. Technique and results of double lung transplantation. Chest Surg Clin North Am 1993; 3:89–111.

4. Schidlow DV, Taussig LM, Knowles MR, Egan TM, et al. Cystic Fibrosis Foundation Consensus Conference report on pulmonary complications of cystic fibrosis. Pediatr Pulmonol 1993; 15:187–198.

5. Schuster SR, McLaughlin FJ, Matthews WJ, Jr, Strieder DJ, Khaw KT, Shwachman H. Management of pneumothorax in cystic fibrosis. J Pediatr Surg 1983; 18:492–497.

6. Spector ML, Stern RC. Pneumothorax in cystic fibrosis: a 26-year experience. Ann Thorac Surg 1989; 47:204–207.

7. Cattaneo SM, Sirak HD, Klassen KP. Recurrent spontaneous pneumothorax in the high-risk patient: management with intrapleural quinacrine. J Thorac Cardiovasc Surg 1973; 66:467–471.

8. Tribble CG, Selden RF, Rodgers BM. Talc poudrage in the treatment of spontaneous pneumothoraces in patients with cystic fibrosis. Ann Surg 1986; 204:677–680.

9. Noppen M, Dhondt E, Mahler T, Malfroot A, Dab I, Vincken W. Successful management of recurrent pneumothorax in cystic fibrosis by localized apical thoracoscopic talc poudrage. Chest 1994; 106:262–264.

10. Nathanson LK, Shimi SM, Wood RAB, Cuschieri A. Videothoracoscopic ligation of bulla and pleurectomy for spontaneous pneumothorax. Ann Thorac Surg 1991; 52:316–319.

11. Torre M, Belloni P. Nd-YAG laser pleurodesis through thoracoscopy: new curative therapy in spontaneous pneumothorax. Ann Thorac Surg 1989; 47:887–889.

12. Murray KD, Matheny RG, Howanitz EP, Myerowitz PD. A limited axillary thoracotomy as primary treatment for recurrent spontaneous pneumothorax. Chest 1993; 103:137–142.

13. Levitsky S, Lapey A, di Sant-Agnese PA. Pulmonary resection for life-threatening hemoptysis in cystic fibrosis. JAMA 1970; 213:125–127.

14. Porter DK, Van Every MJ, Anthracite RF, Mack JW Jr. Massive hemoptysis in cystic fibrosis. Arch Intern Med 1983; 143:287–290.

15. Uflacker R, Kaemmerer A, Neves C, Picon PD. Management of massive hemoptysis by bronchial artery embolization. Radiology 1983; 146:627–634.

16. Fellows KE, Khaw KT, Schuster S, Schwachman H. Bronchial artery embolization in cystic fibrosis: technique and long-term results. J Pediatr 1979; 95:959–963.

17. Cohen AM, Doershuk CF, Stern RC. Bronchial artery embolization to control hemoptysis in cystic fibrosis. Radiology 1990; 175:401–405.

18. Rémy J, Arnaud A, Fardou H, Giraud R, Voisin C. Treatment of hemoptysis by embolization of bronchial arteries. Radiology 1977; 122:33–37.

19. Mearns MB, Hodson CJ, Jackson ADM, et al. Pulmonary resection in cystic fibrosis: results in 23 cases, 1957–1970. Arch Dis Child 1972; 47:499–508.

20. Marmon L, Schidlow D, Palmer J, Balsara RK, Dunn JM. Pulmonary resection for complications of cystic fibrosis. J Pediatr Surg 1983; 18:811–815.

21. Smith MB, Hardin WD, Jr, Dressel DA, Beckerman RC, Moynihan PC. Predicting outcome following pulmonary resection in cystic fibrosis patients. J Pediatr Surg 1991; 26:655–659.

9

Abdominal and General Surgery

FREDERICK J. RESCORLA

Indiana University School of Medicine and
James Whitcomb Riley Hospital for Children
Indianapolis, Indiana

The surgical management of patients with cystic fibrosis (CF) for many years focused on newborns with conditions associated with meconium ileus. As medical management and survival has improved, these children are living longer and many other disorders that occur with advancing age require surgical intervention. In addition, various vascular and intestinal devices are frequently required to allow supportive care. Although some surgical disorders can be managed on an outpatient basis, many of these patients require inpatient hospitalization (Table 1).

I. Meconium Ileus

A. Etiology

Approximately 6%–20% of neonates with CF have intraluminal obstruction of the terminal ileum due to viscid meconium (1–3). Landsteiner initially reported this condition in 1905 after observing an obturator bowel obstruction in a newborn with pathological changes in the pancreas (4). Several other investigators subsequently reported instances of meconium ileus and congenital stenosis of the pancreatic ducts (5,6). Anderson described the histological similarities of

Table 1 General Surgical Indications for Hospitalization in Cystic Fibrosis

Meconium ileus
    Uncomplicated
    Complicated
        Atresia
        Volvulus
        Perforation
        Giant cystic meconium peritonitis
Distal intestinal obstruction syndrome
Intussusception
Appendicitis
Colonic strictures
Cholecystectomy
Biliary dyskinesia
Cholecystitis
Symptomatic cholelithiasis
Gastrostomy jejunostomy placement
    Percutaneous
    Operative
    Fundoplication
Liver-related procedures
    Splenectomy
    Portosystemic shunting
    Transjugular intrahepatic portosystemic shunt (TIPS); radiology department
Rectal prolapse refractory to enzyme adjustments
Hernia repair

the pancreatic lesions in children with meconium ileus and CF (7). The etiology was initially considered a direct result of pancreatic achylia (8), but the severity of the pancreatic disease does not correlate closely with the occurrence of meconium ileus (9). Glanzman and Berger in 1950 described an abnormal protein in meconium that formed a firm jelly (10); other investigators subsequently noted higher protein concentrations in meconium of affected neonates (11). Albumin was described to be the major protein in meconium, with levels five to ten times higher than in normal meconium (12,13). Schutt and Isles in 1968 observed that meconium in affected neonates contained 85% protein, whereas normal meconium contained only 7% protein (14). This high protein content is thought to be due to abnormal pancreatic and intestinal secretions, together with an abnormal concentrating process in the proximal small bowel (9,15). Brock studied the levels of various enzymes and proteins in affected and unaffected fetuses to determine the intestinal site where these changes occurred (15). He noted that albumin (derived from amniotic fluid) and glutamyl-transpeptidase and 5' nucleotidase (produced by the liver) are present in higher concentrations in the meconium of affected fetuses. Aminopeptidase M and alkaline phosphatase, which are secreted at a more distal site, are not present at a higher concentration in affected fetuses, indicating that the abnormal concentrating process occurs at a proximal site and that these latter enzymes are secreted into an already concentrated meconium. This study suggested that the components present in the duodenum and proximal jejunum are abnormally concentrated at this level.

Several interesting observations have been noted in these patients. In one series, families with one child with meconium ileus had an observed occurrence rate of CF in subsequent offspring of 47%, whereas those with a CF child without meconium ileus had a 22.5% incidence of subsequent offspring having CF (16). Two other studies noted that approximately 30% of subsequent CF-affected siblings in families in which the index case had meconium ileus also had meconium ileus (17,18), whereas the rate was 6% when the first affected child did not have meconium ileus.

Meconium ileus can be "uncomplicated" or "complicated." In uncomplicated cases, abnormal meconium causes a simple obturator form of obstruction of the distal ileum (Fig. 1). The bowel proximal to the inspissated meconium dilates and the distal bowel is of small caliber. Complicated cases of meconium ileus include those with associated volvulus, perforation, atresia, and giant cystic meconium peritonitis. Each has a unique clinical presentation and management strategy and are, therefore, discussed separately.

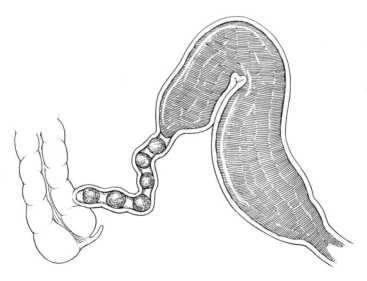

Figure 1 Artist's depiction of uncomplicated meconium ileus with obstructing pellets in the terminal ileum.

B. Uncomplicated Meconium Ileus

Clinical Presentation and Initial Management

In case of uncomplicated or simple meconium ileus, the abnormal thickened meconium causes an ileal obstruction. The distal ileum is filled with meconium pellets and the proximal ileum dilates to 4–6 cm in diameter as it fills with thick puttylike meconium (see Fig. 1). The colon is small ("microcolon") because meconium has not entered it. Neonates with uncomplicated meconium ileus often appear relatively normal for the first day of life. As the proximal bowel fills with air, intestinal secretions, and feedings, the abdomen becomes distended. Emesis, initially clear and later bilious, develops and failure to pass meconium in the first 24 hours is observed.

Neonates with a suspected bowel obstruction should be managed with oral–gastric tube decompression of the stomach and intravenous fluids. Antibiotics are administered after blood cultures are obtained, because sepsis is in the differential diagnosis. Plain abdominal and decubitus radiographs usually demonstrate dilated loops of intestine without air–fluid levels because the viscid meconium prevents an air–fluid interface (Fig. 2). Air mixed with thick meconium in the terminal ileum may create a "soap bubble" appearance in the right lower quadrant ("Neuhauser's sign") (19).

The initial diagnostic test for most neonates with a distal intestinal obstruction is a contrast enema. Some infants whose plain films suggest uncomplicated meconium ileus may be candidates for an initial therapeutic enema. For others, barium is a suitable contrast agent. The enema reveals a microcolon and may demonstrate meconium pellets in the ascending colon and terminal ileum (Fig. 3). This finding excludes meconium plug syndrome, small left colon syndrome, colon atresia, anomalies of rotation, and most cases of Hirschsprung's disease. However, total colonic Hirschsprung's disease may appear very similar to meconium ileus on barium enema. In addition, cases of complicated meconium ileus (atresia and volvulus) can usually be differentiated from uncomplicated meconium ileus if the plain radiographs are nonspecific.

Nonoperative Management

The management of infants with uncomplicated meconium ileus was significantly altered with the introduction of the Gastrografin (diatrizoate meglumine) enema by Helen Noblett in 1969 (20). Before that time, operative removal of the meconium or intestinal resection was required for virtually all of these neonates. Noblett's initial report included four infants successfully given enemas (two with three enemas) consisting of full strength Gastrografin, a hyperosmolar (1900 mosm/L) solution of diatrizoate meglumine with an added wetting agent, 0.1% polysorbate 80 (Tween 80). Noblett's initial criteria are still relevant: (1) adequate intravenous fluid replacement due to the hyperosmolarity of the Gastrografin and (2) a requirement that the infant have no "evidence of compli-

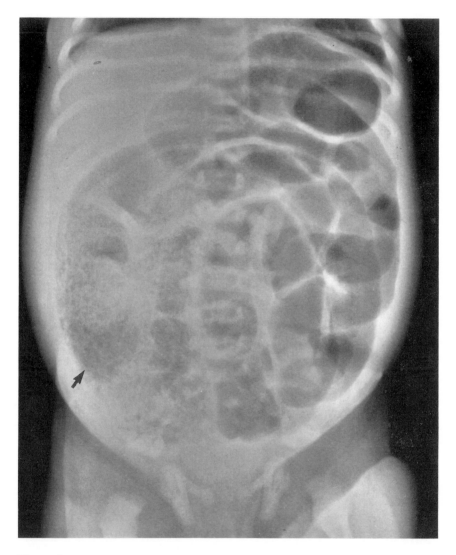

Figure 2 Abdominal radiograph demonstrates small bowel distention with the "soap bubble" appearance (*arrow*) of meconium mixed with air.

cating factors, such as volvulus, gangrene, perforation, peritonitis, or atresia of the small bowel." These initial neonates also received *N*-acetylcysteine 10% (5 mL every 6 hours) per oral gastric tube for 5 days.

The hyperosmolarity of the Gastrografin solution, drawing fluid into the bowel lumen to dislodge the thick meconium, is considered the major factor that

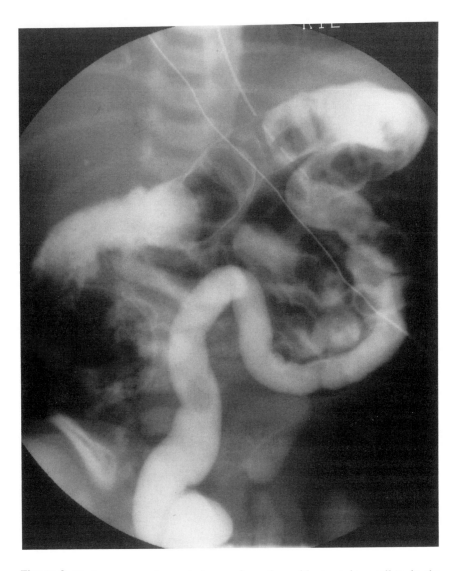

Figure 3 Barium enema demonstrates a microcolon with meconium pellets in the proximal colon.

promotes clearing. Agents without Tween 80 have been effective, and Gastrografin is supplied without this wetting agent as a mixture of diatrizoate meglumine and diatrizoate sodium. Complications observed with Gastrografin have included perforation, necrotizing enterocolitis, shock, and death (21,22). In a follow-up report of 18 patients (14 with successful outcome), Noblett reported two perforations (23), and, in a series of 22 patients (15 with uncomplicated meconium ileus), Ein et al. (21) observed five perforations. Some perforations occur during or immediately after the therapeutic enema and others occur later (12 hours to 2 days), probably when the hypertonic contrast material is flushed proximal to a nearly complete obstruction and draws fluid into the lumen, leading to overdistention of the proximal bowel. In a cumulative review of several reports, the Gastrografin enema was successful in 55% (66 of 121) with an 11% incidence of perforation (2,20,21,23–28). Some radiologists dilute Gastrografin to a lower concentration (2 or 3 parts water to 1 part Gastrografin) to decrease the osmolarity and resultant complications (2,21). Other reported enema solutions have included Tween 80, *N*-acetylcysteine with or without Gastrografin, diatrizoate sodium (Hypaque), and iothalamate meglumine (Conray), although complications have also occurred with these agents (29–32).

My preference is to use Gastrografin diluted 3:1 with water (3 parts water, 1 part Gastrografin). All neonates are appropriately resuscitated before the enema and receive intravenous fluids at 150 mL/kg/day during and after the procedure with careful observation of urine output, heart rate, and blood pressure after the procedure. The dilute Gastrografin is administered per rectum and gently irrigated into the terminal ileum to mix with the inspissated meconium pellets (Fig. 4). Semiliquid meconium usually passes during the first 12 hours after the enema. In some infants, a second or third enema over the following 1–2 days may be required. The use of 5%–10% *N*-acetylcysteine per oral–gastric tube (5–10 mL every 6 hours) may aid in clearing the thick meconium. As the obstruction resolves, the oral–gastric tube is removed and the diet advanced. Confirmatory tests for cystic fibrosis are performed and enzyme replacement instituted. Survival at 1 year in these patients is nearly 100% (33).

Operative Management

Neonates who fail two or three therapeutic enemas require operative intervention. Meconium ileus was generally a fatal condition until 1948 when Hiatt and Wilson described a number of survivors following enterotomy and saline irrigation of the obstructing meconium pellets (34). Several subsequent reports described procedures with temporary ostomies designed to relieve the obstruction, allow postoperative irrigation, maintain intestinal continuity, and allow a simple procedure for ostomy closure. Gross in 1953 reported success with resection of the dilated segment of meconium filled bowel and a Mikulicz enterostomy (Fig. 5A) (35). Bishop and Koop (36) in 1957 described a proximal end-to-distal side ileal anastomosis with distal ostomy after resection of the dilated segment (see Fig. 5B), and, in 1961, Santulli and Blanc (37) reported resection with a side-to-end anastomosis and a proximal enterostomy (see Fig. 5C). All of these ostomies could be closed with an extraperitoneal procedure; however, all had the disadvantage of an ileal resection. The use of resection

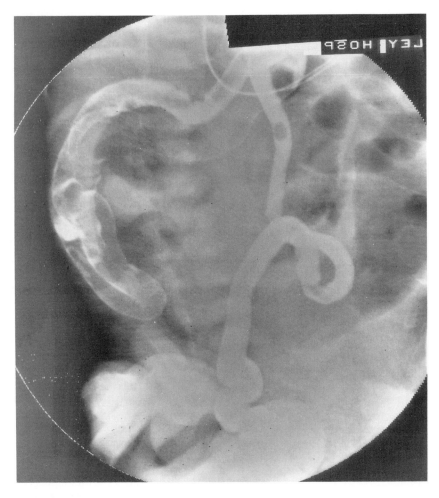

Figure 4 Gastrografin enema demonstrates contrast refluxing into meconium-filled terminal ileum.

with primary anastomosis was reported by Swenson (38) in 1962, but was not widely accepted due to concerns of anastomotic leak. These procedures did, however, improve the survival of babies with meconium ileus. In 1965, Holsclaw et al. (39) reported a survival rate of 72% with the Bishop-Koop procedure. Five years later, O'Neill et al. (40) reported the use of a tube enterostomy with postoperative irrigation, which had the advantage of not involving an intestinal resection or requiring a second procedure (see Fig. 5D).

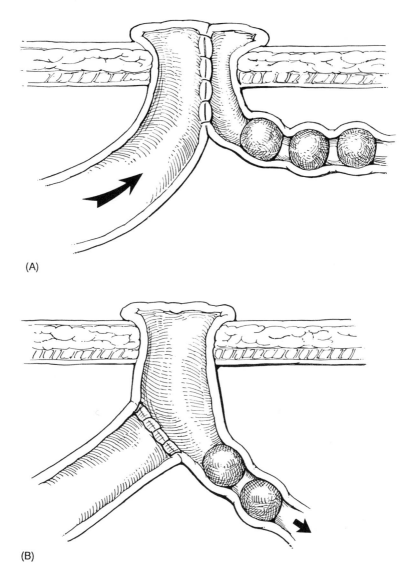

(A)

(B)

Figure 5 Operative procedures used to treat meconium ileus. (A) Resection and Mikulicz enterostomy. (B) Resection and Bishop-Koop enterostomy. (C) Resection and Santulli-Blanc enterostomy. (D) Tube enterostomy.

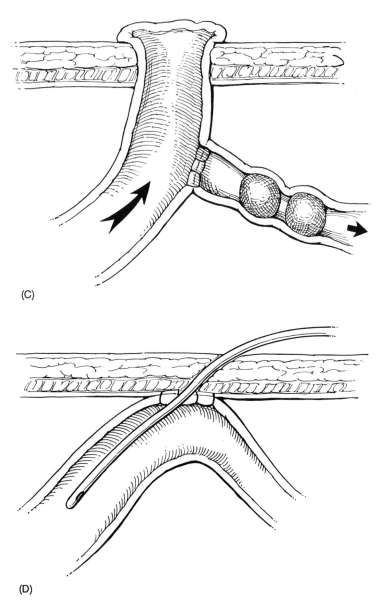

(C)

(D)

Figure 5 Continued

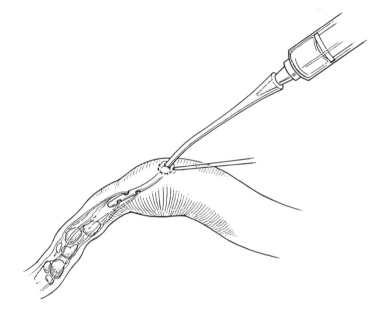

Figure 6   Technique of enterotomy and irrigation.

Enterotomy with irrigation as originally described by Hiatt and Wilson (34) regained popularity in the 1970s and 1980s. Kalayoglu et al. (41) successfully treated 24 neonatal cases with enterotomy and instillation of hydrogen peroxide or *N*-acetylcysteine. Venugopal and Shandling (42) were successful with the same technique in 11 of 12 neonates. Several other investigators have also reported success with this technique (2,27,28) and it appears to be the current standard operative treatment for simple meconium ileus. A pursestring suture is placed on the antimesenteric wall of the ileum and a small soft catheter is inserted through a small enterotomy (Fig. 6). The bowel is then gently irrigated with saline, which is manually mixed with the thick meconium and pellets. The thick meconium is removed through the enterotomy and the pellets are either removed through the enterotomy or flushed into the colon. This is a tedious process and may require several irrigations to break up the thick meconium. If some thick meconium remains within the ileum or pellets in the colon, it is probably worthwhile to use dilute Gastrografin at the conclusion of the procedure to aid in postoperative clearing of the bowel. The appendiceal stump has also been used as a site for irrigation and removal of pellets and thick meconium (43).

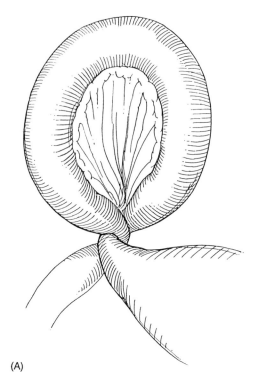

(A)

Figure 7 (A) Volvulus of the distended segment of ileum. (B) Perforation of the ischemic segment of bowel. (C) Ileal atresia may arise when the base of the volvulus becomes ischemic.

C. Complicated Meconium Ileus

Complicated cases of meconium ileus include those associated with volvulus, perforation, ileal atresia, and giant cystic meconium peritonitis. The cause of these complications is thought to be related to the twisting of the heavy meconium-filled bowel (Fig. 7A). This may result in a volvulus, which may perforate (see Fig. 7B), resulting in meconium peritonitis. In some cases, the volvulus become ischemic and liquefies, which, with leakage of meconium, results in a pseudocyst, termed "giant cystic meconium peritonitis." The ischemic base of the volvulus may result in an ileal atresia (Fig. 7C).

Prenatal ultrasonography has allowed detection of some cases of meconium ileus with a mass effect and peritoneal calcifications (44,45). Neonates with complicated meconium peritonitis, particularly perforation or giant cystic meconium peritonitis, often have abdominal distention at birth and bilious gastric aspirate. A mass may be present in cases of volvulus or giant cystic meconium peritonitis. Unusual presentations in neonates with meconium peri-

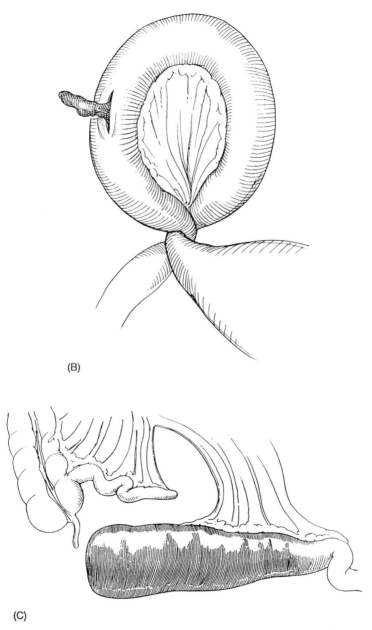

(B)

(C)

tonitis have included a buttock mass (46) or meconium in the vagina from passage through the fallopian tube or in the scrotum from passage through a patent processus vaginalis. Some neonates with a distal atresia may tolerate feedings for the first day of life before abdominal distention develops.

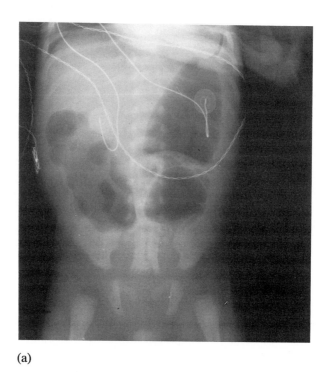

(a)

Figure 8 (a) Radiograph demonstrating distended small bowel in a neonate with ileal atresia. (b) Peritoneal calcifications noted on radiograph of a newborn with abdominal distention and bilious vomiting. Meconium peritonitis was noted at surgery. (c) Barium enema demonstrates a microcolon and failure of contrast to pass retrograde beyond the colon, suggesting ileal atresia in a neonate with meconium ileus and ileal atresia.

Radiographs in complicated meconium ileus usually demonstrate more bowel dilatation than in uncomplicated cases as well as air–fluid levels on decubitus views (Fig. 8a). Intraperitoneal calcifications may develop in neonates with perforations due to intraperitoneal meconium (see Fig. 8b). Cases of giant cystic meconium peritonitis may also have a mass effect from the cyst, which may be filled with fluid. In some cases of atresia, a barium enema may be useful to confirm the diagnosis by demonstrating a microcolon and the failure of contrast to pass retrograde beyond the colon (see Fig. 8c).

Neonates with complicated meconium ileus must be managed operatively. In cases of atresia or volvulus, the procedure of choice is resection of the dilated segment, irrigation of the distal bowel to remove meconium pellets, and then a primary anastomosis. Because the distal bowel is much smaller, an end-to-oblique anastomosis is usually performed by dividing the proximal bowel at a 90-degree angle with respect to the mesentery and the distal bowel at a 45-degree angle (Fig. 9). In cases of meconium ileus with atresia, adequate bowel

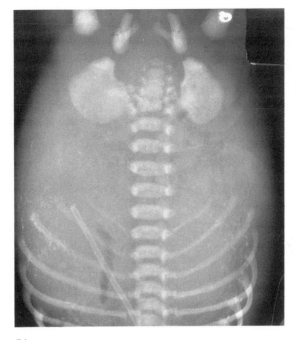

(b)

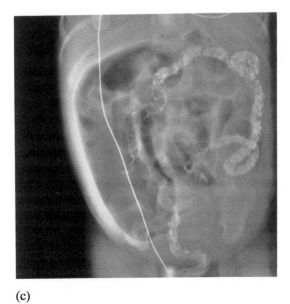

(c)

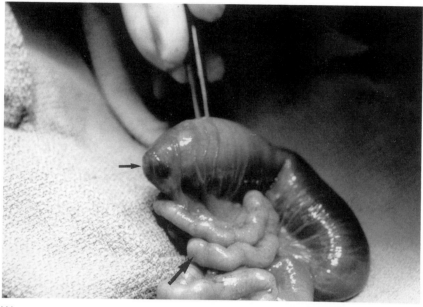

(A)

Figure 9 (A) Operative photo of ileal atresia with blind-ending dilated ileum (*small arrow*). Note the small caliber of terminal ileum with meconium pellets (*large arrow*). (B) Resection of dilated atonic segment with division of the proximal bowel at a 90-degree angle and the distal bowel at a 45-degree angle. (C) Completion of end-oblique anastomosis.

length is usually present, allowing resection of the dilated segment (10–15 cm) because this portion is frequently atonic.

In cases of perforation with meconium peritonitis or giant cystic meconium peritonitis, numerous adhesions are frequently present, making the operative procedure very difficult. The proximal bowel is usually brought out as a temporary stoma. The distal bowel can be closed and left in the abdomen or brought out as a mucous fistula. Enterostomy closure is generally performed 4–6 weeks after the initial procedure. Although most of these patients can be managed with enteral feeds, some require supplementation with parenteral nutrition. The survival of these neonates with complicated meconium ileus is approximately 90% (33).

II. GASTROINTESTINAL DISORDERS

A. Distal Intestinal Obstruction Syndrome

Gastrointestinal problems beyond the newborn period are common. Intestinal obstruction from inspissated bowel contents beyond the neonatal period was

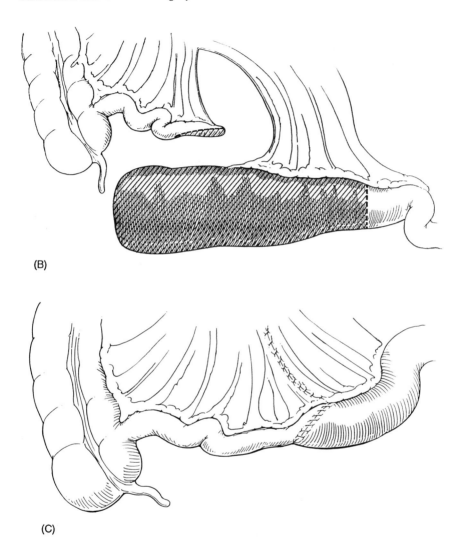

(B)

(C)

initially described by Rasor and Stevenson in 1941 (47). This was subsequently termed "meconium ileus equivalent" (48), although other investigators have preferred the more accurate phrase "distal intestinal obstruction syndrome" (DIOS) (49). These terms are used interchangeably throughout recent reports. This disorder occurs in 2.4%–11% of patients with cystic fibrosis (50,51) in most large series, although has been reported in as high as 37% of patients in other reports (52). It has even been the presenting symptom leading to the diagnosis of cystic fibrosis (53).

The cause of DIOS is unknown, although these patients are more likely to have a history of steatorrhea from pancreatic exocrine insufficiency. Various contributing factors have been proposed (e.g., cessation or a decrease in enzyme therapy, increased activity level or inadequate fluid replacement, particularly in warm weather, thick intestinal mucus, and decreased small intestinal pH with precipitation of proteins).

The clinical presentation nearly always includes crampy abdominal pain with an associated decrease in stool frequency, which may occasionally precede the obstruction. Physical findings usually include a tender mass in the right lower quadrant. This must be differentiated from constipation and intussusception, which are also fairly common in this patient population (50), as well as appendiceal disease, which can occur as a right lower quadrant mass. Plain abdominal radiographs frequently demonstrate large amounts of fecal material with the bubbly, granular appearance that is similar to that of infants with meconium ileus (Fig. 10); many asymptomatic CF patients have similar radiographic findings.

The difficulty and importance of establishing a correct diagnosis is emphasized in one report in which 25% of patients thought to have DIOS actually had other conditions including adhesive bowel obstruction, volvulus, Crohn's disease, and opiate abuse and dependence (54). Computed tomography (CT) has been recommended to aid in the diagnosis and may also occasionally be useful for monitoring therapy (55). Most often, the diagnosis is straightforward, and CT is not needed.

The distal intestinal obstruction syndrome usually responds to nonoperative therapy. If dehydration is present, intravenous fluids should be administered. Gastric decompression may be required in cases with associated vomiting. *N*-acetylcysteine administered rectally or through long intestinal tubes was initially used (56,57) and is still recommended by some authors (50). Maintenance therapy with oral *N*-acetylcysteine has been used to prevent recurrence (58,59). Gastrografin enemas were subsequently reported to clear the obstruction (52). O'Halloran et al. (52) observed success in 81% of episodes with a single dose of oral Gastrografin. Children younger than 8 years old received 50 mL and those older than 8 years received 100 mL, followed by at least four times that volume in water. A second dose resulted in resolution in all but one patient in this series and that child responded to a Gastrografin enema (Fig. 11). Both *N*-acetylcysteine and Gastrografin taste terrible and may not be accepted by the oral route. Nasogastric administration may be more successful.

Success with the use of a balanced salt solution has been reported in patients unresponsive to *N*-acetylcysteine (60,61). These solutions, which include the commercial products GoLYTELY and NuLYTELY, should not be used in the presence of a complete bowel obstruction.

Thus, current options for therapy include (1) enemas of Gastrografin or *N*-acetylcysteine, (2) oral solutions of Gastrografin or *N*-acetylcysteine (30 mL of 20% solution every 4 to 8 hours), and (3) oral or nasogastric balanced lavage solutions. In the absence of a complete obstruction, I prefer to use a balanced

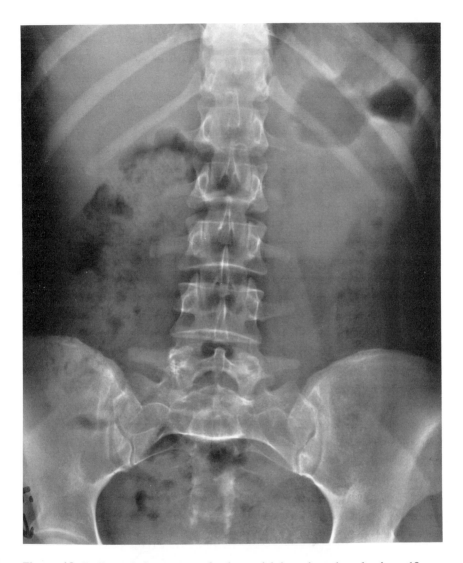

Figure 10 Radiograph demonstrates fecal material throughout the colon in an 18 year old with the distal intestinal obstruction syndrome.

salt solution. The total dose of GoLYTELY is 4–6 L in adults and 2–3 L in children. The fluid must be taken rapidly (20–30 mL/kg/h in children). Children frequently require a nasogastric tube, whereas older patients can usually drink the solution. In the presence of a complete obstruction or with failure of oral solutions, enemas with Gastrografin are used (50). One advantage to using a contrast enema is that it can identify an associated intussusception.

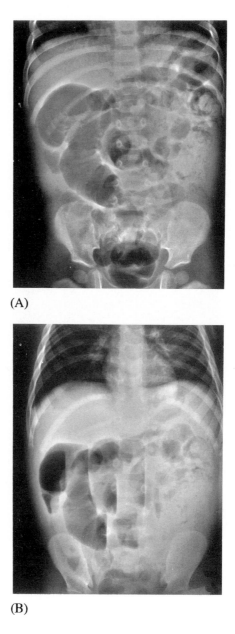

(A)

(B)

Figure 11 Successful treatment of DIOS. (A) Plain abdominal radiograph. (B) Decubitus view demonstrating dilated loops of small bowel with air–fluid levels in a 2-year-old boy. (C) Gastrografin enema demonstrates thickened fecal material in the ascending colon and terminal ileum. (D) Due to failure of resolution, 50 mL of Gastrografin and 200 mL of water was administered by nasogastric tube with resultant passage of Gastrografin into the distal small bowel and resolution of the obstruction.

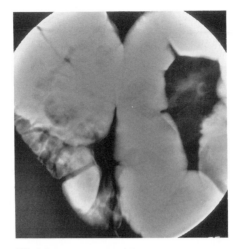

(C)

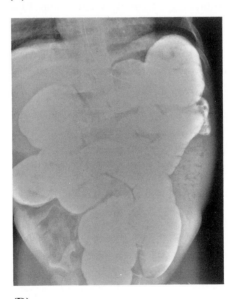

(D)

After successful therapy, adjustment of enzyme replacement as well as regular administration of lactulose may help to prevent recurrence. Cimetidine may have a role by increasing intestinal pH. *N*-acetylcysteine therapy is efficacious, but has the disadvantage of expense and poor taste. In addition, liver injury has been reported with oral and rectal administration of *N*-acetylcysteine and patients on prolonged therapy must be monitored for liver dysfunction (62). The prokinetic agent cisapride (pediatric dose: 0.2 mg/kg three to four times a day; adult dose: 10 mg three times a day) has been shown to decrease symptoms associated with DIOS and to decrease, but not eliminate, the need for intestinal lavage for acute DIOS (63,64).

B. Intussusception

Intussusception occurs in approximately 1% of patients with cystic fibrosis (65) and appears more common in those with DIOS. The most common location is ileocolic but can also be ileoileal and cecocolic. The process presumably occurs when fecal material adheres to the mucosa and serves as a lead point. These patients are older than those with the idiopathic intussusception seen in infancy, with an average age in one series being 9 years old (65).

Common symptoms include abdominal pain, a right lower quadrant mass, and vomiting. Rectal bleeding is reported in only one-fourth of patients, probably due to a large capacity colon and because the intussusceptum remains in the cecum or ascending colon. This can be difficult to differentiate from DIOS, and failure to respond to therapy for DIOS should prompt further studies. Intussusception can be chronic, and the diagnosis can be delayed up to 1 month (66). Although an ultrasound examination may demonstrate the concentric circles characteristic of intussusception, several authors have found this modality unreliable (64,66). A contrast enema demonstrates the defect and is often therapeutic. Intussusception in CF may require operative reduction, perhaps with cececotomy. The appendix should always be removed to eliminate its acting as a lead point or complicating a diagnosis of subsequent episodes of abdominal pain.

C. Appendicitis

Appendicitis with appendiceal abscess can manifest with a similar scenario of pain and a right lower quadrant mass. Due to the chronic nature of the process and obliteration of the appendiceal lumen with thick mucus, perforation and abscess may develop without the typical clinical appearance of appendicitis. One center recently reported three patients with this entity in a 4-year period, emphasizing the atypical presentation (67). The overall 4.9% incidence of appendicitis in a large group of CF patients is not too dissimilar from the incidence of appendicitis in the general population, although other investigators have noted an incidence of only 1%–2% (68). Patients with CF may undergo an appendectomy in the absence of appendicitis due to the diagnostic difficulty of evaluating right lower quadrant pain. In many cases, the appendix is distended with inspissated mucus but without signs of inflammation. Some authors have identified patients with pain from the distended noninflamed appendix that are cured by appendectomy (69). In cases of appendicitis, the process is often delayed in presentation and frequently progresses to perforation and abscess (70,71).

Confirmatory findings may include extrinsic compression of the cecum on contrast enema. A CT scan may demonstrate the abscess, but if no contrast material is in the cecum, it may be difficult to differentiate DIOS from appendiceal abscess. The standard management involves appendectomy and appropriate surgical management of associated peritonitis or abscess.

D. Rectal Prolapse

Rectal prolapse occurs in 11%–30% of patients with cystic fibrosis (64,72,73). The frequency of rectal prolapse in patients with CF in one large study was 11%–12% in those presenting with meconium ileus or respiratory symptoms and 20% in those presenting with gastrointestinal signs (64). It usually occurs between 1 and 3 years of age, frequently before institution of adequate enzyme therapy (72). It can be the presenting feature of CF, and any child with rectal prolapse should have a sweat chloride test. Factors that may contribute to prolapse are frequent bowel movements, colon distention, and increased abdominal pressure due to coughing and lung hyperinflation. Medical therapy with pancreatic enzyme therapy is usually successful, although some children may continue to have episodes until they are 3–5 years of age. In some persistent cases, operative therapy may be necessary. In one large series, 9% of patients required operative intervention (73). Injection therapy with hypertonic saline (30%), 50% dextrose, or 5% phenol in almond oil is frequently successful (74). If this fails, an operative procedure may be required. I prefer a posterior rectopexy with obliteration of the presacral space (75). This can be performed through an abdominal or a posterior sagittal approach.

E. Colonic Strictures

Colon strictures in children with cystic fibrosis were originally described by Smyth et al. in 1994 (76). This initial report identified five patients with marked thickening of the ascending colon wall and stricture occurring within 12–15 months of a change to high-dose enzyme supplementation. Several other reports have followed, confirming the association of these strictures with high-dose pancreatic enzymes (77). Nine patients with this disorder have undergone treatment at this author's institution between 1992 and 1994. Although various theories have been proposed, the exact mechanism of this process is unknown. The clinical presentation nearly always includes abdominal pain and either obstructive symptoms or diarrhea, which may be bloody. In the original report by Smyth et al. (76), persistent symptoms after treatment of presumed DIOS prompted further investigation. In others, diarrhea has been a more prominent feature, and, unfortunately, may be perceived by the family as an indication to increase supplemental enzymes even further. Occasionally, acute distention with a complete obstruction may be the presenting symptom.

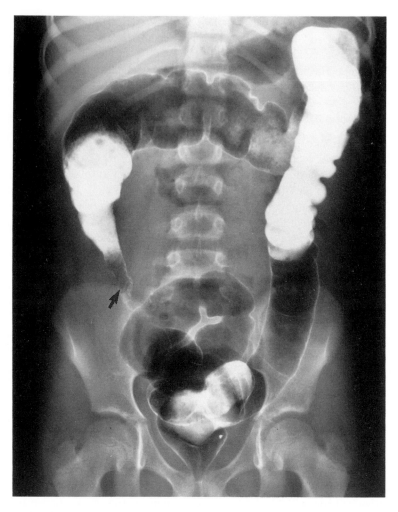

Figure 12 Colonic strictures. Barium enema demonstrates loss of haustral markings in the distal descending colon and a stricture in the ascending colon (*arrow*).

Stevens et al. (78) retrospectively reviewed the pancreatic enzyme history of the nine patients at our institution and compared them to those of 258 nonaffected patients. The affected patients took significantly greater amounts of supplemental pancreatic enzymes in the year prior to the diagnosis of colonic stricture than did their unaffected counterparts. The age range of reported cases is between 2 and 14 years, with the average being between 5 and 7 years.

Failure of response to standard treatment of DIOS or persistence of diarrhea should prompt further evaluation. Plain abdominal radiographs may demonstrate colon thickening and small bowel dilatation, but may also be unremarkable. The most useful test is a barium enema (Fig. 12). This can demonstrate mucosal irregularity, nodular thickening of the wall, and loss of haustral marking. In one reported case, the entire colon was foreshortened (79). At the time of clinical presentation, strictures are usually identified. Although the initial report identified strictures in the ascending colon (76), subsequent reports have identified pancolonic involvement (77) as well as disease in the sigmoid colon and rectum without ascending colon involvement (78).

Ultrasound may be useful in demonstrating thickening of the colon wall as well as peritoneal fluid, which, in several cases, has been to be chylous ascites (77,78). Computed tomography scans can also demonstrate the abnormality but are not necessary. Colonoscopy may occasionally be useful if Crohn's disease is in the differential diagnosis.

If the diagnosis is established before stricture formation, observation with decreased enzyme supplementation may be possible; however, nearly all reported cases have required operative intervention. If obstructive symptoms are present, surgical resection is required. A gentle mechanical bowel preparation is administered for several days before surgery and enteral antibiotics are administered the day before surgery. The goal of operative management is resection of the involved bowel with a primary anastomosis. In cases of complete obstruction, pancolonic involvement, or rectal involvement, this may not be feasible and the child may require an ostomy. At the time of exploration, the involved bowel is thickened, noncomplaint, foreshortened, and may have thickened mesentery. "Creeping fat," characteristic of Crohn's disease, is not seen.

Microscopic examination reveals a mild inflammatory infiltrate in the mucosa with thickening of the submucosa. The absence of mucosal ulcers, transmural granulomas, or fissures differentiates this process from Crohn's disease. Review of specimens at the author's institution demonstrated hyperplasia of the submucosal and intermyenteric plexuses (78).

F. Gallbladder Disease

Gallbladder abnormalities are detected in many patients with CF (80). This can include microgallbladder containing thick colorless "white bile" with occlusion of the cystic duct or radiolucent gallstones, which are noted in 12%–27% of patients with CF (81–83). Recent studies have demonstrated that these are not typical cholesterol stones (80). In addition, the use of ursodeoxycholic acid to dissolve gallstones has not been very effective on the stones in CF patients (84). Although may patients with CF and either gallbladder sludge or stones are asymptomatic, approximately 4% of CF patients have classical symptoms of cholecystitis (85). In addition, biliary dyskinesia, a disorder attributed to abnormalities of motor function in the biliary drainage system, may occur in CF patients. Cholecystectomy, optimally by a laparoscopic technique, is the procedure of choice for symptomatic gallbladder disease (86,87). Rarely, conversion to an open procedure may be required. The anesthesiologist should be prepared for the anesthetic management of patients with CF as well as laparoscopy because the air in the peritoneal cavity required for the procedure can impede diaphragm excursion. The lessened postoperative pain and pulmonary compromise with the laparoscopic technique compared with classical laparotomy have made this an ideal procedure for the patient with CF.

III. Inguinal Hernia, Hydrocele, Undescended Testes, and Absence of Vas Deferens

An increased incidence of inguinal hernia, hydrocele, and undescended testes in male children with cystic fibrosis was noted in several early studies (88,89). Due to this increased incidence, some children undergo surgical repair of one of these defects before the diagnosis of CF is given or symptoms of CF occur (90). The absence of the vas deferens in CF has been well documented (e.g., 91) and, if this is observed at surgery, appropriate diagnostic evaluation for CF is indicated (88–90).

IV. Feeding Tubes and Vascular Access

A. Feeding Tubes and Gastroesophageal Reflux

Many CF patients are given supplemental enteral nutrition. Although nasogastric, nasoduodenal, or nasojejunal tubes may be useful for short-term feeding, direct access is more practical for long-term use and avoids the various drawbacks of nasal tubes. The current standard of gastrostomy tube placement generally involves either percutaneous endoscopic placement by a surgeon or gastroenterologist, or fluoroscopically guided placement by a radiologist. I prefer endoscopic guidance to allow visualization of the tube within the stomach and determination of the distance between the inner portion of the tube, which holds the stomach up to the abdominal wall, and the external portion of the tube. This tube can be placed under general anesthesia in children or with intravenous sedation and local anesthesia in older patients.

Intravenous antibiotics are administered just before the procedure and for 24 hours as prophylaxis because the tube track through the abdominal wall can be contaminated with oral flora. Feedings are usually held for 24 hours after the procedure and then resumed. Numerous commercial devices are available. I prefer to place a gastrostomy tube button device with the percutaneous endoscopic technique (One Step Button, Surgitek, Racine, WI) (92). This device protrudes only 3–4 mm and is very comfortable and easily hidden under clothing. Patients can receive bolus feedings or night infusions, depending on patient and physician preference. Jejunostomy tubes are used in some centers. I prefer to use gastrostomy tubes.

The relationship of gastroesophageal reflux (GER) to a feeding gastrostomy has been debated for years. Actually, the chance of GER developing after gastrostomy tube placement is relatively low. The incidence of GER after a gastrostomy is thought to be highest in children with neurological impairment. Some studies have noted a 25%–44% incidence of GER after placement of a gastrostomy tube (with negative preoperative studies) (93–95) in these children, whereas a more recent study has noted the level to be only 14% (96). In a large series, Gauderer observed that 12.8% of patients required subsequent Nissen fundoplication (97). In most studies, the incidence of subsequent GER in neurologically normal children is less than that of neurologically impaired children.

In view of these data, if reflux symptoms occurring before gastrostomy are not severe or are medically controlled, I simply place a gastrostomy tube. If reflux symptoms are severe and unresponsive to medical management, an antireflux procedure may be necessary, but this is unusual. In addition, many children improve after restoration of their nutritional status (97). If severe reflux appears after placement of a gastrostomy tube, an antireflux procedure can be performed at that time without any added difficulty related to the presence of the gastrostomy tube.

Gastroesophageal reflux has been noted in association with CF by several authors (98–101), and Barrett's esophagus has also been reported (102). Symptoms consistent with reflux should be documented and esophagitis treated medically. Surgical intervention is rarely needed, but if esophagitis is unresponsive to medical management or is associated with Barrett's esophagus, an antireflux procedure should be considered. Although various procedures have been used, the Nissen fundoplication is probably the most widely used. This can be performed by a standard open surgical technique or with the use of laparoscopy. Chronic lung disease has been associated with a higher failure rate of fundoplications (103).

B. Vascular Access

Long-term vascular access is frequently needed for intravenous antibiotics in children and adults with CF. The initial management usually involves peripheral sites, but, as these become less accessible, longer term catheters may be useful. The insertion of percutaneously placed long catheters in the antecubital space, which may be advanced into the basilic or cephalic vein and thence centrally into the superior vena cava, may be used for as long as 2–3 weeks. This allows convenient administration of antibiotics in an outpatient setting.

Percutaneously placed temporary central catheters may also be useful. However, the physician must be cognizant of the hyperinflated lung and risk of pneumothorax when the subclavian vein is used (104). Other central sites for temporary lines include the internal jugular vein and femoral vein; however, these have considerable disadvantages in terms of patient comfort.

Long-term catheters may be useful in patients with recurring episodes of infection. The options include tunneled central lines or the use of subcutaneous ports. The sites of access for percutaneous placement of these catheters include the subclavian vein, internal jugular vein, or femoral vein. In rare cases, a direct cutdown over a more peripheral vein (cephalic, external jugular, saphenous) may be useful, allowing the catheter to pass into the more central vein and then on into the superior or inferior vena cava. The catheter exit sites or port sites are the anterior chest wall or, with the femoral site, the lower abdomen or leg depending on the patient's preference. These can be placed under general or local anesthesia depending on the patient's age and pulmonary status.

The use of subcutaneous ports compared with external lines is often preferable in terms of patient convenience. In addition, several large studies have documented the long-term efficacy of ports with infection rates being the same (105, 106) of lower (107) than external catheters. The safety and efficacy of ports in patients with CF have been documented in several studies (108–110). Sola et al. noted an increased rate of thrombotic complications with ports in CF patients and recommended aspirin prophylaxis as long as there is no evidence of liver disease or bleeding disorders (111). The author's institution has not routinely recommended this added therapy.

References

1. Park RW, Grand RJ. Gastrointestinal manifestations of cystic fibrosis: a review. Gastroenterology 1981; 81:1143–1161.
2. Rescorla FJ, Grosfeld JL, West KW, Vane DW. Changing patterns of treatment and survival in neonates with meconium ileus. Arch Surg 1989; 124:837–840.
3. Donnison AB, Shwachman H, Gross RE. Review of 164 children with meconium ileus seen at the Children's Hospital Medical Center, Boston. Pediatrics 1966; 37:833–850.
4. Landsteiner K. Darmverschluss durch eingedictes Meconium Pankreatitis. Zentralbl Allg Pathol 1905; 16:903–907.
5. Kornblith BA, Otani S. Meconium ileus with congenital stenosis of the main pancreatic duct. Am J Pathol 1929; 5:249–262.
6. Hurwitt ES, Arnheim EE. Meconium ileus associated with stenosis of the pancreatic ducts. Am J Dis Child 1942; 64:443–454.
7. Anderson DH. Cystic fibrosis of the pancreas and its relation to celiac disease. Am J Dis Child 1938; 56:344–399.
8. Farber SJ. The relation of pancreatic achylia to meconium ileus. J Pediatr 1944; 24:387–392.
9. Thomaidis TS, Arey JB. The intestinal lesions in cystic fibrosis of the pancreas. J Pediatr 1963; 63:444–453.

10. Glanzmann VE, Berger H. Uber Mekoniumileus. Ann Pediatr 1950; 175:33.
11. Buchanan DJ, Rapoport S. Chemical comparison of normal meconium and meconium from a patient with meconium ileus. Pediatrics 1952; 9:304–310.
12. Rule AH, Baran DT, Schwachman H. Quantitative determination of water soluble proteins in meconium. Pediatrics 1970; 45:847–850.
13. Ryley HC, Neale L, Brogan TD. Plasma proteins in meconium from normal infants and from babies with cystic fibrosis. Arch Dis Child 1974; 49:901–904.
14. Schutt WH, Isles TE. Protein in meconium from meconium ileus. Arch Dis Child 1968; 43:178–181.
15. Brock D. A comparative study of microvillar enzyme activities in the prenatal diagnosis of cystic fibrosis. Prenat Diagn 1985; 5:129–134.
16. Mornet E, Simon-Bouy B, Serre JL, et al. Genetic differences between cystic fibrosis with and without meconium ileus. Lancet 1988; 1:376–378.
17. Allan JL, Robbie M, Phelan PD, Danks DM. Familial occurrence of meconium ileus. Eur J Pediatr 1981; 135:291–292.
18. Kerem E, Corey M, Kerem B, Durie P, Tsui LC, Levison H. Clinical and genetic comparisons of patients with cystic fibrosis, with or without meconium ileus. J Pediatr 1989; 114:767–773.
19. Neuhauser EBD. Roentgen changes associated with pancreatic insufficiency in early life. Radiology 1946; 46:319–328.
20. Noblett HR. Treatment of uncomplicated meconium ileus by Gastrografin enema: a preliminary report. J Pediatr Surg 1969; 4:190–197.
21. Ein SH, Shandling B, Reilly BJ, Stephens CA. Bowel perforation with nonoperative treatment of meconium ileus. J Pediatr Surg 1987; 22:146–147.
22. Rowe MI, Furst J, Altman DH, Poole CA. The neonatal response to Gastrografin enema. Pediatrics 1971; 48:49.
23. Noblett H. Meconium ileus. In: Ravitch MM, Welch KJ, Benson CD, Aberdeen E, Randolph JG, eds. Pediatric Surgery. 3rd ed. Chicago: Year Book 1979:943–952.
24. Wagget J, Bishop HC, Koop CE. Experience with Gastrografin enema in the treatment of meconium ileus. J Pediatr Surg 1970; 5:649–654.
25. Lillie JG, Chrispin AR. Investigation and management of neonatal obstruction by Gastrografin enema. Ann Radiol (Paris) 1972; 15:237–241.
26. Mabogunje OA, Wang CI, Mahour GH. Improved survival of neonates with meconium ileus. Arch Surg 1982; 117:37.
27. Nguyen LT, Youssef S, Guttman FM, Laberge JM, Albert D, Doody D. Meconium ileus: is a stoma necessary? J Pediatr Surg 1986; 21:766–768.
28. Caniano DA, Beaver BL. Meconium ileus: a fifteen year experience with forty-two neonates. Surgery 1987; 102:699–703.
29. Grantmyre EB, Butler GJ, Gillis DA. Necrotizing enterocolitis after Renografin 76 treatment of meconium ileus. Am J Radiol 1981; 136:990–991.
30. Bowring AC, Jones FC, Kern IB. The use of solvents in the intestinal manifestations of mucoviscidosis. J Pediatr Surg 1970; 5:338–343.
31. Shaw A. Safety of *N*-acetylcysteine in the treatment of meconium obstruction in the newborn. J Pediatr Surg 1969; 4:119–125.
32. Stringer DA. Congenital and developmental anomalies of the small bowel. In: Stringer DA, ed. Pediatric Gastrointestinal Imaging. Philadelphia: BC Decker, 1989:259–262.
33. Rescorla FJ, Grosfeld JL. Contemporary management of meconium ileus. World J Surg 1993; 17:318–325.

34. Hiatt RB, Wilson PE. Celiac syndrome: Therapy of meconium ileus: report of eight cases with a review of the literature. Surg Gynecol Obstet 1948; 87:317–327.
35. Gross RE. The Surgery of Infancy and Childhood. Philadelphia: WB Saunders, 1953;175–191.
36. Bishop HC, Koop CE. Management of meconium ileus: resection, Roux-en-Y anastomosis and ileostomy irrigation with pancreatic enzymes. Ann Surg 1957; 145:410–414.
37. Santulli TV, Blanc WA. Congenital atresia of the intestine: pathogenesis and treatment. Ann Surg 1961; 154:939–948.
38. Swenson O. Pediatric Surgery. 2nd ed. East Norwalk, CT: Appleton & Lange, 1962.
39. Holsclaw DS, Eckstein HB, Nixon HH. Meconium ileus. Am J Dis Child 1965; 109:101–113.
40. O'Neill JA, Grosfeld JL, Boles ET, Clatworthy NW Jr. Surgical treatment of meconium ileus. Am J Surg 1970; 119:99–105.
41. Kalayoglu M. Sieber WK, Rodnan JB, Kiesewetter WB. Meconium ileus: a critical review of treatment and eventual prognosis. J. Pediatr Surg 1971; 6:290–300.
42. Venugopal S, Shandling B. Meconium ileus: laparotomy without resection, anastomosis or enterostomy. J Pediatr Surg 1979; 14:715–718.
43. Fitzgerald R. Colon K. Use of the appendix stump in the treatment of meconium ileus. J Pediatr Surg. 1989; 24:899–900.
44. Fleischer AC, Davis FJ, Campbell L. Sonographic detection of a meconium-containing mass in a fetus: a case report. J Clin Ultrasound 1983; 11:103.
45. Goldstein RB, Fill RA, Callen PW. Sonographic diagnosis of meconium ileus in utero. J Ultrasound Med. 1987; 6:663–666.
46. West DK, Touloukian RJ. Meconium pseudocyst presenting as a buttock mass. J Pediatr Surg 1988; 23:864–865.
47. Rasor R, Stevenson C. Cystic fibrosis of the pancreas, a case history. Rocky Mt Med J 1941; 38:218–220.
48. Jensen K. Meconium ileus equivalent in a 15 year old patient with mucoviscidosis. Acta Paediatr Scand 1962; 51:344–348.
49. Cleghorn GJ, Forstner GG, Stringer DA, Durie PR. Treatment of distal intestinal obstruction syndrome in cystic fibrosis with a balanced intestinal lavage solution. Lancet 1986; 1:8–11.
50. Rubinstein S, Moss R, Lewiston N. Constipation and meconium ileus equivalent in patients with cystic fibrosis. Pediatrics 1986; 78:473–479.
51. Matseshe J, Go V, DiMagno E. Meconium ileus equivalent complicating cystic fibrosis in post neonatal children and young adults. Gastroenterology 1977; 72:732–736.
52. O'Halloran SM, Gilbert J, McKendrick OM, Carty HML, Heaf DP. Gastrografin in acute meconium ileus equivalent. Arch Dis Child 1986; 1128–1130.
53. Holsclaw D, Rocmans C, Shwachman H. Abdominal complaints and appendiceal changes leading to the diagnosis of cystic fibrosis. J Pediatr Surg 1974; 9:867–873.
54. Dalzell AM, Heaf DP, Carty H. Pathology mimicking distal intestinal obstruction syndrome in cystic fibrosis. Arch Dis Child 1990; 65:540–541.
55. Moody AR, Haddock JA, Given-Wilson R, Adam EJ. CT monitoring of therapy for meconium ileus. J Comput Assist Tomogr 1990; 14:1010–1012.

56. Synder W, Gwinn J, Landin B, Assay L. Fecal retention in children with cystic fibrosis, report of three cases. Pediatrics 1964; 34:72–77.

57. Sigler R, Reeves H, Lynn H, Burke E. Cystic fibrosis with fecal retention (meconium ileus equivalent): report of two cases. Mayo Clin Proc 1965; 40:477–480.

58. Lillibridge C, Docter J, Eidelman S. Oral administration of *N*-acetylcysteine in the prophylaxis of "meconium ileus equivalent." J Pediatr 1967; 71:887–889.

59. Hodson M, Mearns M, Batten J. Meconium ileus equivalent in adults with cystic fibrosis of pancreas: a report of six cases. BMJ 1976; 2:790–791.

60. Cleghorn GJ, Forstner GG, Stringer DA, Durie PR. Treatment of distal intestinal obstruction syndrome in cystic fibrosis with a balanced intestinal lavage solution. Lancet 1986; 1:8–11.

61. Khoshoo V, Udall JN, Jr. Meconium ileus equivalent in children and adults. Am J Gastroenterol 1994; 89:153–157.

62. Bailey DJ, Andres JM. Liver injury after oral and rectal administration of *N*-acetylcysteine for meconium ileus equivalent in a patient with cystic fibrosis. Pediatrics 1987; 79:281–282.

63. Koletzko S, Corey M, Ellis L, Spino M, Stringer DA, Durie PR. Effects of cisapride in patients with cystic fibrosis and distal intestinal obstruction syndrome. J Pediatr 1990; 117:815–822.

64. Littlewood JM. Gastrointestinal complications. Br Med Bull 1992; 48:847–859.

65. Holsclaw D, Rosmans C, Shwachman H. Intussusception in patients with cystic fibrosis. Pediatrics 1971; 48:51

66. Webb AK, Khan A. Chronic intussusception in a young adult with cystic fibrosis. J R Soc Med 1989; 82(suppl 16):47–48.

67. Martens M, DeBoeck K, VanDerSteen K, Smet M, Eggermont E. A right lower quadrant mass in cystic fibrosis: a diagnostic challenge. Eur J Pediatr 1992; 151:329–331.

68. Holsclaw DS, Hobboushe C. Occult appendiceal abscess complicating cystic fibrosis. J Pediatr Surg 1976; 11:217–220.

69. Coughlin JP, Gauderer MW, Stern RC, Doershuk CF, Izant RJ, Zollinger RM. The spectrum of appendiceal disease in cystic fibrosis. J Pediatr Surg 1990; 25:835–839.

70. McCarthy VP, Mischler EH, Chernick MS, di Sant'Agnese P. Appendiceal abscess in cystic fibrosis. Gastroenterology 1984; 86:564–568.

71. Shields MD, Levison H, Reisman JJ, Durie PR, Canny GJ. Appendicitis in cystic fibrosis. Arch Dis Child 1990; 65:307–310.

72. Stern R, Izant RJ, Boat TF, Wood RE, Matthews LW, Doershuk CF. Treatment and prognosis of rectal prolapse in cystic fibrosis. Gastroenterology 1986; 82:707–710.

73. McIntosh R. Cystic fibrosis of the pancreas in patients over ten years of age. Acta Pediatr Scand 1954; 100(suppl):471–480.

74. Wyllie GG. The injection treatment of rectal prolapse. J Pediatr Surg 1979; 14:62–64.

75. Ashcraft KW, Garred JL, Holder TM, Amoury RA, Sharp RJ, Murphy JP. Rectal prolapse: 17-year experience with the posterior repair and suspension. J Pediatr Surg 1990; 25:992–995.

76. Smyth RL, vanVelzen D, Smyth AR, Lloyd DA, Heaf DP. Strictures of ascending colon in cystic fibrosis and high-strength pancreatic enzymes. Lancet 1994; 343:85–86.

77. Pettei MJ, Leonidas JC, Levine JJ, Gorvoy JD. Pancolonic disease in cystic fibrosis and high-dose pancreatic enzyme therapy. J Pediatr 1994; 125:587–589.

78. Stevens J, Chong S, West K, Collins M, Maguiness K. Colonic strictures in cystic fibrosis patients on very high-dose pancreatic enzyme supplementation (abstr). Pediatr Pulmonol 1994; (suppl 10):275.

79. Zerin JM, Kuhn-Fulton J, White SJ, et al. Colonic strictures in children with cystic fibrosis. Radiology 1995; 194:223–266.

80. Angelico M, Gandin C, Canuzzi P, Bertasi S, Cantafora A, DeSantis A, Quattrucci S, Antonelli M. Gallstones in cystic fibrosis: a critical reappraisal. Hepatology 1991; 14:768–775.

81. L'Heureux PR, Isenberg JN, Sharp HL, Warwick WJ. Gallbladder disease in cystic fibrosis. AJR Am J Roentgonel 1977; 128:953–956.

82. Isenberg JN. Cystic fibrosis: its influence on the liver, biliary tree and bile salt metabolism. Semin Liver Dis 1982; 2:302–313.

83. Shwachman H, Kowalski M, Khaw K-T. Cystic fibrosis: a new outlook. Medicine 1977; 56:129–149.

84. Colombo C, Bertolini E, Assaiso ML, Bettinardi N, et al. Failure of ursodeoxycholic acid to dissolve radiolucent gallstones in patients with cystic fibrosis. Acta Paediatr 1993; 82:562–565.

85. Stern RC, Rothstein FC, Doershuk CF. Treatment and prognosis of symptomatic gallbladder disease in patients with cystic fibrosis. J Pediatr Gastroenterol Nutr 1986; 5:35–42.

86. Anagnostopoulos D, Tsagari N, Noussia-Arvanitaki S. Gallbladder disease in patients with cystic fibrosis. Eur J Pediatr Surg 1993; 3:348–351.

87. Williams SGJ, Westaby D, Tanner MS, Mowat AP. Liver and biliary problems in cystic fibrosis. Br Med Bull 1992; 48:877–892.

88. Wang CI, Kwok S, Edelbrock H. Inguinal hernia, hydrocele and other genitourinary abnormalities in boys with cystic fibrosis and their male siblings. Am J Dis Child 1970; 119:236–237.

89. Holsclaw DS, Shwachman H. Increased incidence of inguinal hernia, hydrocele and undescended testicles in males with cystic fibrosis. Pediatrics 1971; 3:442–445.

90. Goshen R, Kerem E, Shoshani T, Kerem BS, Feigen E, Zamir O, Yahau Y. Cystic fibrosis manifested as undescended testis and absence of vas deferens. Pediatrics 1992; 90:982–983.

91. Rigot JM, Lafitte JJ, Dumur V, et al. Cystic fibrosis and congenital absence of the vas deferens. N Engl J Med 1991; 325:64–65.

92. Treem WR, Etienne NL, Hyams JS. Percutaneous endoscopic placement of the "button" gastrostomy tube as the initial procedure in infants and children. J Pediatr Gastroenterol 1993; 17:382–386.

93. Jolley SG, Smith El, Tunnell WB. Protective antireflux operation with feeding gastrostomy. Ann Surg 1985; 201:736–740.

94. Mollitt DL, Golladay EJ, Seibert JJ. Symptomatic gastroesophageal reflux following gastrostomy in neurologically impaired patients. Pediatrics 1985; 75:1124–1126.

95. Grunow JE, Al-Hafidh AS, Tunnell NP. Gastroesophageal reflux following percutaneous endoscopic gastrostomy in children. J Pediatr Surg 1989; 24:42–45.
96. Wheatley MJ, Wesley JR, Tkach DM, Coran AB. Long-term follow-up of brain-damaged children requiring feeding gastrostomy: should an antireflux procedure always be performed? J Pediatr Surg 1991; 26:301–305.
97. Gauderer M. Percutaneous endoscopic gastrostomy: a 10 year experience with 220 children. J. Pediatr Surg 1991; 226:288–294.
98. Cucchiara S, Santamaria F, Andreotti MR, et al. Mechanisms of gastroesophageal reflux in cystic fibrosis. Arch Dis Child 1991;66:617–622.
99. Orenstein SR, Orenstein DM. Gastroesophageal reflux and respiratory disease in children. J Pediatr 1988; 112:847–858.
100. Vandenplas Y, Diericx A, Blecker U, et al. Esophageal pH monitoring data during chest physiotherapy. J Pediatr Gastroenterol Nurt 1991; 13:23–26.
101. Davidson AGF, Wong LTK. Gastroesophageal reflux in cystic fibrosis. Pediatr Pulmonol 1991; 56:99–100.
102. Hassall E, Israel DM, Davidson AGF, Wong LTK. Barrett's esophagus in children with cystic fibrosis: not a coincidental association. Am J Gastroenterol 1993; 88:1934–1938.
103. Taylor LA, Weiner T, Lacey SR, Azizkhan RG. Chronic lung disease is the leading risk factor correlating with the failure (wrap disruption) of antireflux procedures in children. J Pediatr Surg 1994;,29(2):161–164.
104. Morris JB, Occhionero ME, Gauderer MWL, Stern RC, Doershuk CF. Totally implantable vascular access devices in cystic fibrosis: a four year experience with fifty-eight patients. J Pediatr 1990; 117:82–85.
105. Keung YK, Watkins K, Chen SC, Groshen S, Silberman H, Douer D. Comparative study of infectious complications of different types of chronic central venous access devices. Cancer 1994; 74:2832–2837.
106. Wiener ES, McGuire P, Stolar CJH, Rich RH, Albo VC, Ablin AR, Betcher DL, Sitarz AL, Buckley JD, Krailo MD, Versteeg C, Hammond GD. The CCSG prospective study of venous access devices: an analysis of insertions and causes for removal. J Pediatr Surg 1992; 27:155–164.
107. Mirro J Jr, Rao BN, Kumar M, Rafferty M, Hancock M, Austin BA, Fairclough D, Lobe TE. A comparison of placement techniques and complications of external-ized catheters and implantable port use in children with cancer. J Pediatr Surg 1990; 25:120–124.
108. Cassey J, Ford WDA, O'Brien LO, Martin AJ. Totally implantable system for venous access in children with cystic fibrosis. Clin Pediatr 1988; 27:91–95.
109. Ball ABS, Duncan FR, Foster FJ, Davidson TI, Watkins RM, Hodson ME. Long term venous access using a totally implantable drug delivery system in patients with cystic fibrosis and bronchiectasis. Respir Med 1989; 83:429–431.
110. Stead RJ, Davidson TI, Duncan FR, Hodson M, Batten JC. Use of a totally implantable system for venous access in cystic fibrosis. Thorax 1987; 42:149–150.
111. Sola JE, Stone MM, Wise B, Colombani PM. A typical thrombotic and septic complications of totally implantable venous access devices in patients with cystic fibrosis. Pediatr Pulmonol 1992; 14:239–242.

10

Intensive Care

JOHN C. STEVENS and HOWARD EIGEN

Indiana University School of Medicine and
James Whitcomb Riley Hospital for Children
Indianapolis, Indiana

I. Introduction

The clinical course in patients with cystic fibrosis (CF) is well delineated, with
approximately 95% succumbing to a gradual but persistent deterioration in
respiratory function. Early studies demonstrated that, when patients reached the
terminal stage of their respiratory disease, assisted ventilation was futile (1–3).
Given this outlook, the indications to admit a CF patient to the intensive care
unit (ICU) were fairly narrow. However, with the advent of improved techniques of assisted ventilation and successful lung and liver transplantation, and
with the extended longevity of CF patients and the consequential development
of other nonrespiratory life-threatening complications, the indications for ICU
treatment have expanded to encompass a wide variety of conditions (Table 1).
This chapter reviews these indications and describes their current treatment
regimens. For nearly all of these indications, there are no clearly defined criteria
for ICU admission. Intensive care units are intense units, where decisions are
made and aggressive treatment is carried out at a much more rapid pace than
most CF physicians and families are used to or comfortable with. The decision
to admit or transfer a patient to the ICU is based on the primary physician's

Table 1 Possible Indications for Admission or Transfer
to the Intensive Care Unit in Cystic Fibrosis

Acute respiratory failure
Severe bronchospasm
Severe electrolyte abnormalities
Massive hemoptysis
Liver failure
Massive hematemesis
Postoperative complications
Chronic respiratory failure awaiting transplantation
Trauma

level of comfort with the adequacy of care on a standard hospital unit, the relationship of the primary physician with the ICU staff, and the feelings of the patient and family.

II. General CF Care

Regardless of the problem prompting ICU admission, the patient must continue to receive appropriate general CF care, including pancreatic enzymes with any nonelemental oral or enteral feeds, chest physical therapy with or without aerosol treatments, and careful attention to electrolyte balance.

Many patients with CF have been treated well in ICUs for their pulmonary surgery or liver transplantation, only to have major setbacks from bowel obstruction, because pancreatic enzymes were not resumed, or from hypomagnesemic seizures, because the CF patient's propensity for development of hypomagnesemia was not kept in mind.

III. Acute Respiratory Failure

Cystic fibrosis pulmonary disease often progresses to severe hypoxemia and hypercapnia. Davis and di Sant'Agnese reviewed the outcome of 46 CF patients, aged 1 month to 31 years, who underwent 51 episodes of assisted ventilation for respiratory failure during the 1970s. They found that 69% percent of patients died while receiving mechanical ventilation and three patients lived longer than 1 year (3). Other studies of this era found a similar outcome with mechanical ventilation (1,2).

Despite these dismal early reports, it is apparent that some CF patients with respiratory failure are candidates for assisted ventilation (Table 2). A review of patients who received assisted ventilation at three CF centers in the late 1980s found 73% of patients younger than 1 year of age at the time of

Table 2 Indications for Assisted Ventilation in CF

Respiratory failure in infancy
Acute respiratory failure in a patient with mild or moderate lung disease
Pretransplantation (selected patients)
Transient reversible pulmonary complication with any level of underlying lung disease
  (e.g., bilateral pneumothorax)

mechanical ventilation were alive 0.5 to 7 years later (4,5). The improved survival rate was thought to be related to improvements in techniques and equipment for mechanical ventilation of infants and better antibiotics (5). However, the possibility that some of these patients might have survived without assisted ventilation must also be considered.

The CF patients with mild lung disease who have a reversible cause of their respiratory failure are likely to have a good outcome with assisted ventilation (3–5). Reversible processes include trauma, pneumothorax, severe bronchospasm, seizures with apnea, viral pneumonia, pertussis, upper airway obstruction, and postoperative pulmonary complications.

Short-term assisted ventilation has been used successfully in some patients awaiting lung transplantation (6,7). Recently, noninvasive mechanical ventilation using nasal intermittent positive pressure ventilation has also been successful in CF patients awaiting lung transplantation (8–10).

A. Treatment of Respiratory Failure

The basic approach to respiratory failure in the CF patient is to treat the underlying cause, while being very aggressive with airway clearance techniques, antibiotics, maintaining adequate nutrition, providing supplemental oxygen as needed, and intervening with mechanical ventilation when indicated (Table 3).

Inhaled bronchodilators are often used in the treatment of CF, although the bronchodilator response in CF patients is variable (11–17) and, at times, may be negative, resulting in reduced flows (18,19). Nevertheless, increasing

Table 3 Treatment of Respiratory Failure in CF

Supplemental oxygen
Frequent percussion and postural drainage
Broad antibiotic coverage (when possible, based on recent cultures)
Inhaled bronchodilators
Adequate nutrition
Mucolytics
Ventilatory muscle stimulation (e.g., theophylline)
Ventilation—when indicated

Table 4 Bronchodilator Drugs for Cystic Fibrosis ICU Care

Drug	Dose	Frequency (q__hr)	Side effects
Albuterol			Increased heart rate
Intermittent	2.5–5 mg	Up to 1–2 h	
Continuous	1mL of 0.5% solution in 4mL normal saline	continuous	
Atropine	0.4–1.0 mg	6–8 h	Increased heart rate, dry secretions
Ipratropium			Increased heart rate, dry secretions
Metered dose inhaler	2 puffs	6–8 h	
Nebulized	75–250μg		

respiratory distress justifies a trial of frequent nebulized bronchodilators such as albuterol or terbutaline. The doses are similar to those used in treating asthma. We have successfully used anticholinergic agents such as atropine and ipratropium bromide after an inadequate response to inhaled beta-agonists. Atropine is given in a dose of 0.4 to 1.0 mg nebulized every 6 to 8 hours while carefully monitoring for side effects, including tachyarrhythmias and excessive drying of pulmonary secretions. Ipratropium bromide is associated with fewer side effects and can be given by metered dose inhaler at two inhalations (36 μg) every 6 to 8 hours. A nebulized form is available and the dose suggested for use in asthmatic children is 75–250 mg (20). Table 4 lists the major bronchodilators used for patients with CF in the ICU.

Maximizing pulmonary secretion clearance with chest physiotherapy is a critical component of the treatment of severe pulmonary exacerbations in CF patients. These patients often tolerate only partial treatments, and shorter sessions can then be ordered. Overly aggressive therapy can mobilized a large amount of very viscid secretions from the peripheral to the central airways, potentially obstructing large areas of the lung and causing even greater distress and further deterioration of arterial blood gas values. A number of new approaches to airway clearance, such as positive expiratory pressure (PEP) mask therapy, the Therapy Vest, autogenic drainage, and the Flutter valve have become available recently; however, their use during respiratory failure has not been reported. We rely on manual segmental percussion and postural drainage for CF patients who are acutely ill.

Airway clearance is often impeded by thick and tenacious secretions. The mucolytic *N*-acetylcysteine has been used in a dose of 1–2 mL of 10% solution inhaled before percussion and postural drainage. However, acetylcysteine often causes bronchospasm, and so is rarely used in our institution. The newest mucolytic, human recombinant DNase (alpha dornase), is readily available and can be used to thin pulmonary secretions. Although shown in one study to be safe, DNase appears no more effective than placebo in very sick patients (21), and there are anecdotal reports of patients with severe disease having trouble handling the large amounts of acutely mobilized secretions. The recommended dose is 2.5 mg inhaled once or twice a day.

To account for the changing patterns of antimicrobial resistance, we typically obtain sputum cultures at admission and repeat them to identify newly resistant organisms if improvement is suboptimal or if the patient takes an unexpected downturn. On admission, we typically treat with two antibiotics that are effective in vitro against the predominant organisms from the most recent culture. This typically includes an aminoglycoside and a semisynthetic penicillin or third-generation cephalosporin. Dosages and dosing intervals are adjusted according to pharmacokinetic parameters (see Chapter 11). When treating with tobramycin or gentamicin, we aim for a peak level of 8–10 µg/mL and a trough of less than 2 µg/mL. In recent years, an increasing number of patients with advanced lung disease have harbored methicillin-resistant *Staphylococcus aureus* in their pulmonary secretions. We therefore add vancomycin empirically to the treatment regimen if the patient is not responding to initial therapy. Atypical mycobacterial infections and allergic bronchopulmonary aspergillosis also need to be considered if a patient is not responding to the treatment regimen. These problems are discussed in Chapter 4.

Cystic fibrosis patients may have a resting energy expenditure of up to 150% of normal (22–24). With respiratory distress, energy expenditure is even greater at a time when caloric intake is often poor. Maintaining adequate nutrition is extremely important in facilitating recovery. Supplemental nutrition can be provided by nasogastric tube feedings or by central hyperalimentation. To avoid the need for supplemental pancreatic enzymes with enteral feedings, elemental formulas such as Vital HN (Ross Laboratories) or Tolerex (Norwich Eaton) are typically used. Some centers use the less expensive nonelemental formulas, and simply add enzymes to the bottle or bag of formula. In the ICU, this feeding would be given in a continuous drip at a rate to meet 100% of the recommended daily caloric allowance for the patient. If the patient is able to eat by mouth, a high-calorie, high-fat, high-protein diet is supplied to provided extra calories.

Cystic fibrosis patients often become very hypoxemic during severe pulmonary exacerbations. Humidified oxygen is provided to maintain adequate oxygen saturation and to decrease the work of breathing. So as not to suppress respiratory drive in CF patients with advanced lung disease and chronic carbon dioxide retention, oxygen saturation should be maintained between 88% and 92% (see Chapter 4). If chronic carbon dioxide retention is not a problem, oxygen saturations of 92%–93% or greater are generally acceptable, depending on the patient's work of breathing. We monitor $Paco_2$ frequently and, when possible, adjust oxygen delivery to prevent a dangerously rapid increase in $Paco_2$ (see Chapter 14).

Right heart failure, secondary to pulmonary hypertension (cor pulmonale), occurs in approximately 25% of patients with cystic fibrosis and severe respiratory failure. The mainstay of prevention and therapy for cor pulmonale and heart failure is providing adequate oxygenation. Diuretics may be used if the patient has fluid retention, but they can decrease right heart filling, causing further decrease in pulmonary perfusion. Cardiac glycosides are generally not indicated, because they do little to augment right heart function and may precipitate arrhythmias.

When the patient has progressive hypoxemia, hypercapnia, or acidosis, despite the aggressive therapy described, and meets one of the criteria in Table 2, it may be reasonable to initiate assisted ventilation. The salient features in ventilation of the CF patient with advanced lung disease and severe airway obstruction are listed in Table 5. Intubation should be done by an experienced operator, because these patients become hypoxemic rapidly and are often difficult to ventilate using a mask and bag. An induction using rapid onset, short-acting sedatives and neuromuscular blocking agents is carried out. This is followed by intubation with a relatively large, cuffed endotracheal tube to facilitate removal of secretions and to help prevent air leak, despite the high pressures needed to ventilate the low-compliance lungs. We use volume ventilation to ensure consistent tidal volume. The rate and tidal volume are adjusted to maintain some level of spontaneous ventilation, which maintains tone in the patient's respiratory muscles and facilitates weaning. It is helpful to use pressure support to facilitate this and to increase comfort. Allowing spontaneous breaths to be taken easily relieves anxiety and permits more effective coughing. We use moderate sedation and avoid neuromuscular blockade whenever possible. Because of severe airway obstruction, these patients have a markedly prolonged expiratory phase; therefore, we use a short inspiratory time and a long expiratory time. The objective is to have expiratory flow cease before initiation of the next breath. Tidal volume is adjusted to control $Paco_2$ at the

Table 5 Salient Features of Ventilation of CF Patients

Use large endotracheal tube
Provide volume ventilation
Provide pressure support
Avoid paralysis and heavy sedation
Allow complete exhalation
Maximize mean airway pressure
Maximize airway clearance
Extubate as soon as possible

desired levels, while taking into account that overdistention of the lung increases the likelihood of pneumothorax.

Typically, for a teenager or adult, this translates into a rate of 10–15 breaths per minute and a tidal volume of 12–15 mL/kg. Physicians should be alert for the development of pneumothorax. Any sudden deterioration in respiratory status, especially if accompanied by a decrease in blood pressure, is strongly suggestive of an air leak. We always keep a chest tube at the bedside when caring for such patients in case the need arises to evacuate air from the chest.

Airway secretions can be cleared much more effectively by a patient's cough than by a nurse's or respiratory therapist's suctioning of an endotracheal tube. Therefore, patients should be encouraged to cough, and heavy sedation and paralysis should be avoided if possible. Extubation should be undertaken as soon as the patient can tolerate discontinuation of supplemental ventilation. In patients who have chest, back, or abdominal pain (e.g., after surgery or trauma), adequate analgesia must be provided to allow for deep breaths and strong coughing.

Noninvasive nasal ventilation has been successfully employed with CF patients by using either the conventional volume ventilator or the bilevel positive airway pressure system (BiPAP Respironics Inc.) with a tight-fitting nasal mask. These systems, initially designed to treat obstructive sleep apnea, have been successfully used to treat respiratory failure in patients with chronic obstructive pulmonary disease and cystic fibrosis, especially as a bridge to lung transplantation (8–10,25). They deliver positive pressure to the airway throughout the respiratory cycle, with greater assisting pressure during inspiration than expiration. The positive pressure on inspiration helps diminish the work required of the inspiratory muscles, and the lower level of positive pressure during expiration serves to stent airways open. The advantages of nasal ventilation over conventional endotracheal ventilation include improved pulmonary toilet by maintaining the patient's cough, lessened airway trauma, and allowing of the patients to eat, drink, and move about freely so that they maintain overall physical condition. It is often difficult to initiate this therapy in patients with severe respiratory compromise because they may feel the nasal mask is oppressive or "suffocating." The constant attendance of a familiar physician or respiratory therapist is often helpful while the system is adjusted. Typically, use of the BiPAP system is initiated with low pressure settings (e.g., inspiratory pressure of 6 cm H_2O/expiratory pressure 2 cm) and a short duration of wearing the nasal mask (e.g., 10–15 minutes per hour). It is important to have a tight-fitting but comfortable nasal mask. The duration of use is gradually increased and the pressure settings fine tuned to optimize ventilation and oxygenation. Supplemental oxygen can be added if the BiPAP alone does not result in adequate oxygen saturations.

IV. Severe Bronchospasm

Although up to 95% of CF patients have a significant response to bronchodilator at some time, severe wheezing similar to status asthmaticus develops in only a very small percentage of older patients (12). Severe wheezing is occasionally seen in CF infants and may require ICU treatment. The specific indications for transfer or admission to the ICU are listed in Table 6. Generally, the patient with a very high oxygen requirement of greater than or equal to 0.60 FIO_2 or with a rapidly increasing oxygen requirement should be observed in the ICU. A "normal" or elevated $PaCO_2$ is also very concerning. Patients who are tachypneic should have a low $PaCO_2$. A $PaCO_2$ in the normal or elevated range indicates that the patient is tiring and needs close monitoring, including serial blood gas analyses. Another indicator of the severity of asthma is the frequency of bronchodilator treatments. At our institution, if treatments are required more frequently than every 3 hours, the patient is transferred to the ICU. Many patients with CF who are terminally ill have O_2 requirements that are greater than or equal to 0.60 FIO_2, $PaCO_2$ greater than 40 mmHg, and bronchodilator treatments more frequently than every 3 hours. These patients, who have arrived at this stage gradually, should **not** be in the ICU (see Chapter 14).

The ICU treatment regimen for status asthmaticus in the CF patient is listed in Table 7. Warmed humidified oxygen should be administered to keep O_2 saturations in the mid 92%–95% range unless a lower oxygen saturation of 88%–92% is warranted because of chronic hypercapnia. We generally use albuterol in a dose of 2.5 to 5 mg every 1 to 2 hours. If the patient is in marked distress, especially with an abnormal $PaCO_2$, a continuous aerosol of albuterol or terbutaline can be used. Albuterol is administered continuously by diluting 1.0 mL of albuterol 0.5% with 4 mL of normal saline and refilling the nebulizer when it is empty. This is continued until an adequate response is seen and the patient can tolerate reduction in treatment to once an hour.

Beta-agonists given by inhalation or by intravenous infusion increase ventilation–perfusion mismatch, which worsens hypoxemia. Albuterol administration can also cause hypokalemia, warranting careful monitoring of serum potassium.

Table 6 ICU Admission Criteria for CF Patient with Acute Wheezing

FIO_2 > 0.60
$PaCO_2$ > 40 mm Hg
Frequent arterial blood gas measurements
Bronchodilator treatments needed every 3 hours or more

Table 7 ICU Measures for CF Status Asthmaticus

Warm humidified oxygen
Albuterol treatments Q2 to continuous
Intravenous methylprednisolone
Intravenous aminophylline
Chest physical therapy as tolerated
Intravenous antibiotics
Continuous pulse–oxygen monitoring
Frequent arterial blood gas measurements

To decrease the inflammatory component of the attack, intravenous corticosteroids, typically methylprednisolone, are used. Patients are given a bolus of 2 mg/kg and then given 0.5–1 mg/kg every 6 hours. Although the benefit of aminophylline in treatment of status asthmaticus has been questioned in recent years (26,27), a trial seems warranted for a patient in severe acute distress. Aminophylline may help in this setting by dilating bronchi, improving ventilatory muscle function, providing mild diuresis, decreasing dyspnea, or providing a combination of these effects. Patients are given a bolus of 5–6 mg/kg followed by a continuous intravenous infusion of 0.8–1.0 mg/kg/h. The rate is adjusted to achieve a serum concentration of 10–15 mg/dL.

The CF patient in status asthmaticus needs concurrent treatment with chest physiotherapy and appropriate intravenous antibiotics (Chapter 4).

The patient's respiratory status needs to be assessed frequently by physical examination and arterial blood gas analysis. We use continuous pulse oximetry in all patients requiring aerosol therapy more frequently than every 3 hours. If the patient's condition deteriorates despite the treatment described, consideration should be given to the use of intravenous terbutaline. Terbutaline is given as a continuous infusion at a dose of 0.1–0.25 μg/kg/min. We monitor the patient for the development of tachycardia, cardiac dysrhythmias, and hypokalemia. Patients in whom respiratory failure develops, despite intensive therapy, are usually candidates for assisted ventilation.

V. Severe Electrolyte Abnormalities

Cystic fibrosis patients are prone to development of severe electrolyte abnormalities, often with dehydration. The acute form is most often seen in young infants exposed to high environmental temperature. Prolonged exposure to environmental heat can lead to dehydration and hypoelectrolytemia because of excessive salt loss from sweating (31,32). In the most severe form, this is manifested as heat stroke, defined as a body temperature above 40.6°C associated with a central nervous system disturbance. Untreated heat stroke can lead to shock, seizures, kidney and liver failure, respiratory insufficiency, disseminated intravascular coagulopathy, and eventually death (33,34). Treatment consists of cooling the patient and replacement of current and ongoing fluid and electrolyte losses. Cooling the patient with the use of an ice bath and skin massage to facilitate heat exchange is commonly used. Inadequate or delayed cooling is highly correlated with poor outcome in the treatment of heat stroke (34,35). It is important to differentiate heat stroke from infectious febrile illnesses. In heat stroke, the hypothalamic thermostat is set properly, but, because of high environmental temperatures, overbundling, or lack of sweating, the patient cannot transfer heat to the environment adequately. In these cases, cooling the skin makes good physiological sense. In febrile infectious illnesses, it is the setpoint of the hypothalamic thermostat that is altered, and removing heat from the skin serves only to increase metabolic heat production with shivering and nonshivering thermogenesis, thus making the patient more uncomfortable and increasing energy expenditure. Aspirin or acetaminophen can lower the hypothalamic setpoint and lower temperature in these patients.

The second form of electrolyte abnormality seen in CF patients is hypoelectrolytemia with metabolic alkalosis without dehydration (36–38). A number of CF infants at our institution were seen with such a presentation during the summer. The condition is thought to be secondary to a chronic negative salt balance. Treatment is by intravenous or oral electrolytes and fluid replacement. CF patients are also at increased risk for hypomagnesemia, a problem that is discussed in Chapter 6.

VI. Hemoptysis

Hemoptysis is seen in as many as 60% of CF patients. Usually, however, this amounts to little more than blood streaking of the sputum. Five percent of CF patients experience at least one episode of massive hemoptysis, with expectoration of more than 250 mL of blood in a 24-hour period (39). Holsclaw et al. reported 19 CF patients with massive hemoptysis, of whom, 32% died from asphyxiation and exsanguination with their first episode (40). In contrast, Stern et al. found that none of 69 patients died as a direct result of massive hemoptysis (41). However, because of the risk of death, physicians should be quick to evaluate and manage massive hemoptysis. Only in very unusual cases does this require ICU care (Table 8). In these rare cases, the objective of ICU care is to prevent patients from exsanguinating or drowning in their own blood. In rare instances, this may require prompt endotracheal intubation, with the isolation of one lung by placing the endotracheal tube into the main stem bronchus on the side opposite the bleeding. This may need to be done using a rigid bronchoscope to control the bleeding and to allow for adequate suctioning of the airway.

Table 8 Indications for ICU Admission for CF Patients with Hemoptysis

Acute decrease in SaO_2 to < 90%, despite supplemental oxygen
Hemodynamic instability (inability to maintain blood pressure despite blood
   transfusions)

Localization of the bleeding site may be important if invasive treatment (angiography, single-lung intubation, lobectomy) is needed. History and physical examination occasionally provide clues to the site of bleeding. Patients may report localized gurgling, warmth or discomfort just prior to hemoptysis and can occasionally point accurately to the side of the bleeding. Auscultation may reveal new focal findings such as coarse crackles or rhonchi. A chest roentgenogram may show a new infiltrate or demonstrate an area of marked bronchiectasis that oftentimes is the source of bleeding. Bronchoscopy may be useful for localizing the site of bleeding. However, in some cases, the only bronchoscopic findings are streaks of blood along many bronchi. With active bleeding, the bronchoscopist may see only a mass of blood welling up out the lower airways. In either of these cases, it may be impossible to localize the bleeding source. Bronchoscopy is best done with a flexible fiberscope if the bleeding is not immediately life threatening. Because the flexible scope has limited suctioning capacity and is of no use in controlling the airway, it should not be used during brisk, life-threatening bleeding. Instead, the evaluation should be carried out using a rigid bronchoscope so that the airway can be controlled and blood and secretions can be suctioned in large quantities. However, with massive bleeding, it may be difficult to delineate the source with either flexible or rigid bronchoscopy because of poor visualization, and it may be best to delay bronchoscopy until after major bleeding has ceased.

Selective bronchial angiography may reveal the source of bleeding as dye escaping from the vessel. If such a finding is absent, angiography usually shows areas of markedly dilated, tortuous bronchial vessels that can be assumed to be the source of bleeding (42). Evaluation of hemoptysis at the time of presentation should also include an investigation for medications that may be interfering with coagulation such as aspirin, nonsteroidal antiinflammatory drugs (NSAIDs), and penicillin. With the CF patient's propensity for fat malabsorption, vitamin K should be given empirically. A sputum culture should be obtained to evaluate the sensitivities of the patient's predominant organisms. A complete blood count, platelet count, and blood typing should be drawn at presentation to evaluate the degree of blood loss and to prepare for transfusion if needed. The treatment of massive hemoptysis is listed in Table 9, demonstrating conservative to most aggressive therapies (43). The less invasive steps are discussed at greater length in Chapter 4.

Table 9 Possible Therapeutic Measures for Massive Hemoptysis

Bed rest, with bathroom privileges
Elimination of contributory drugs
Antibiotics
Transfusion for severe blood loss
Therapy with vitamin K (empirical), 5 mg, intramuscularly
Intravenous Pitressin, 20 units, infused over 20 min, followed by 0.2 units/minute, continuously[a]
Intravenous Premarin, 10–25 mg infused over 10–15 minutes every 4–6 hours[a]
Arterial embolization[a]
Endobronchial tamponade[a]
Local pulmonary resection[a]

[a]ICU care required

If the patient has a life-threatening episode, in addition to initiation of the conservative measures, intravenous Pitressin with 20 units of vasopressin can be infused over 20 minutes followed by a continuous infusion of 0.2 units/minute; and desmopressin 4 μg bolus followed by 0.3 μg/kg over 12 hours may be tried (44). Intravenous Premarin in a dose of 10–25 mg over 10–15 minutes every 4–6 hours for three to four doses may also be tried (45).

Arterial embolization has also been successfully used in CF patients with massive hemoptysis (47–49). It does, however, have some serious side effects, which include organ infarction, and should only be performed by an experienced interventional radiographer.

If these measures are not successful in controlling life-threatening hemoptysis, bronchoscopy with endobronchial tamponade with a catheter and balloon system followed by iced saline lavage or topical alpha-agonists may be used (50).

In rare cases, the measures described fail to control massive hemoptysis and local pulmonary resection is indicated. Localization of the bleeding site must be established before surgery, and candidates for this procedure should have adequate baseline lung function (51,52). Lung resection should be undertaken only in desperation.

VII. Hepatic Failure

Up to 25% of CF patients have hepatic steatosis and focal biliary cirrhosis (50–53). However, liver disease often does not become clinically apparent until this has progressed to severe cirrhosis. In fact, the incidence of clinically manifest liver disease in CF is only 2%–5% (53–56) and appears to increase with age (57) until the teenage years. The initial feature of advanced liver disease is often hepatosplenomegaly or acute gastrointestinal bleeding from esophageal varices.

Table 10 ICU Admission Indications in CF Hepatic Failure

Massive esophageal variceal bleeding
Pleural effusion and ascites with severe respiratory compromise
Encephalopathy

Liver failure may also be complicated by ascites, pleural effusion, hypoalbuminemia, clotting dysfunction, jaundice, hypersplenism, and encephalopathy. The complications of liver failure that may precipitate ICU admission are listed in Table 10.

Severe portal hypertension with bleeding from esophageal varices is one of the main reasons CF patients with hepatic failure need the ICU. In the study by Stern et al., 13 of 15 patients older than 18 years of age with clinical hepatic disease had portal hypertension, and six had variceal bleeding (54). Treatment of variceal bleeding should be aggressive. In most cases, endoscopic sclerotherapy controls the bleeding. Only rarely should intravenous vasopressin or esophageal balloon tamponade be required (55,56). If vasopressin is required, it is given intravenously, with 20 units infused over 20 minutes, followed by a continuous 0.2 units/minute infusion. Emergency portosystemic shunt can also be considered if the measures described fail to control the bleeding and for persistent hypersplenism, but outcome has not been good in the face of significant lung disease in CF patients. The role of the transjugular intrahepatic portosystemic shunting (TIPS) procedure for acutely bleeding CF patients has not been established.

Ascites may complicate acute or chronic CF liver disease and may be accompanied by pleural effusion. Both ascites and pleural effusion can lead to respiratory compromise, especially in the patient with severe underlying lung disease. Treatment consists of diuretics, intravenous albumin, and pleural or peritoneal tap to remove fluid; supplemental oxygen; and proceeding with aggressive pulmonary treatment with intravenous antibiotics, bronchodilators, and chest physiotherapy.

Encephalopathy is rarely seen with CF liver disease. Treatment involves reduction of colonic ammonia production and absorption with poorly absorbed antibiotics (e.g., neomycin and purgatives such as lactulose). In patients awaiting liver transplantation, continuous venovenous hemofiltration may halt progression of the encephalopathy (60).

VIII. Postoperative Complications

Cystic fibrosis patients often need to undergo surgical procedures for treatment of various conditions related to their disease such as nasal polyposis, pneumothorax, bowel obstruction, appendiceal disease, and need for central vascular access. They may also require surgery for problems unrelated to CF, such as trauma. The reported complications of surgery and general anesthesia in CF patients are variable but appear to have lessened over the years. (28,29,61,62). A recent report showed 3% morbidity and 0.5% mortality rates. The majority of the most serious postoperative complications are pulmonary, including pneumothorax, atelectasis, and respiratory failure. To reduce the incidence and severity of pulmonary complications, it is helpful to admit CF patients to the ICU after any major surgical procedure or any procedure during which respiratory difficulties were encountered (30). Treatment in the ICU would consist of close monitoring of oxygen saturation, $PaCO_2$, and respiratory effort, and vigorous airway clearance techniques, in addition to appropriate antibiotic coverage.

References

1. Stern RC, Boat TF, Doerschuk CF, Tucker AS, Primiano FP, Matthews LW. Course of cystic fibrosis in 95 patients. J Pediatr 1976; 89:406–411.

2. Lloyd-Still JD, Khaw, K-T, Shwachman J. Severe respiratory disease in infants with cystic fibrosis. Pediatrics 1974; 53:678–682.

3. Davis PB, di Sant'Agnese PA. Assisted ventilation for patients with cystic fibrosis. JAMA 1978; 239:1851–1854.

4. Ackerman V, Eigen H, Newth C. A positive outcome of mechanical ventilation in young cystic fibrosis patients with acute respiratory compromise (abstr). Pediatr Pulmonol 1987; 1:132.

5. Garland JS, Chan YM, Kelly KJ, Rice TB. Outcome of infants with cystic fibrosis requiring mechanical ventilation for respiratory failure. Chest 1989; 96:136–138.

6. Shennib H, Noirclerc, Ernst P, Metras D, Mulder DS, Giudicelli R, Lebel F, Dumon J. Double-lung transplantation for cystic fibrosis. Ann Thorac Surg 1992; 54:27–32.

7. Massard G, Shennib H, Metras D, et al. Double-lung transplantation in mechanically ventilated patients with cystic fibrosis. Ann Thorac Surg 1993; 55:1087–1092.

8. Hodson ME, Madden BP, Steven MH, Tsang VT, Yacoub MH. Non-invasive mechanical ventilation for cystic fibrosis patients—a potential bridge to transplantation. Eur Respir J 1991; 4:524–527.

9. Padman, R, Von Nesson S, Goodill J, Inselman L. Non-invasive mechanical ventilation for cystic fibrosis patients with end stage disease (abstr). Pediatr Pulmonol 1992; 8:297.

10. Padman R, Lawless S, Von Nessen S. Use of BiPAP by nasal mask in the treatment of respiratory insufficiency in pediatric patients: preliminary investigation. Pediatr Pulmonol 1994; 17:119–123.

11. Ormederod LP, Thomson RA, Anderson CM, Stableforth DE. Reversible airway obstruction in cystic fibrosis. Thorax 1980; 35:768–772.

12. Hordvik NL, Konig P, Morris D, Kreutz C, Bavbero GJ. A longitudinal study of bronchodilator responsiveness in cystic fibrosis. Am Rev Respir Dis 1985; 131:889–893.

13. Eggleston PA, Rosenstein BJ, Stackhouse CM, Alexander MF. Airway hyperreactivity in cystic fibrosis. Chest 1988; 94:360–365.
14. Kattan M, Mansell A, Levison H, Grey M, Krastins I. Response to aerosol salbutamol, SCH 1000 and placebo in cystic fibrosis. Thorax 1980; 35:531–535.
15. Hiatt P, Eigen H, Yu P, Tepper RS. Bronchodilator responsiveness in infants and young children with cystic fibrosis. Am Rev Respir Dis 1988; 137:119–122.
16. Sanchez I, Holbrow J, Chernick V. Acute bronchodilator response to a combination of beta-adrenergic and anticholinergic agents in patients with cystic fibrosis. J Pediatr 1992; 120:486–488.
17. Pattishall EN. Longitudinal response of pulmonary function to bronchodilators in cystic fibrosis. Pediatr Pulmonol 1990; 9:80–85.
18. Landau LI, Phelan PD. The variable effect of a bronchodilating agent on pulmonary function in cystic fibrosis. J Pediatr 1973; 82:863–868.
19. Zach MS, Oberwaldner B, Forche G, Polgar G. Bronchodilators increase airway instability in cystic fibrosis. Am Rev Respir Dis 1985; 131:537–543.
20. Davis A. Vickerson F, Worsley G, Mindorff C, Kazim F, Levison H. Determination of dose–response relationship for nebulized ipratropium in asthmatic children. J Pediatr 1984; 105:1002–10005.
21. Wilmott R. A phase II double blind, multicenter study of the safety and efficacy of aerosolized recombinant human DNase I (rh DNase) in hospitalized patients with CF experiencing acute pulmonary exacerbations (abstr). Pediatr Pulmonol 1993; 16(suppl 9):154.
22. Vaisman N, Pencharz PB, Corey M, Canny GJ, Hahn E. Energy expenditure in cystic fibrosis. J Pediatr 1987; 111:496–500.
23. Buchdahl RM, Cox M, Fulleylove C, et al. Increased resting energy expenditure in cystic fibrosis. J Appl Physiol 1988; 64:1810–1816.
24. Grunow JE, Azcue MP, Berall G, Pencharz PB. Energy expenditure in cystic fibrosis during activities of daily living. J Pediatr 1993; 122:243–246.
25. Waldhorn RE. Nocturnal nasal intermittent positive pressure ventilation with bilevel positive airway pressure (BiPAP) in respiratory failure. Chest 1992; 101:516–521.
26. DiGiulio GA, Kercsmar CM, Krug SE, Alpert SE, Marx CM. Hospital treatment of asthma: lack of benefit from theophylline given in addition to nebulized albuterol and intravenously administered corticosteroid. J Pediatr 1993; 122:464–469.
27. Carter E, Curz M, Chesrown S, Sheih G, Reilly K, Hendeles L. Efficacy of intravenously administered theophylline in children hospitalized with severe asthma. J Pediatr 1993; 122:470–476.
28. Reilly JS, Kenna MA, Stool SE, Bluestone CD. Nasal surgery in children with cystic fibrosis: complications and risk management. Laryngoscope 1985; 95:1491–1493.
29. Olsen MM, Gauderer MW, Girz MK, Izant RS Jr. Surgery in patients with cystic fibrosis. J Pediatr Surg 1987; 22:613–618.
30. Cole RR, Cotton RT. Preventing postoperative complications in the adult cystic fibrosis patient. Int J Pediatr Otolaryngol 1990; 18:263–269.
31. Kessler WR, Andersen DH. Heat prostration in fibrocystic disease of the pancreas and other conditions. Pediatrics 1951; 8:648–655.
32. di Sant'Agnese PA. Salt depletion in cold weather in infants with cystic fibrosis of the pancreas. JAMA 1960; 172:2014–2021.

33. Ramsey CB, Holbrook PR. Heat syndromes. In: Holbrook PR, ed. Textbook of Pediatric Critical Care. Philadelphia: WB Saunders, 1993:1039–1047.
34. Knochel, JP. Heat stroke and related heat stress disorders. Dis Mon 1989; 35:306–377.
35. O'Donnell TF Jr. Acute heat stress: epidemiologic, biochemical, renal and coagulation studies. JAMA 1975; 234:824–828.
36. Beckerman RC, Taussig LM. Hypoelectrolytemia and metabolic alkalosis in infants with cystic fibrosis. Pediatrics 1979; 63:580–583.
37. Forsyth JS, Gillies DNR, Wilson SGF. Cystic fibrosis presenting with chronic electrolyte depletion, metabolic alkalosis and hyperaldosteronism. Scott Med J 1982; 27:333–335.
38. Ruddy R, Anolik R, Scanlin TF. Hypoelectrolytemia as a presentation and complication of cystic fibrosis. Clin Pediatr 1982; 21:367–369.
39. di Sant'Agnese PA, Davis PB. Cystic fibrosis in adults. Am J Med 1979; 66:121–132.
40. Holsclaw DS, Grand RJ, Shwachman H. Massive hemoptysis in cystic fibrosis. J Pediatr 1970; 76:829–838.
41. Stern RC, Wood RE, Boat TF, Matthews LW, Tucker AS, Doershuk CF. Treatment and prognosis of massive hemoptysis in cystic fibrosis. Am Rev Respir Dis 1978; 117:825–828.
42. Cohen AM, Doerschuk CF, Stern RC. Bronchial artery embolization to control hemoptysis in cystic fibrosis. Radiology 1990; 175:401–405.
43. Schidlow DV, Taussig LM, Knowles MR. Cystic Fibrosis Foundation Consensus Conference report on pulmonary complications of cystic fibrosis. Pediatr Pulmonol 1993; 15:187–198.
44. Magee G, Williams MH Jr. Treatment of massive hemoptysis with intravenous Pitressin. Lung 1982; 160:165–169.
45. Popper J. The use of Premarin IV in hemoptysis. Dis Chest 1960; 37:659–660.
46. Fellows KE, Khaw KT, Schuster S, et al. Bronchial artery embolization in cystic fibrosis: technique and long term results. J Pediatr 1979; 95:959–963.
47. Sweezey NB, Fellows KE. Bronchial artery embolization for severe hemoptysis in cystic fibrosis. Chest 1990; 97:1322–1326.
48. Porter DK, Van Every MJ, Anthraule RF, Mack JW. Massive hemoptysis in cystic fibrosis. Arch Intern Med 1983; 143:287–290.
49. Fellows KE, Stigol L, Schuster S, et al. Selective bronchial angiography in patients with cystic fibrosis and massive hemoptysis. Radiology 1975; 114:551–556.
50. Swersky RB, Chang JB, Wisoff BG, Gorvoy J. Endobronchial balloon tamponade of hemoptysis in patients with cystic fibrosis. Ann Thorac Surg 1979; 27:262–264.
51. Levitsky S, Lapey A, di Sant' Agnese PA. Pulmonary resection for life-threatening hemoptysis in cystic fibrosis. JAMA 1970; 213:125–127.
52. Porter DK, Van Every MJ, Mack JW Jr. Emergency lobectomy for massive hemoptysis in cystic fibrosis. J Thorac Cardiovasc Surg 1983; 86:409–411.
53. Roy CC, Weber AM, Morin CL, Lepage G, Brisson G, Yousef I, Lasalle R. Hepatobiliary disease in cystic fibrosis: a survey of current issues and concepts. J Pediatr Gastroenterol 1982; 1:469–478.
54. Stern RC, Stevens DP, Boat TF, Doerschuk CF, Izant RJ, Matthews LW. Symptomatic hepatic disease in cystic fibrosis: incidence, course, and outcome of partial systemic shunting. Gastroenterology 1976; 70:645–649.

55. Scott-Jupp R, Lama M, Tanner MS. Prevalence of liver disease in cystic fibrosis. Arch Dis Child 1991; 66:698–701.
56. Schwarz HP, Kraemer R, Thurnheer U, Rossi E. Liver involvement in cystic fibrosis Helv Paediatr Acta 1978; 33:351–364.
57. Durie PR. Cystic fibrosis: gastrointestinal and hepatic complications and their management. Semin Paediatr Gastroenterol Nutr 1993; 4:3–9.
58. Tanner MS. Current clinical management of hepatic problems in cystic fibrosis. J R Soc Med 1986; 79:38–43.
59. Fitzgerald JF. Gastrointestinal bleeding in infants and children. In: Sugawa C, Shumon BM, Lucas CE, eds. Gastrointestinal Bleeding. New York: Igaku-Shoin Medical Publishers, 1992:51–63.
60. Treem WR. Hepatic failure. In: Walker AW, Durie PR, Hamilton JR, Walker-Smith JA, Watkins JB. Pediatric Gastrointestinal Disease. Pathophysiology, Diagnosis, Management. Philadelphia: BC Decker, 1991:146–192.
61. Salanitre E, Klonymus D, Rackow H. Anesthetic experience in children with cystic fibrosis of the pancreas. Anesthesiology 1964; 25:801–807.
62. Doershuk CF, Reys AL, Regan AG, Matthews LW. Anesthesia and surgery in cystic fibrosis. Anesth Analg 1972; 51:413–421.

11

Clinical Pharmacokinetics: Concepts to Practice

MICHAEL D. REED

Case Western Reserve University
School of Medicine and
Rainbow Babies and Childrens Hospital
Cleveland, Ohio

MICHAEL SPINO

Apotex, Inc.
Weston, Ontario, Canada, and
Hospital for Sick Children
Toronto, Ontario, Canada

I. Introduction

Cystic fibrosis (CF) is an unusual disease in that, after equal doses of many drugs, serum concentrations are inexplicably low. These lower concentrations can be attributed to a larger apparent volume of distribution and enhanced body clearance, but the underlying physiology behind these altered pharmacokinetics remains an enigma. Specific testing reveals some degree of functional impairment of all the major organs associated with drug disposition, including the gastrointestinal tract, the heart, the liver, and the kidney. In patients with other diseases who experience impairment of organ function, drug elimination is decreased, resulting in drug accumulation—the opposite of what is observed in CF patients. The reasons for these differences in drug disposition remain unknown and may not be defined until the metabolic consequences of the abnormal CFTR proteins are understood more fully. Despite incomplete understanding of drug disposition differences in CF patients, drug therapy will continue to play an important role in the management of CF patients until a cure for this genetic disorder is achieved. The application of clinical pharmacokinetic principles to the care of these patients allows the design of optimal pharmacotherapeutic regimens for each patient. Pharmacokinetic data permit identification of the drug dose needed to achieve the desired clinical effect in an individual while minimizing the likelihood of associated adverse effects. In this chapter, the fundamental concepts of clinical pharmacokinetics and their application to the care of patients with CF are reviewed.

II. Clinical Pharmacokinetics: Important Concepts for the Clinician

Pharmacokinetics is the quantitative assessment of each component of the disposition profile of a drug, which is a function of the interplay of its absorption, distribution, metabolism, and excretion. The mathematic description of these processes depends on the ability to determine drug concentrations in various body fluids. Drug concentrations are plotted as "best-fit" lines drawn through the concentration–time values, and numeric values define the important dynamic processes of absorption, distribution, and elimination (clearance).

Clinical pharmacokinetics can be used to control drug concentrations at any time after any dose. The utility of this practice assumes a direct relationship between the drug concentration in blood (serum or plasma) and well-defined pharmacological or toxicological effects. A clear relationship between concentration and effect does not always exist, however, and in only a few cases have well-designed clinical studies demonstrated a clear relationship between serum drug concentration and measurable clinical outcomes (1). For these drugs, peak and trough serum drug concentrations are targeted to specific values by careful adjustment of dose and frequency of administration. The controversy surrounding a target concentration strategy for drug dosing is discussed in subsequent paragraphs.

A. Absorption

Most drugs achieve their pharmacological effect by binding to and modulating a physiological receptor. To gain access in sufficient quantity to the receptor site, a drug must be absorbed from the site of administration into the systemic circulation and distributed to its sites of action. Thus, absorption becomes tremendously important when drugs are administered via any route of drug administration, including the intravenous (IV) route.

Bioavailability describes the total amount of drug that is "absorbed" into the systemic circulation through any route of administration. Bioavailability encompasses both the rate and overall extent of drug absorption. Bioavailability is calculated by comparing the ratio of the area under the drug concentration time curve (AUC) for a drug given by two different routes of drug administration. The AUC is a measure of the amount of drug in the body. A drug's "absolute bioavailability" is calculated by comparing the AUC after extravascular administration (e.g., orally, intramuscularly) with the AUC determined after IV administration. This evaluation is termed "absolute bioavailability" because it is assumed that drug bioavailability after IV administration is 100% (i.e., all drug given via the IV route is absorbed into the systemic circulation). Although this assumption is correct for most drugs used clinically, some exceptions apply. For example, the IV formulation of some drugs are prodrug salts of the parent drug. Some drugs are not chemically stable or sufficiently soluble to permit formulation as an IV drug product. In such circumstances, chemical modification of the parent compound with different esters may produce a chemically stable and clinically acceptable drug product. An example of this phenomenon that may be important for CF patients is chloramphenicol. Chloramphenicol succinate for IV administration is an inactive prodrug that requires cleavage of the succinate ester by nonspecific plasma esterases to liberate active chloramphenicol. As a result of the variability of the enzymatic cleavage process, the total IV dose administered may not result in 100% of the dose being liberated as active chloramphenicol (Fig. 1).

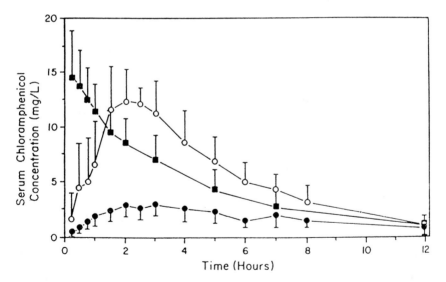

Figure 1 Chloramphenicol serum concentration–time curve after administration of three different pharmaceutical formulations to CF patients in the absence of pancreatic enzyme replacement. Data presented as numeric plot of the mean (± SD) serum concentration vs time for chloramphenicol after intravenous chloramphenicol-succinate ($n = 10$) (■), oral chloramphenicol base as the capsule ($n = 10$) (○), and oral chloramphenicol-palmitate suspension ($n = 8$) (●) administration without concurrent exogenous pancreatic enzyme replacement. (From Ref. 2, used with permission.)

Table 1 Factors Influencing Drug Absorption

Physicochemical factors

Molecular weight
Degree of ionization under physiological conditions
Product formulation characteristics
    Disintegration and dissolution rates for solid dosage forms
    Drug-release characteristics for time-release preparations
Cosolutes and complex formation

Patient factors

Surface area available for absorption
Gastric and duodenal pH
Gastric emptying time
Bile salt pool size
Bacterial colonization of the gastrointestinal tract
Presence and extent of underlying diseases
Presence or absence of metabolic pathways or enzymes necessary for biotransformation

The physicochemical and physiological factors that influence absorption are outlined in Table 1. For most patients, clinically available drug formulations possess many of the desirable physicochemical attributes fostering adequate drug absorption including low molecular weight, relative degrees of lipid solubility, and chemical stability and limited degree of ionization at physiological and pathophysiological pH. However, in patients with CF, these factors have added importance. Disease-induced compromise of exocrine pancreatic function and bile salt dynamics can have a profound effect on the bioavailability of certain drugs. Furthermore, exogenous supplementation of pancreatic enzymes or bile salts can also influence absorption characteristics of labile drugs. These factors outlined in Table 1 influence the rate and extent of drug absorption following any means of extravascular drug administration (e.g., intramuscular, topical, patch application).

A prime example of prodrug pharmacokinetics and the influences of pancreatic insufficiency and pancreatic enzyme replacement therapy on drug disposition involves chloramphenicol (2). The absorption characteristics of the three different formulations of chloramphenicol in CF patients is shown in Figure 1. The amount of drug absorbed into systemic circulation was greatest when administered as the oral capsule formulation (mean AUC 79.6 μg · hr/mL) rather than as either the IV prodrug formulation (55.6 μg · hr/mL) or the oral palmitate prodrug suspension (49.7 μg · hr/mL). The bioavailability of the oral prodrug suspension increased markedly when coadministered with exogenous pancreatic supplementation (49.7 vs 32.5 μg · hr/mL). This latter finding was expected because palmitate esters require pancreatic enzyme to cleave the ester and liberate active drug. Despite the average increase in chloramphenicol bioavailability when given with pancreatic enzymes, overall bioavailability was highly variable with the suspension formulation. Such differences in disease-induced alterations in drug bioavailability should be considered in any patient who is responding poorly to normally effective oral drug doses or who manifests unexpected serum drug concentrations.

B. Clinical Significance of Drug Bioavailability

The pharmacokinetic parameter estimate of bioavailability (F) provides information on the amount of drug absorbed into systemic circulation following a given route of drug administration. Assuming that the published F for a drug is the absolute F, this value can be used as a conversion factor defining the oral dose needed to achieve the same amount of drug in the body as achieved with IV dosing. If a drug's oral bioavailability is 1 (i.e., 100%), the oral and IV dose would be identical; if the F of the drug is 50%, the oral (or intramuscular) dose required would be twice the IV dose.

A low F (e.g., 40%–60%) is not necessarily bad. Rather, the clinician must simply adjust the oral dose upward if concentrations similar to IV drug dosing are desired. A limitation to large oral doses for drugs with relatively low F is gastrointestinal intolerance such as diarrhea from unabsorbed drug (e.g., ampicillin).

Differences in peak drug concentration between oral and IV dosing are expected. The peak drug concentration for most drugs is lower and occurs later after oral dosing. Some experts consider the peak drug concentration to be an important determinant of antibacterial activity for antibiotics; high peak concentrations may enhance tissue diffusion into diseased areas, especially those with a poor blood supply (e.g., sputum). Only limited data address the importance of the peak drug concentration to drug effect in treating infectious diseases (3). Nevertheless, if a high peak concentration is desired, the formulation must have a rapid absorption rate. The faster the absorption rate, the faster and higher the resultant peak serum drug concentration. Similarly, higher peak serum drug concentrations are achieved by IV drug administration with a bolus or short-term infusion (<5 minutes) than with longer infusions (e.g., 30–60 minutes). The potential value of the higher peak concentration after IV dosing must be weighed against the possibility of a higher risk of toxicity.

C. Volume of Distribution

Once absorbed into the systematic circulation, a drug is distributed throughout the body, achieving an equilibrium among body "compartments." The extent to which a drug diffuses out of the blood and into these other compartments depends on physicochemical characteristics similar to those that influence absorption (see Table 1). For example, a drug with a positive charge at physiological pH may distribute extensively in the body but not into the central nervous system.

An understanding of in vivo distribution characteristics is important in the selection of a specific drug and dose to be given. The pharmacokinetic parameter volume of distribution (Vd) is a proportionality constant that relates the amount of drug in the body to the amount in blood (serum or plasma). Because the estimate of this parameter does not conform to any real physiological volume, it is most appropriately termed the apparent Vd. Although it is tempting for investigators and clinicians to correlate the Vd of a drug with known physiological volumes, such correlations are inaccurate. Any assumption of preferential distribution to specific anatomical sites based on the size of Vd alone is erroneous and can lead to errant clinical decisions regarding the selection of one drug over another.

The extent to which a drug is bound to circulating plasma proteins influences the distribution characteristics of the drug. Only the free, non–protein-bound drug can be distributed from the vascular space into other body fluids and tissues. However, the binding of drugs to proteins is reversible, dynamic, and in a state of equilibrium. As a molecule leaves the circulation to go to another compartment or bind to a receptor, equilibrium is reestablished. Thus, the simplistic in vitro state is not representative of the complex in vivo state, and a drug (e.g., antibiotic) that is 10% unbound is not twice as active as one that is 5% unbound.

Drug protein binding is influenced by a number of variables, including patient age, certain diseases, and the presence of displacing substances, such as bilirubin or other highly protein bound (>95%) drugs. A number of studies have demonstrated that plasma protein binding for many drugs is not significantly different in CF patients than in unaffected individuals. The mean percent bound for acidic drugs such as cloxacillin is the same as that observed in unaffected subjects (4). However, the range of values in CF patients in most cases is broader, indicating that although the average may be the same, some CF patients are likely to have higher free fractions than non-CF patients. These drugs are acidic and are bound mainly to albumin. Because some CF patients have low albumin concentrations, a lower percent of bound drug may be anticipated. However, unless albumin concentrations decline to below 2g/dL, there is little or no noticeable effect on drug–protein binding (5).

Drug interactions involving the displacement of one drug by another occur rarely and, even then, only under specific circumstances (5,6). A clinically important displacement interaction usually involves two drugs with affinity for the same protein (e.g., albumin) and protein-binding sites and high degrees of protein binding (>95%) and low volumes of distribution (<10 L). When a displacement interaction occurs, the increase in free drug concentration is transitory and equilibrium is quickly reestablished. Thus, for a clinically important interaction to occur, the rate of drug elimination of the displaced drug must be slow, fostering body accumulation of the displaced agent in excess of the redistribution (5). For these reasons, very few drug–drug interactions between most highly bound drugs lead to clinical consequences. Examples of drugs for which clinically important drug–drug protein displacement interactions may occur include lidocaine, midazolam, and verapamil.

Basic drugs have been less well studied in CF patients. Considering that basic drugs are also bound to circulatory components, notably lipoproteins and alpha-1-acid glycoprotein, they are more likely to be affected by disease. It is probable that high concentrations of disease-associated acute-phase reactants (e.g., lipoproteins) will displace basic drugs from their alpha-1-acid glycoprotein binding sites.

D. Clinical Significance of the Volume of Distribution

The Vd is one of the most important pharmacokinetic characteristics for determining the correct dose of a drug for an individual patient. Defining the Vd for a drug allows the clinician to determine the exact drug dose needed to achieve a specific target concentration in blood. Knowledge of the age-predicted Vd (in L/kg) allows the clinician to extrapolate this population-based value to the individual patient to initiate a pharmacological regimen [i.e., drug dose (mg/kg) = (desired drug concentration in blood mg/L) × (Vd L/kg)]. Population-based Vd values for various drugs can be obtained from review articles and most clinical pharmacology textbooks.

E. Elimination Half-Life

The elimination half-life ($t_{1/2}$) is the time required for the drug concentration to decrease by one-half. Most often calculated as a serum or plasma t 1/2, that is, the time required for the concentration of drug in serum or plasma to decrease by 50%, the $t_{1/2}$ can be calculated in any biological fluid (e.g., cerebrospinal fluid). Importantly, the $t_{1/2}$ value pertains to the biological fluid for which it was determined and does not necessarily denote excretion of 50% of all the drug from the body. In contrast, the body clearance (Cl) of a drug refers to drug removal from the body. For drugs that follow first-order elimination, the $t_{1/2}$ is a constant value inherent to the drug in question and independent of the drug concentration. Thus, the time required for the serum drug concentration to decrease from 250 to 125 mg/L would be the same time required for the serum drug concentration to fall from 2 to 1 mg/L. First-order pharmacokinetics implies proportionality, for example, doubling the dose doubles the drug concentration in the body. Most drugs used clinically exhibit first-order disposition characteristics. In contrast, some drugs exhibit nonlinear pharmacokinetic characteristics, wherein serum drug concentrations change disproportionately to changes in dose, that is, zero-order disposition characteristics. Drugs commonly used that display zero-order characteristics include aspirin and phenytoin. One common reason for the greater than expected increase in serum drug concentration is that saturation of enzymes are responsible for metabolism and elimination (e.g., Michaelis-Menten kinetics).

F. Clinical Significance of Elimination Half-Life

The elimination $t_{1/2}$ is an important pharmacokinetic parameter for the clinician. The $t_{1/2}$ can be used to determine the time required to achieve steady-state concentrations, that is, when the rate of drug administration in and the rate of drug elimination from the body achieve equilibrium. With repeated administration of the same dose at a constant interval (e.g., every 4 hours), approximately 90% of steady-state drug concentrations are achieved after three drug half-lives and 96% of steady-state drug concentrations after five half-lives. Because usual target serum drug concentrations used to guide drug dosing are based on steady-state drug concentrations, knowledge of the $t_{1/2}$ of a drug can assist in determining the proper time for obtaining blood samples. Furthermore, when possible and in the absence of drug toxicity, it is usually prudent to assess a patient's response to drug therapy under steady-state conditions when drug effect reflects maximum total amount of drug in the body, rather than after first dose administration.

Elimination $t_{1/2}$ is also important in defining the dosing interval for drug administration. The elimination $t_{1/2}$ defines the time required for a serum drug concentration to decline before the next dose is needed. Thus, for a drug like tobramycin with a usual $t_{1/2}$ of 2 hours, it can be predicted that, in 4 hours, the trough concentration will be below 2 mg/L if, at the end of a 30-minute infusion, the peak serum concentration was 8 mg/L (i.e., two half-lives). If the concentration declines to 1 mg/L before administering the next dose, then drug administration every 6 hours should achieve the desired goal.

The $t_{1/2}$ is related to the reciprocal of the elimination rate constant (K) by the formula, $(t_{1/2} = 0.693/K)$. Therefore, K is a hybrid constant and is directly proportional to the Vd and inversely proportional to the CL. In CF, it is common for many drugs to have both an increased Vd and increased CL. The result may be no change in $t_{1/2}$, even though the drug is being eliminated from the body more rapidly than in normal subjects. Thus, it is best to use CL to calculate altered dose requirements, particularly in CF patients.

G. Body Clearance

The overall rate of drug removal from the body is described by the pharmacokinetic parameter estimate of body clearance (CL). The CL of a drug is the summation of all mechanisms involved in removing the drug from the body. Thus, body CL is the sum of renal clearance (CL r), hepatic clearance (CL h), biliary clearance (CL b), pulmonary clearance (CL pul), and so on. For most drugs, the kidney or the liver accounts for the majority of drug removal from the body.

Clearance describes the volume of drug removed per unit of time, as reflected in the units of clearance (mL/min), which may be "corrected" for body size (e.g., mL/min/kg or mL/min/m^2). The kidney has been well studied as an organ of drug clearance. Drug is removed via the kidney mainly by two mechanisms, filtration and secretion. Some drugs are also partially metabolized by the kidney, but this is usually a minor pathway. The glomerulus filters only the drug that is not bound to plasma protein ("free drug"). Once the drug is in the tubule, it may be reabsorbed into the renal tubular cell and back into the efferent arteriole of the nephron and into systemic circulation. Thus, renal clearance is the summation of filtration plus secretion minus reabsorption. For example, if a drug is minimally bound to plasma proteins (<10%) and is completely eliminated from the body via glomerular filtration rate (GFR) with little to no hepatic biotransformation, the CL value should approximate the GFR. Such is the case with the aminoglycosides. Drugs that undergo filtration and tubular secretion (e.g., ticarcillin, piperacillin) have clearance values in excess of the GFR.

H. Clinical Significance of Body Clearance

Knowledge of organ flow rates (e.g., hepatic blood flow) and organ function (e.g., glomerular filtration rate) along with an understanding of the metabolic disposition of a drug allows direct comparison of clearance rates in the absence and presence of disease. Such correlations can be used to adjust drug dosing intervals in patients with major organ dysfunction (e.g., renal compromise). Body CL determines the dosing requirements. A patient with a high CL requires more drug to maintain the same amount of drug in the body, similar serum drug concentrations, and presumably the same pharmacological effect or duration of effect than a patient with a low drug CL.

Dose requirements can be determined if the drug CL and the average steady-state drug concentration (Css) are known: dose = (CL) × (Css). Using the example of an aminoglycoside (e.g., tobramycin), dose requirements for an individual patient can be estimated before obtaining serum tobramycin concentrations. For example, if the patient's estimated GFR is 100 mL/min and the desired average steady-state serum tobramycin concentration is 4 mg/L, then dose = (0.1 L/min) × (4 mg/L) = 0.4 mg/min = 24 mg/hr, or approximately 200 mg administered every 8 hours.

III. Drug Disposition in Patients with Cystic Fibrosis

The pharmacokinetics of a number of drugs have been shown to be different in CF patients compared with unaffected individuals. In 1975, Jusko and colleagues described differences in the disposition profile of orally administered dicloxacillin in CF patients compared with a group of healthy volunteers (7). These investigators described a significantly decreased dicloxacillin AUC with resultant increased plasma clearance and renal clearance. Since the publication of this first description of a difference in drug disposition in CF patients, a number of laboratories have performed careful pharmacological studies that clearly demonstrate differences in drug disposition in CF patients compared with unaffected control subjects) (8–10). The drugs that have been studied represent a diverse group of compounds that rely on the kidney, the liver, or both as their primary route of drug elimination.

As listed in Table 2, the most common differences in drug disposition characteristics in CF patients involve an increased apparent Vd, an increased body CL, and a resultant decrease in serum drug concentrations. These differences appear paradoxical in view of known CF-associated pathophysiological conditions, such as cor pulmonale and focal biliary cirrhosis, which would be expected to impair rather than increase drug elimination (11). The mechanisms responsible for these disease-specific differences in drug disposition are unknown. Attempts to identify alterations in the functional capacity of the kidney in CF patients have revealed little or no increased renal function (12) except in some studies in patients who were fed high-fat diets (13). Following resumption of a normal diet, the measured glomerular filtration rate decreased to normal values. However, it is clear that there is wider variation in clearance values among CF patients than among unaffected individuals. The possibility of a link between the genetic defect in CF and the observed enhanced biotransformation of some drugs was suggested by some investigators as an explanation for these differences (10,14).

A. Clinical Significance of Altered Drug Disposition in CF Patients

The differences observed in the pharmacokinetic disposition of many drugs in CF patients (see Table 2) have led to the common clinical practice of empirically increasing drug doses for these patients. For drugs with apparent serum concentration–effect relationships (e.g., the aminoglycosides), such an approach to drug dosing appears warranted. Increased individual doses, possibly given more frequently, are necessary to overcome these disease-related differences in pharmacokinetic behavior and to achieve serum aminoglycoside concentrations in CF patients similar to those targeted in non-CF patients.

Table 2 Pharmacokinetic Differences of Selected Drugs in Cystic Fibrosis Patients as Compared with Unaffected Control Subjects

Pharmacokinetic parameter estimate	Drug	Differences compared with unaffected controls
Bioavailability	Acetaminophen	No difference
	Chloramphenicol	Decreased
	Ciprofloxacin	No difference
	Ibuprofen	Increased
Volume of distribution	Aminoglycosides[a]	Increased
	Azlocillin	Increased
	Cefoperazone	Increased
	Ceftazidime	Increased
	Cimetidine	Increased
	Ciprofloxacin	No difference
	Cloxacillin	Increased
	Furosemide	Increased
	Ibuprofen	Increased
	Methicillin	No difference
	Piperacillin	Increased
	Theophylline	Increased
	Ticarcillin	Increased
Protein binding	Cefoperazone	No difference
	Cefsulodin	No difference
	Ceftazidime	No difference
	Cloxacillin	No difference
	Dicloxacillin	No difference
	Gentamicin	No difference
	Theophylline	Decreased
Body clearance	Acetaminophen	Increased
	Aminoglycosides	Increased
	Azlocillin	Increased
	Cefoperazone	Increased
	Ceftazidime	Increased
	Cimetidine	Increased
	Ciprofloxacin	No difference
	Cloxacillin	Increased
	Dicloxacillin	Increased
	Furosemide	Increased
	Ibuprofen	Increased
	Methicillin	Increased
	Piperacillin	Increased
	Sulfamethoxazole	Increased
	Theophylline	Increased
	Ticarcillin	Increased
	Trimethoprim	Increased

[a]Gentamicin, tobramycin, amikacin.

The routine monitoring of serum aminoglycoside concentrations to guide drug dosing has been demonstrated not to be necessary in most clinical situations (1,15). Recent reviews of decades of published experience appropriately question the clinical practice of routinely monitoring serum aminoglycoside concentrations in most patients. However, the known disease-specific differences in aminoglycoside disposition and the great variability observed in CF patients necessitate that serum concentrations be monitored to assist the clinician in rapidly attaining target serum aminoglycoside concentrations.

More recent data, both in CF (16) and non-CF patients (17,18) clearly demonstrate the efficacy and safety of once-daily aminoglycoside dosing. Peak serum drug concentrations (20–60 mg/L) far in excess of customary targets (e.g., 8–12 mg/L) have been described with no increased incidence of nephrotoxicity or ototoxicity. These data raise questions about routinely targeting peak drug concentrations of 8–12 mg/L and the routine practice of simply addressing an absolute serum drug concentration while ignoring the time that the serum drug concentration exceeds certain values.

Even less is known about the clinical importance of disease-altered disposition for drugs that are not subject to routine serum drug concentration monitoring (e.g. beta-lactam antibiotics, colistin, acetaminophen, and furosemide). Nevertheless, it is common practice to increase the dose of many of these drugs empirically in CF patients, particularly beta-lactam antibiotics, coincident with increased aminoglycoside dosing. Such practice has been used for decades without serious critique, fostered by the exceptional safety profile of the beta-lactam antibiotics. One short-term study was unable to demonstrate any difference between approximately 2 weeks of high-dose or conventional-dose ceftazidime monotherapy in a group of CF patients admitted to the hospital for treatment of acute pulmonary exacerbation (19). However, this study must be interpreted with caution because it evaluated only a brief period in the therapy of a lifelong process. Long-term evaluation is necessary to define any real differences between drug dose regimes that use conventional doses and those that adjust doses for known differences in pharmacokinetic behavior.

B. When to Obtain the Serum Drug Concentration

For aminoglycosides, drug distribution is essentially complete 30 minutes after completion of the 30-minute IV infusion. For this reason, peak aminoglycoside concentrations are best determined 30 minutes after completion of the 30-minute infusion. If the aminoglycoside is infused over 1 hour, the peak serum concentration should be obtained immediately upon completion of the 1-hour infusion. If the infusion time is anytime between 30 and 60 minutes, the peak should be obtained at 1 hour after the beginning of the infusion. As stated previously, the time for distribution to be essentially complete differs for individual drugs as well as after different routes of administration for the same drug (e.g., for aminoglycosides, approximately 30 minutes after a 30-minute IV infusion, immediately upon completion of a 1-hour infusion, or 1 hour after intramuscular injection). For digoxin, distribution is much slower, approximately 4–6 hours to ensure near complete distribution before obtaining a blood sample. Whenever a question arises, the clinician should consult the clinical pharmacy, pharmacology service, or clinical laboratory.

C. Clinical Application of Pharmacokinetic Principles

The strategy of a target concentration–effect relationship is the foundation of clinical pharmacokinetic practice. This strategy relates specific responses (e.g., therapeutic and toxic) to specified concentrations of drug in a biological fluid (e.g., blood). This approach evolved from the recognition that pharmacological and toxicological responses of a drug correlated much better with the concentration of the drugs in a biological fluid than with the absolute dose administered. A number of excellent reviews and commentaries state that serum concentration–therapeutic effect relationships purported for some drugs that are routinely monitored (e.g., aminoglycosides and vancomycin) are questionable (1,15,20). Although there is little doubt that a relationship exists between drug concentration and effect, it is much more complex than originally believed and more difficult to quantify with present technology. Furthermore, for most drugs used in clinical practice, no clear line of demarcation exists between efficacy and toxicity, and, usually, these important endpoints cannot be determined with precision.

Notwithstanding these difficult obstacles, adjusting drug doses to a desired concentration is perceived to be superior than administering a common dose to all patients, because it avoids the problem of variable absorption and disposition. Until more specific data are available regarding serum drug concentration–effect relationships, it seems reasonable to use pharmacokinetic principles to guide drug dosing in CF patients. Using pharmacokinetic parameters, the clinician can accurately and easily determined the dose of a given drug necessary to achieve the desired target concentration. The following case illustrates the application of these principles.

Case

A 30-kg 8-year-old boy with CF is hospitalized with an acute pulmonary exacerbation. His last course of intravenous antibiotics was 3 months before. The antibiotic regimen most effective in his previous care was ceftazidime and tobramycin. His medical record is not available to obtain previous antibiotic doses associated with desired clinical effect and desired serum tobramycin concentrations. The house physician initiates antibiotic therapy with 1500 mg of ceftazidime IV infused over 15 minutes every 8 hours and 75 mg of tobramycin IV infused over 30 minutes every 8 hours.

What Is the Expected Peak Serum Tobramycin Concentration After the First Dose?

Because the patient was not receiving tobramycin at home, the initial peak serum concentration can be estimated by dividing the dose administered by the estimated volume of distribution. An age- and disease-appropriate estimate of the patient's tobramycin Vd can be obtained from the literature (Table 3):

Table 3 Average Values for Volume of Distribution and Body Clearance for Selected Drugs Studied in Patients with Cystic Fibrosis[a]

	Pharmacokinetic parameter	
Drug	Vd (L/kg)	CL (mL/min/1.73 m²)
Penicillins		
Cloxacillin	0.14	255
Methicillin	NA	512
Ticarcillin	0.23	90[a]
Piperacillin		
Cephalosporins		
Cefoperazone	0.17	76
Cefsulodin	0.24	120
Ceftazidime	0.24	135
Aminoglycosides		
Amikacin	0.31	130
Gentamicin	0.31	120
Netilimicin	0.31	110
Tobramycin	0.31	120
Quinolones		
Ciprofloxacin	2.4	620
Other drugs		
Furosemide	0.33	265[b]
Aztreonam	0.25	127
Imipenem	0.3	225
Theophylline	0.6	72
Cimetidine	1.9	19
Sulfamethoxazole	0.21	22
Trimethoprim	1.7	180
Chloramphenicol	1.0	60[b]

[a]Values shown in this table obtained from Ref. 10 and individual publications. Data are average values that may be useful in initial dose calculations in patients with cystic fibrosis.
[b]Body clearance value expressed as mL/min.

approximate Vd = approximately 0.3 L/kg. The tobramycin Vd in this patient is (30 kg body weight) × (0.3 L/kg) = 9 L. Assuming instantaneous drug distribution, the estimated peak serum tobramycin concentration can be calculated from (dose) × (F) / Vd = 75 mg / 9 L = 8.3 mg/L. Because the dose was given intravenously, the bioavailability (F) is assumed to be 100%. This estimate of the peak serum tobramycin concentration will most likely overestimate the true peak because some drug is eliminated from the body during the 30-minute intravenous infusion and during the time it takes for the drug to be distributed in the body. If the elimination half-life of the drug is known for the patient or from a literature estimate, the amount of drug eliminated during the 30-minute infusion and 30-minute distribution phase could be estimated.

Knowledge of the Vd of a drug allows the clinician to easily calculate any dose to achieve a desired serum drug concentration: (dose) × (F) = (desired serum concentration minus any residual serum concentration from previous doses) × (drug Vd). Thus, if a peak serum tobramycin concentration of 10 mg/L is desired, the estimated initial dose would be (10 mg/L minus zero because no drug is yet in the patient's body) × (9 L) = 90 mg. In this 30-kg child, the dose would be 3 mg tobramycin/kg.

What Are Serum Tobramycin Concentrations at Steady State?

Steady-state condition is reached when the rates of drug administration and drug elimination are equal. The time to steady-state conditions can be estimated from the elimination half-life. In one $t_{1/2}$, 50% of steady state is achieved; in two $t_{1/2}$s, 75%; three $t_{1/2}$s, 87.5%; in four $t_{1/2}$s, 93.75%. After approximately five $t_{1/2}$s, steady-state conditions have been achieved. Estimated tobramycin $t_{1/2}$ in CF patients without renal compromise approximates 1.75 to 2 hours; thus, greater than 96% of steady-state conditions should be achieved within 8 hours. Furthermore, use of the $t_{1/2}$ allows the trough serum drug concentration to be estimated. If the patient's estimated peak serum tobramycin concentration is 10 mg/L, this serum concentration halves every 2 hours, providing an estimate of an 8-hour trough concentration of approximately 0.625 mg/L (after four $t_{1/2}$s). Thus, a dose of 90 mg administered IV over 30 minutes every 8 hours should produced peak serum tobramycin concentrations of 10 mg/L and trough concentrations of 0.6 mg/L.

How Can Tobramycin Therapy Be Individualized in This Patient?

Using a literature estimate of the average tobramycin Vd in CF patients of 0.3 L/kg, the initial dose can be calculated as described, dose = (desired concentration minus residual drug concentration) × (Vd) = (10 mg/L) × (9 L) = 90 mg. Recognizing that the Vd is a literature estimate, the actual patient tobramycin Vd, $t_{1/2}$, and body CL can be calculated by analysis of two blood samples obtained after this first dose—a peak obtained when drug distribution is expected to be complete, 30 minutes after a 30-minute intravenous infusion, and a trough concentration obtained just before the next scheduled dose, for example, 8 hours later. Drug $t_{1/2}$ can be estimated from these two points as the time it takes for the serum concentration to decrease to half. This can be quickly estimated or plotted on graph paper and more accurately defined. Assuming the tobramycin $t_{1/2}$ in the patient is 2 hours, the elimination rate constant Kd can be calculated from $t_{1/2} = 0.693/Kd$; the Vd can be estimated as dose/peak concentration; and the body clearance (Cl) can be estimated from CL = (Kd) × (Vd). To obtain the most accurate estimate of the Vd, the peak concentration used in the stated ratio should be the concentration obtained by "back extrapolation" to time zero, that is, assuming the drug was administered as a rapid bolus infusion, using the $t_{1/2}$ to estimate the amount of drug lost during the infusion. With these patient-specific pharmacokinetic parameter estimates, serum drug concentrations after any dose at any time can be calculated with a high degree of accuracy.

IV. Conclusion

Cystic fibrosis is a genetic disorder with unique effects on drug disposition. Patients with CF metabolize many drugs faster and eliminate many drugs more rapidly from their body than unaffected individuals. Moreover, the Vd for most drugs in CF patients is larger than in non-CF patients. The reasons for these differences are unknown. Similarly, the ultimate impact of these differences on the overall care of CF patients remains to be defined. Nevertheless, it seems reasonable to target drug doses in CF patients to achieve similar amounts and concentrations as obtained in non-CF patients who are receiving the same drugs for similar reasons. This chapter discusses the principles of applied clinical pharmacokinetics and how this tool can be applied to optimize drug therapy in patients. Published average Vd and CL data for many drugs in CF patients are listed in Table 3. These parameter estimates can be used to enhance the patient's benefit from their drug therapy.

References

1. Tange SM, et al. Therapeutic drug monitoring in pediatrics: a need for improvement. J Clin Pharmacol 1994; 34:200–214.
2. Dickenson CJ, et al. The effect of exocrine pancreatic function on chloramphenicol pharmacokinetics in cystic fibrosis. Pediatr Res 1988; 23:388–392.
3. LeBel M, Spino M. Pulse dosing versus continuous infusion of antibiotics. Clin Pharmacokinet 1988; 14:71–95.
4. Spino M, et al. Cloxacillin absorption and disposition in cystic fibrosis. J Pediatr 1984; 105:829–835.

5. Sansom LN, Evans AM. What is the true clinical significance of plasma protein binding displacement interactions? Drug Safety 1995; 12:227–233.
6. MacKichan JJ. Protein binding displacement interactions: fact or fiction? Clin Pharmacokinet 1989; 16:65–73.
7. Jusko WJ, et al. Enhanced renal excretion of dicloxacillin in patients with cystic fibrosis. Pediatrics 1975; 56:1038–1044.
8. de Groot R, Smith AL. Antibiotic pharmacokinetics in cystic fibrosis: differences and clinical significance. Clin Pharmacokinet 1987; 13:228–253.
9. Prandota J. Clinical pharmacology of antibiotics and other drugs in cystic fibrosis. Drugs 1988; 35:542–578.
10. Spino M. Pharmacokinetics of drugs in cystic fibrosis. Clin Rev Allergy 1981; 9:169–210.
11. Kearns GL, et al. Enhanced hepatic drug clearance in patients with cystic fibrosis. J Pediatr 1990; 117:972–979.
12. Spino M, et al. Assessment of glomerular filtration and effective renal plasma flow in cystic fibrosis. J Pediatr 1985; 107:64–70.
13. Strandvik B, et al. Effect of renal function of essential fatty acid supplementation in cystic fibrosis. J Pediatr 1989; 115:242–250.
14. Knoppert DC, et al. Cystic fibrosis: enhanced theophylline metabolism may be linked to the disease. Clin Pharmacol Ther 1988; 44:254–264.
15. McCormack JP, Jewesson PJ. A critical reevaluation of the "therapeutic range" of aminoglycosides. Clin Infect Dis 1992; 14:320–329.
16. Powell SH, et al. Once-daily vs continuous aminoglycoside dosing: efficacy and toxicity in animal and clinical studies of gentamicin, netilmicin and tobramycin. J Infect Dis 1983; 147:918–932.
17. Rotschafer JC, Rybak MJ. Single daily dosing of aminoglycosides: a commentary. Ann Pharmacother 1994; 28:797–801.
18. Elhanan K, et al. Gentamicin once-daily vs thrice-daily in children. J Antimicrob Chemother 1995; 35:327–332.
19. Reed MD, et al. Randomized double-blind evaluation of ceftazidime dose ranging in hospitalized patients with cystic fibrosis. Antimicrob Agents Chemother 1987; 31:698–702.
20. Cantu TG, et al. Serum vancomycin concentrations: reappraisal of their clinical value. Clin Infect Dis 1994; 18:533–543.

12

Special Considerations for the Hospitalized Adult

PAMELA B. DAVIS

Case Western Reserve University School of Medicine
and Rainbow Babies and Childrens Hospital
Cleveland, Ohio

I. Introduction

More and more patients with cystic fibrosis (CF) survive to adulthood. Whereas in 1969, only 8% of CF patients were adults, in 1994, more than one-third of all CF patients reported to the national CF data registry were older than age 18 years. In some of the long-established CF centers in the United States, as in our center in Cleveland, more than half the patients are adults. Because patients become more ill as they age (the death rate is at least threefold higher for patients older than 21 years of age compared with those younger than 10 years of age), it is not surprising that these patients account for many of the CF hospital admissions. A total of 34.2% of adults aged 18–71 years (compared with 24.6% of children aged 0–17 years) had one to two hospitalizations in 1994, and 13.4% of adults (and 5.3% of children) had three or more admissions in that year. Many of the same considerations that apply to children with CF in the hospital apply to adults as well. However, some complications are more prevalent or more severe in adults. Some issues, such as the reproductive complications, arise only in the adult age range. As any patient ages, degenerative changes and other complications of age may enter the clinical picture. Psychosocial issues differ as well in the adult age range. This chapter discusses

319

complications of CF that are more prevalent and more severe in older patients, addresses the issues raised by the CF patient reaching reproductive age, discusses the relation of diseases prevalent in adulthood to CF patients, and touches upon the psychosocial complications of CF in adults, especially as they relate to hospitalized patients.

II. Lung Disease

A. The Pathophysiological Process and Its Implications for the Hospitalized Adult

Recent evidence indicates that patients with CF from the very earliest days in infancy have an inflammatory process in the lung, and there is some evidence that this occurs (or can persist) in the absence of demonstrable infection (1,2). However, even infants have pathogens recovered from cultures of lung aspirates, the sputum, or the "deep" posterior pharynx after cough (3). As time goes by, the patient with CF has an ever-increasing probability of being colonized by gram-negative bacteria, especially *Pseudomonas aeruginosa*. The adult with CF, thus, has had 20 years or more of ongoing inflammation and infection in the lung, and the damage wreaked by this process may be severe. Some of the complications of the CF lung disease appear to be time dependent as well as dependent on the severity of the lung disease. For example, in an autopsy series, patients with CF had increasing amounts of anatomical emphysema the older they were at death (4). However, a recent study of predictors of mortality in patients with CF showed that for any given level of pulmonary function assessed by the forced vital capacity (FVC) or the forced expiratory volume in 1 second (FEV_1), the 2-year mortality rate is less for older patients than for younger patients (5). In addition, for any given FEV_1 and age, female patients had mortality rates double those of males. On the other hand, poorer nutritional-state, expressed as weight for height, was a stronger predictor of mortality in adults than in children. Thus, it is clear that the disease processes that contribute to mortality differ in adults and children, but exactly how this occurs and what the therapeutic implications should be are unclear.

Although adults with CF generally have more severe disease than children, within the adult age group, it is difficult to detect clear age-related trends in illness severity. The death rate is statistically similar in all age groups of persons older than 21 years. The presence of two organisms—*P. aeruginosa* (6,7) and *Burkholderia cepacia* (8)—in sputum has been associated with poorer pulmonary status. Both of these are more prevalent in adults. Approximately 80% of CF patients older than age 20 years are colonized with *P. aeruginosa*, compared with less than one-third younger than age 5 years, and the proportion does not change as age increases in the adult age range. *B. cepacia* is more than four times more prevalent in persons older than age 11 years than in younger patients, but the proportion of patients colonized does not change with age in the teenage years and beyond. The prevalence of *Staphylococcus aureus* and *Haemophilus influenzae* in sputum cultures, on the other hand, appears to decline with increasing age (3). In one series, the presence of *S. aureus* in sputum was actually a favorable prognostic indicator (9). Thus, as patients with CF age, the prevalence of bacteria associated with worsening lung function (i.e., *P. aeruginosa* and *B. cepacia*) increases, and the bacterial colonization associated with more favorable outcomes recedes. Moreover, adults with CF acquire other potential pathogens with greater frequency than children. Nontuberculous mycobacteria may be quite frequent in adults (10,11), and *Aspergillus fumigatus* (and host reactions to it) is also seen in variable proportions of older patients, depending on the geographic locale (12–14). Because the lung disease is the dominant reason for hospitalization among patients with CF, and because a cornerstone of treatment is antibiotic therapy of presumed pathogens in the lung, the changing sputum flora affects the in-hospital treatment of adults. The need for antistaphylococcal therapy may decrease, but the prevalence of resistant *Pseudomonas* species and the presence of other pathogens may predispose the adult to longer hospitalizations with more intense antibiotic treatment. Sometimes, the antibiotics required for treatment of resistant organisms are more toxic and cannot be safely given at home. For example, colistin is a drug to which most *P. aeruginosa* pathogens are sensitive, but besides the potential nephrotoxicity, it can produce neurological disturbances, including paresthesias, numbness, and vertigo (15). These symptoms are not necessarily indications to discontinue the drug, but do mark the patient for careful monitoring. In addition, patients with these symptoms usually cannot keep up with home intravenous antibiotic dosing. Thus, colistin treatment is better given in the hospital. Moreover, as the lung disease advances, hospitalizations are required more frequently.

The social situations of young adults may affect hospitalization rates as well. When children live with their parents, there are caretakers at home who are often quite familiar with the medical regimen, the needs of the patient, and the need for intensive bronchial drainage. In addition, the parents are usually responsible individuals dedicated to the care of their children. As young people mature and begin to live away from home in college dormitories or on their own, the social support system locally available is often limited, and the potential caretakers are neither sophisticated in medical care nor dedicated to the patient. Therefore, to be assured of adequate execution of a course of treatment for pulmonary exacerbation, a young adult may require hospitalization, whereas a child with parent caretakers may not.

Adults are also represented disproportionately among candidates for lung transplantation. More than 300 transplants have been done in patients with CF in the United States, most of them in young adults, and 300 patients were on the waiting list in 1994 (16). Maintaining patients as viable transplant candidates may require many hospitalizations, and the requirements of different transplant centers may entrain the specifics of antibiotic treatment, nutritional repletion, exercise programs, and other therapeutic modalities. In addition, mechanical ventilation is sometimes offered as a short-term bridge to transplant (17), although under other circumstances mechanical ventilation is usually not undertaken for patients with relentless respiratory failure unresponsive to maximal conventional treatment (18).

Some complications of the CF lung disease are also more prevalent in older patients. These include massive hemoptysis, pneumothorax, and right heart failure. Whether these complications are simply more prevalent with increasing severity of disease, or whether time in addition to severity can be implicated in their pathogenesis cannot be ascertained with certainty from the available information

B. Complications

Hemoptysis

Massive hemoptysis (>240 mL of blood expectorated in 24 hours) is seen in fewer than 0.4% of children younger than 15 years, in 1.5% of patients aged 16–20 years, and in more than 2.5% of patients older than 21 years (3). Blood streaks in the sputum are common in adults with CF and are not cause for alarm (19). Massive hemoptysis, however, is cause for hospitalization and observation, and may require supportive care such as volume expansion or transfusion. In addition, treatment of the underlying respiratory infection is indicated. Especially if the patient lives alone, it may not be possible to ensure safety at home, so adults are often best hospitalized until it is clear that the crisis is past. Massive hemoptysis is caused by systemic arterial bleeding from dilated, tortuous bronchial arteries that develop with bronchiectasis. Bleeding may be brisk and even rapidly fatal, although this is rare. Although massive hemoptysis is frightening and there are reports of patients dying during such an episode (20), patients with massive hemoptysis as a group have no higher mortality rate than other patients with disease of comparable severity (21). Nevertheless, the complication is at best worrisome and at worst life-threatening, and may be especially dangerous in an adult patient living alone, so an attempt at definitive treatment is often made. If the bleeding vessel can be located angiographically and the spinal artery does not take off above it, embolization of the bleeding vessel can be attempted and is often curative (22,23). If a single site is responsible for the bleeding and the disease elsewhere is mild, resection may be effective (24). The remaining lobes often deteriorate, however, and the complication may recur at another site. Ordinarily, it is difficult to localize the site of bleeding by bronchoscopy, and angiography may also be ambiguous. For this reason, embolism of large and tortuous vessels is sometimes undertaken without clear demonstration of the bleeding site, or conservative management may be pursued.

Pneumothorax

Pneumothorax is another pulmonary complication more prevalent in adults. In 1990, it was reported in fewer than 0.3% of patients younger than age 15 years but in more than 1% of patients older than age 16 years (3). This complication has been described as ominous, with median survival from first pneumothorax estimated at 29.9 months (25) and with occurrence always necessitating hospitalization (17). The management of this complication has changed substantially with the advent of lung transplantation to treat the CF lung disease. Before transplantation, was an option, because the probability of recurrence of pneumothorax was approximately 50%, the initial episode of pneumothorax was usually treated definitively, with chemical or, preferably, surgical pleurodesis. By eliminating the potential space between the visceral and parietal pleura, this treatment reduced the chance that the lung would collapse, even if rupture of subpleural blebs occurred. However, separating a lung that is densely adherent to the chest wall to remove it for transplant is always difficult and often bloody, and the patient may not survive. So, pleural sclerosis is a relative contraindication to transplant. Thus, in patients who might be candidates for transplant, the most conservative treatment of pneumothorax is often elected (26). Small pneumothoraces may be observed; larger ones may be treated with tube thoracostomy (17).

Right Heart Failure

Frank right heart failure is a grim prognostic sign, with median survival of only 8 months from its appearance (27). Even patients with mild to moderate disease may have some signs of right heart strain on echocardiography, and the more severe the lung disease, the more prevalent and severe the echocardiographic abnormalities (28). Pulmonary artery pressure correlates with oxygenation in several series (29,30). Therefore, it is likely that frank failure represents the accumulation of insults from relative hypoxemia over many years. Treatment focuses on treating the underlying lung disease. Therapies directed at relieving pulmonary hypertension (except for oxygen, the best pulmonary vasodilator) have met with only limited success. Usually, patients with frank right heart failure are sick enough to be hospitalized, where careful monitoring of electrolytes during diuresis and aggressive treatment of the lung disease are undertaken.

Arthritis

Arthritis may complicate the lung disease of cystic fibrosis, and the prevalence of this complaint seems to be higher in older patients, although the percentage is still well under 5%. Two CF-specific mechanisms have been proposed. The first is hypertrophic pulmonary osteoarthropathy, an inflammatory condition related to clubbing. Patients with this condition suffer periosteal elevation and inflammation along the distal long bones, such as the femur, the tibia and fibula, and the ulna and radius. Occasionally, the inflammatory process extends into the adjacent joints, and effusions develop in the knees, ankles, wrists, and occasionally other joints. Warmth and erythema that are more prominent over the adjacent long bones than the joint itself are characteristic of this disorder, and, usually, bone scan demonstrates increased uptake in the same area. When the process has been repeated several times, the repeated episodes of periosteal elevation and mineralization leave a layered appearance on plain film of the distal long bones. Sometimes, the flare-ups of hypertrophic pulmonary osteoarthropathy coincide with pulmonary exacerbations and subside with treatment of the lung disease, but usually the addition of nonsteroidal antiinflammatory therapy is warranted as well. Because the flare-ups often accompany pulmonary exacerbations and subside in a few days with treatment of the lung disease, they often occur in conjunction with hospitalization.

The second mechanism of joint disease in cystic fibrosis patients is immune complex disease. Although as many as 30% of adult patients have circulating immune complexes, the pathophysiological significance of these immune complexes per se is unclear. However, in a series of eight patients with episodic arthropathy, six had elevated ^{125}I-C1q binding compared with only one of 12 control patients, and synovial biopsies of patients with active joint inflammation showed intimal deposition of IgG, IgM, C3, and C1q in one patient. Seven of these patients had frank effusions, and all of them had circulating immune complexes. The eighth patient had only arthropathy without frank inflammation and did not have circulating immune complexes detected. Flare-ups of arthritis were associated with pulmonary exacerbations. This form of arthritis is episodic and self-limited, is not associated with radiographic changes in the long bones and joints, and does not progress (31). Thus, it seems likely that, as in Crohn's disease, Reiter's syndrome, or psoriasis, circulating immune complexes may contribute to arthritis in CF.

Nasal Polyposis

Almost all patients with CF, children and adults alike, have roentgenographic abnormalities of the paranasal sinuses. Sometimes, the rhinosinusitis is also manifest by the development of nasal polyps, which occur in children and young adults and are sometimes resistant to medical management with nasal antiinflammatory agents. Resection is undertaken, often as an outpatient procedure or with only a brief inpatient stay. Keeping the nasal passages clear following polypectomy may be attempted with nasal steroids, but, in more than 50% of patients, the polyps recur and repeated resections may be necessary.

III. Gastrointestinal Complications

A. Pancreatic Disease

Pancreatic insufficiency is one of the most common complications of cystic fibrosis and is present in approximately 80% of patients at diagnosis. It is often severely symptomatic in children, and the presence or absence of pancreatic insufficiency dominates the growth patterns of patients with CF in the first 6 years of life (32). After that time, growth and weight-for-height can be more closely related to the pulmonary status than the pancreatic status, presumably because of the caloric demands of chronic infection and inflammation, and the anorexia sometimes associated with chronic illness. Many patients are born with little or no pancreatic function; for the others, the pancreatic disease is progressive throughout life. Patients who are initially pancreatic sufficient may become insufficient with the passage of time. For some patients, the progressive loss of pancreatic function is marked by episodes of pancreatitis. These episodes often require hospitalization for intravenous hydration and pain control. By adulthood, more than 90% of patients have pancreatic insufficiency (19). Paradoxically, anecdotal and clinical experience indicates that the symptoms from pancreatic insufficiency diminish in older patients. Whether this is due to learned behaviors in taking enzymes appropriately or avoiding foods that are noxious, or whether this is due to physiological factors is uncertain. However, in patients who have ignored nutritional advice, difficulties from chronic nutritional deficiencies may arise in adulthood. For example, failure to take water-miscible vitamin E may lead to peripheral neuropathy over a period of years (33). Treatment of pancreatic insufficiency has improved markedly in the last decade with the introduction of pancreatic enzyme supplements packaged in microspheres, which permit the enzymes to survive the acid of the stomach and be released in the small bowel where the pH is more favorable and where digestion and absorption of nutrients occurs. However, because of the impaired pancreatic bicarbonate secretion, even under these more favorable circumstances, the pH in the CF gut is below the optimum for pancreatic enzyme activity, and digestion and nutrient absorption ordinarily remain imperfect. For patients whose nutritional status is of concern, administration of H_2-blockers to limit the amount of gastric acid that needs to be neutralized can be quite effective (34,35). However, the long-term consequences of these drugs are unknown. Nevertheless, data on the fatty acid composition of membrane proteins indicate that even after treatment, patients with CF and pancreatic insufficiency differ significantly from normal subjects, and serum carotene levels often remain below normal as well (36). As patients with CF live longer, previously unrecognized complications associated with prolonged subtle nutritional deficiencies may begin to emerge. Although pancreatic insufficiency per se is rarely a cause of hospitalization for patients with CF, its complications may require hospital treatment.

B. Gallstones

Gallstones are more frequent in older patients than in children. Of the patients reported to the Cystic Fibrosis Foundation (CFF) Data Registry in 1994, 0.1% of those younger than 20 years and 0.7% of those older than 21 years had gallbladder disease (16). Presumably, these data reflect incidence of acute symptoms during that year, because, in most series, the prevalence of gallstones ranges from 8% to 30% (37,38). Gallstones have been considered to be a complication of pancreatic insufficiency, based on a study that indicated that cholesterol gallstones arose in CF as a consequence of bile acid malabsorption related to pancreatic insufficiency (39). However, gallstones probably arise because of a confluence of many different factors. Several recent studies have failed to confirm the original observations of Roy et al. (40,41); furthermore, study of the CF mouse has revealed that abnormalities of the gallbladder in animals lacking CFTR are not necessarily coupled to pancreatic insufficiency (42). Recent studies suggest that the radiolucent stones produced in CF patients are not composed predominantly of cholesterol, but that protein is a major component (43). In addition, gallstones are observed in CF patients without pancreatic insufficiency, and the vigorous treatment of pancreatic insufficiency in clinics around the world has not influenced the prevalence of gallstones. Whatever the origin of the stones, if they are associated with symptoms, resection is indicated. However, most of the stones are asymptomatic. For these patients, two schools of thought exist. It can be argued that the asymptomatic stone might never be troublesome and therefore should be left alone. On the other hand, CF patients have lung disease that deteriorates with time, making surgery at a later time (especially under urgent conditions) almost surely more hazardous than elective surgery when stones are discovered. Thus, some physicians recommend resection. Hospitalization is usually brief with modern techniques of cholecystectomy. There is not yet enough experience with medical therapy for gallstones in CF, but the initial results are encouraging (44).

C. Diabetes

The endocrine pancreatic insufficiency that complicates exocrine pancreatic disease becomes more overt in older patients. Hyperglycemia and frank diabetes occur much more frequently in older patients. Before age 10 years, fewer than 0.5% of persons with CF have diabetes treated with insulin compared with 12% of those older than age 26 years (3). Glucose intolerance often becomes evident during a hospitalization in adult patients, presumably due to the effects of metabolic stress on glucose tolerance. Pregnancy may also be a precipitating factor. Diabetes may also be precipitated as an adverse effect of treatment in CF. In a recent long-term trial of alternate day prednisone therapy, the group receiving 2 mg/kg on alternate days was terminated early because of an unacceptable incidence of glucose abnormalities (45). This result emphasizes the contribution of corticosteroid therapy to the manifestation of symptomatic glucose intolerance, and it also shows that the predilection for development of diabetes exists in younger CF patients. Sometimes, when the stress is alleviated, glucose intolerance recedes. Usually, however, the course of diabetes is inexorable, and care must be taken with all subsequent stresses to control hyperglycemia and its complications. Pulmonary function in untreated diabetic CF patients deteriorates more rapidly than in control subjects and tends to improve after initiation of insulin therapy (46). Insulin therapy should therefore be initiated promptly once diabetes is recognized. In general, patients with CF suffer the osmotic complications of diabetes and rarely does ketoacidosis develop, so diabetes per se rarely accounts for hospital admission, after the initial admission for the institution of insulin therapy. The secondary consequences of diabetes (e.g., retinopathy, nephropathy, microangiopathy) have been thought to be rare in patients with CF, perhaps because the hypoinsulinemia results from loss of islet cells, glucagon levels are low rather than high, and the genetic predisposition to diabetes and the environmental insults that initiate it are usually absent in CF. However, such complications definitely occur (47). It is also possible that not enough patients with CF have survived long enough with frank diabetes for the secondary complications to become manifest in a large number of patients. The results of the Diabetes Complications Control Trial, which link the development of diabetic complications in the non-CF patient closely to blood sugar levels (48), suggest that sustained hyperglycemia may result in complications over time in patients with CF as well. For that reason, and because of the suggestion that insulin therapy is salutary for the course of the lung disease, attempts to control the blood sugar closely may be warranted. This may be more difficult but even more important during the stress of hospitalization.

D. Intestinal Obstruction

Intestinal obstruction, common in the neonatal period as meconium ileus, is less frequent later in childhood. As patients become older, however, distal intestinal obstruction syndrome (DIOS; previously called "meconium ileus equivalent") becomes more frequent. In one series, more than 20% of adults had intestinal obstruction at some point in their adult course (19). Rubenstein et al. (49) reported that patients older than 30 years of age have prevalence of intestinal obstruction of 27%. Nearly all the patients with this complication have pancreatic insufficiency (50), so this complication is sometimes classified as a complication of the pancreatic lesion of CF. However, anecdotal experience is that intestinal obstruction does develop in patients with pancreatic sufficiency (who are few in the adult age group), and that the untreated CF "knockout" mouse, which produces pancreatic enzymes and has minimal pancreatic lesions, dies of intestinal obstruction either in the neonatal period (presumably the murine equivalent of meconium ileus) or at approximately the time of weaning (presumably the murine equivalent of distal intestinal obstruction syndrome) (42). The failure to secrete fluid into the gut, combined with the abnormal fecal stream caused by maldigestion and malabsorption, is probably the most common cause of the obstruction. Clearly, changes in gut motility or mechanical obstructions can also contribute, and some physicians relate these episodes to dietary indiscretion or changes in the use of pancreatic enzyme supplements, but, for most episodes, no distinct precipitating event can be identified. The obstruction often takes the form of high fecal impaction, but sometimes a piece of stool becomes densely adherent to the bowel wall and serves as a lead point for intussusception. Recently, intestinal strictures were reported as a possible complication of high-dose pancreatic enzyme therapy in patients with CF, and this problem could clearly predispose the patient to intestinal obstruction, but the preponderance of cases of stricture is in the younger (toddler) age group. The symptoms of intestinal obstruction (i.e., crampy abdominal pain, fewer bowel movements, occasionally vomiting, and often a right lower quadrant mass) must also be distinguished from those of appendicitis or abscess, particularly in persons in whom the full symptom complex is masked by the antibiotics taken for the lung disease. A patient in whom this complication has been identified previously and who can recognize the early symptoms may use GoLYTELY or similar agents very early in the course to prevent the development of full obstruction. However, if there is any suspicion of intussusception, if air–fluid levels are present on plain film, or if obstruction appears to be complete, hospitalization for enemas with Hypaque or Gastrografin is prudent. If intussusception is present, the enema may reduce it. If not, hypertonic contrast material, by drawing water into the gut and dislodging the inspissated stool, can flush out the obstruction. To be successful, the hypertonic contrast material must fully penetrate the obstructing stool, which usually requires its reaching the terminal ileum. Attention to fluid and electrolyte balance is essential during treatment with osmotic agents because substantial amounts of water and electrolyte can pool in a distended gut. Surgery, which was once the primary therapy for this complication, should be a last resort. Manipulation of the inflamed gut often leads to adhesions, conferring on the patient mechanical problems in addition to the biochemical ones that led to the obstruction in the first place. In addition, because the obstruction is often at the ileocecal junction, resection often involves the ileum. This, then, compromises the absorptive surface of the gut, a deficiency that patients with CF, pancreatic insufficiency, maldigestion, and malabsorption can ill afford. Nevertheless, occasionally, there is no alternative and resection is lifesaving.

Because of the urgency of the situation and the potential for dehydration and electrolyte imbalance during treatment, hospitalization is indicated for all but the mildest cases of intestinal obstruction in adults and children.

E. Liver Disease

When it first became clear that treatment could alter the course of CF and that patients would survive into the third and fourth decades with fastidious and aggressive pulmonary care, CF clinicians predicted that biliary cirrhosis would become more prevalent and more severe, and would itself claim more lives. This has not occurred. Patients with liver disease have usually declared themselves by their teenage years. The prevalence of cirrhosis does not increase substantially after patients become 11–15 years of age (3). One clinic reports that 25% of adults with CF have abnormal liver function by the criteria of hepatomegaly or abnormal liver function tests, and the subgroup of these patients studied further had significant abnormalities on endoscopic retrograde cholangiography, ultrasound, and hepatobiliary scintigraphy, suggesting that subclinical liver disease may be more common than previously thought in adults (51). Liver disease is a potentially fatal complication of CF, because of bleeding from esophageal varices, rupture of a massive spleen, or very rarely, hepatocellular failure. Adults with liver disease require close attention and careful management, often in the hospital during acute episodes. Sclerosis of the varices or shunting of the blood flow away from the portal system, with or without splenectomy, may be successful (52). Portosystemic shunting is possible in some patients, without laparotomy, via interventional radiology with the transjugular intrahepatic portosystemic shunting (TIPS) procedure (53). This procedure avoids the extensive abdominal scarring seen with laparotomy and thus does not preclude future liver transplantation. Because there is little hepatocellular disease in patients with CF, shunts may have fewer complications than they do in patients with other types of liver disease in which hepatic encephalopathy often complicates the postoperative course of patients undergoing shunt. Liver transplantation has also become an option for patients with CF (54). Both shunting procedures and transplantation require extended hospitalization. Data are sparse on the efficacy of these different treatments in patients with CF because of the rarity of severe liver disease and the diversity of approaches that have been taken for this complication. There has been interest in ursodeoxycholic acid as prophylactic treatment of developing liver disease (44,55,56).

IV. The Sweat Defect

The sweat defect is present throughout life and does not change with age. However, the clinical implications of this defect are most evident in infancy and among adolescents and adults who exercise heavily in hot weather. In patients engaged in physical labor (e.g., construction workers, mail carriers) or sports, who pursue these activities without adequate attention to fluid and salt repletion, heat prostration can develop, which can be fatal if fluid and salt are not replaced rapidly. This condition is a true medical emergency and repletion of fluid and salt should not be delayed for transport to a center. Ordinarily, replenishment with fluid and electrolytes begins with at least 15 mL/kg of normal saline administered over the first 30 minutes, with slower repletion to follow. It is better to avoid the complication altogether by maintaining adequate fluid and salt intake during heavy or prolonged exercise.

V. Reproduction

A. Fertility

Ordinarily, fertility or lack thereof is not an important consideration for CF patients until puberty, when questions about reproduction arise. Besides the obvious reproductive issue of propagating an abnormal gene, the CF disease process results in infertility in both males and females.

Because patients with CF are homozygous for the abnormal CF gene, all their offspring will have at least one abnormal gene for CF. The odds of having a child with CF then depend on the odds of the spouse having an abnormal gene for CF. In the white American population, assuming a negative family history, the odds of being a CF heterozygote are approximately 1 in 25. Thus, the odds of a CF patient having a child with CF are one in fifty ($1/25 \times 1/2$), compared with the 1/2500 chance of a white child of parents of unknown CF genetic status having a CF child. Currently, the genetic status of the fetus can be ascertained with near certainty. It is too soon to determine how this change in the information available to prospective CF parents will influence their reproductive decisions.

More than 98% of CF males are sterile due to the absence or atrophy of the vas deferens, leading to a functional vasectomy (57). Cystic fibrosis accounts for 1%–2% of male sterility, and the presence of mutations in the CFTR protein is associated with congenital bilateral absence of the vas deferens, even in patients who do not have CF. Although the exact mechanism is not known, it is presumed that sludging of secretions in the vas early in fetal life leads to plugging and then resorption of the abnormal structure. Alternatively, it is possible that this structure fails to develop at all in most men with CF. Although libido and sexual performance are normal (assuming the patient is not severely ill), spermatozoa do not reach the ejaculate, and the patient is sterile. However, a few men have spermatozoa in the semen and can father children. For this reason, semen analysis is prudent for all CF males before they become sexually active.

Married couples in which the husband has CF have many options for child rearing. Adoption is possible and has been pursued. The wife may undergo artificial insemination with spermatozoa from an anonymous donor. The possibility of recovery of spermatozoa from the testes of the male partner for insemination of the wife has been raised, but some couples prefer to reduce the risk of transmitting the abnormal gene for CF and use spermatozoa from an anonymous donor. Rarely do the male reproductive complications provoke hospitalization themselves, but they may bring male patients with CF to medical attention, and the psychosocial implications of infertility may complicate the management of the disease, both in hospitalized patients and in outpatients.

Women with CF appear to be less fertile than healthy women of comparable age. Estimates of the relative fertility have been at 20%–25% of normal, although this number is difficult to estimate because of the conscious decision of many women with CF to avoid pregnancy. Several factors probably contribute to this relative infertility. The relative underweight of many women with CF can lead to anovulatory cycles and cessation of menses. In addition, the cervical mucus of women with CF has reduced water content compared with normal mucus and may be more difficult for spermatozoa to penetrate. In addition, the mucus does not undergo the usual midcycle thinning, which presumably facilitates fertilization of the released egg around the time of ovulation (58).

B. Contraception

Because pregnancy is sometimes difficult for the woman with CF and the prospect of raising a child may be difficult to contemplate for either a man or woman with CF, many sexually active patients with CF require contraception. Cystic fibrosis itself is not adequate birth control, nor does it protect against sexually transmitted diseases (STDs). Condoms protect against STDs, but are not quite as successful as other methods for contraception. Birth control pills (BCPs), particularly with the number of placebo pills decreased from seven to four per month, are effective. (Decreasing the number of placebo days is done because of the theoretical interference of antibiotics with BCP efficacy.) Surgical sterilization is the most effective method and is chosen by many CF patients. The safest contraception for a woman with CF is for her partner to have a vasectomy. However, these couples must understand that if the wife later dies of CF, her husband might regret having been sterilized.

C. Pregnancy

Despite their reduced fertility, women with CF can become pregnant, either in the normal course of events or with medical assistance, and deliver healthy children. It is possible to obviate the difficulties of spermatozoa penetrating the cervical plug by artificial insemination with the husband's semen placed beyond the cervical os, and some couples have sought in vitro fertilization. In 1994, 135 pregnancies in 3632 women aged 15–41 years were reported to the CFF data registry. Of these, 58 resulted in a live birth in 1994 and 50 were still in progress at the end of 1994 (16). The women reported as pregnant were more likely to be nonwhite and less likely to have pancreatic insufficiency or diabetes mellitus, but their pulmonary function was similar to that of nonpregnant women with CF. A Canadian series showed patients who became pregnant had similar demographics in some respects but differed in others. Pancreatic sufficiency was more prevalent in pregnant women than in all CF women, and the average nutritional status was excellent. In this series, the pulmonary function was only mildly impaired and no patient had had right heart failure before pregnancy (59). In several series, except for the expected 2% incidence of offspring with CF, no increase in birth defects has been reported, even for mothers treated intensively with antibiotics during pregnancy (59–61). The number of completed pregnancies studied (fewer than 200), however, is too small to detect even fairly common complications of intensive drug treatment. In any case, most physicians try to select the least teratogenic medications compatible with adequate treatment of the mother, and many drugs commonly used in CF have little teratogenic potential (e.g., pancreatic enzyme supplements, vitamins, beta-adrenergic agents, inhaled steroids, or inhaled antibiotics). The penicillins and cephalosporins also appear to have low teratogenic potential. Aminoglycosides should be used with caution because of the potential impact on the fetal kidneys and the eighth nerve, but many women have been given aminoglycosides, with monitoring of maternal blood levels, without detectable ill effects in the fetus. Tetracycline and chloramphenicol should be avoided. The mother's clinical status should be monitored closely, however, and appropriate treatment should not be withheld for fear of harming the fetus. Surprisingly, in the 1990 CFF data registry, there was no more use of any of the reported therapeutic modalities and no more hospital days among the pregnant women than among the nonpregnant adult women (62). The variability of these measures is great, however, and more data may allow trends to be detected.

Pregnancy is not without hazard to women with CF and their infants. In combined series, the perinatal death rate is 8.6% compared with less than 4% for unselected pregnancies, and preterm delivery is reported in 22.8% compared with less than 10% in unselected pregnancies (62). In general, series that selected CF mothers with mild lung disease had fewer perinatal deaths and preterm deliveries: these rates approximate those of the unselected population (59,63). Women reported to the CFF Data Registry in 1990 who carried their babies to full term were more likely to have mild pulmonary disease than either nonpregnant women or pregnant women who delivered prematurely or underwent therapeutic abortion (62). Thus, although women with all levels of pulmonary function became pregnant, pulmonary status was related to pregnancy outcome. Particularly at risk are women with right heart strain, who may not tolerate the 50% increase in blood volume that is characteristic of the second trimester. The discomforts of the third trimester, with possible compromise of diaphragm excursion by the gravid uterus and the stimulus to ventilation that progesterone provides, are somehow less troublesome.

The impact of pregnancy on the mother with CF seems to depend on the pregravid pulmonary status, and perhaps on nutritional status as well. In the early series of Cohen et al. (60), heart failure developed in 13% of mothers and 18% died. However, among pregnant CF patients reported to the data registry in 1994, none died in that year, and, in a recent Canadian series, of 38 pregnancies (59), there was no heart failure and only one death within 2 years of delivery. In the Canadian series, lung function declined in the postpartum period, but no more so than was expected for nonpregnant CF patients with similar baseline pulmonary function. Weight for height and blood gases did not change significantly with pregnancy and delivery. The pregravid pulmonary and nutritional status of the patients in this particular series was excellent. In other series that have included patients with more severe lung disease, those with mild disease have fared well and those with severe disease have fared more poorly. Maintenance of good nutrition is of particular importance to the CF patient during pregnancy. The recommended weight gain of 25–28 lb for a normal pregnancy should be the goal for CF pregnancies as well, with vigorous oral supplementation if necessary. Patients with CF and pancreatic insufficiency, even when treated with pancreatic enzyme supplements and vitamins, have abnormal fatty acid composition of lipid membranes in the direction of mild essential fatty acid deficiency. Additional nutritional stresses, such as those of pregnancy, should be met with vigorous measures to maintain the nutritional state as near normal as possible. The excellent results of pregnancy reported by Canny et al. (59) occurred in a population in which only half were pancreatic insufficient.

Labor and delivery may be taxing in a patient with CF, particularly if there is preexisting cardiovascular compromise, if anesthesia is required, or if cesarean section is performed and there is pain with breathing. However, patients who have tolerated the second-trimester increase in blood volume can usually be taken through labor and delivery without untoward events. The pulmonary and nutritional status should be evaluated after delivery and treatment initiated as indicated.

D. Breast Feeding

Breast feeding is possible and the salt content of the milk is apparently normal (64), in contrast to earlier fears. However, the metabolic demands of breast feeding are considerable, and, unless the nutritional status is robust, the advantages of breast feeding probably do not outweigh the potential for nutritional compromise and fatigue in the mother. Therefore, many physicians recommend that the postpartum period in a CF mother be devoted to nutritional recovery and limit the nutritional drain by recommending bottle feeding of the infant.

VI. Diseases Common in Non-CF Adults

The two major killers of Americans are coronary artery disease and cancer. As CF patients reach the adult age range more regularly, it is to be expected that they will encounter these extremely common diseases of American middle and old age. Coronary atherosclerosis is associated with hypertension, diabetes, a family history of heart disease, and hypercholesterolemia. However, patients with CF, especially those with pancreatic insufficiency, tend to have very low cholesterol levels (65), and, in general, the degree of atherosclerosis observed at postmortem examination is less than expected for age. In addition, the chronic salt loss in the sweat probably accounts for the fact that blood pressure is statistically significantly lower in patients with CF than in control subjects (66,67). A number of years ago, reduced tendency toward hypertension was even proposed as part of the putative "heterozygote advantage" that might explain the high prevalence of a lethal gene line (68). Thus, these two factors would tend to reduce the development of heart disease in CF patients. On the other hand, diabetes, which is prevalent in CF, might enhance it. In any event, there are no available data on comment on the incidence of myocardial infarction, angina, or coronary artery disease in older patients with CF.

Cancer is another prominent killer of adults. Early reports suggested some increase in the cancer risk in patients with CF. Recent epidemiological data from a large number of patient-years at risk indicate that, overall, cancer rates are not increased, but the investigators found a significant sixfold excess of gastrointestinal cancers in CF (69). These cancers occurred at a median age of 29 years. Some were discovered at necropsy, which suggests that the panoply of gastrointestinal symptoms associated with CF itself may mask the symptoms of intestinal cancer. However, from the entire CF data registry for 5 years, only 28 total cancers and eight gastrointestinal cancers (five colon and small intestine, one rectum, one liver, one biliary) were reported, so cancer remains a rare event in patients with CF (69). Clearly, if cancer is identified, it warrants hospitalization and definitive treatment.

VII. Psychosocial Complications

Adults with cystic fibrosis face all the pressures of the modern world, plus reproductive difficulties, infirmity, disability, the consequent limitations on career choices, activities, and finances, and the near certainty of early death. Given these difficulties, the personal successes of this population are remarkable. Of 6045 patients older than age 18 years reported to the CF Foundation Data Registry in 1994, only 20.6% listed themselves as unemployed, whereas 32.5% worked full time and 17.2% worked part time. Five percent characterized themselves as full-time homemakers and 17.4% as students. Sixty-eight percent reported some sort of private health insurance. Some 1670 patients reported that they had finished high school or had the equivalent of a high school diploma, and 2327 reported some college education. The high school graduation rate is twice the national average. On the social side, 26.6% of those older than 18 years are married, 5.3% are divorced or separated, and 4.6% are living with a partner (16). Several studies remark on the strikingly normal psychological adjustment and psychosocial functioning of young adults with CF and their families (70–72).

Some of this success may be attributable to the psychosocial support provided for these patients by the center networks and center personnel, and a good deal of this occurs during hospitalization, which is often a time for addressing nonmedical problems. For a CF center to be accredited by the Cystic Fibrosis Foundation, some network of psychosocial support, usually a social worker backed up by psychologists and psychiatrists as needed, must be in place. Availability of vocational rehabilitation may also assist patients with CF. Often, these services are accessed while the patient is in the hospital and are continued on an outpatient basis. Access to psychosocial support is a critical part of hospitalization for adult patients with CF.

As for any fatal disease, as the patient gets sicker, dealing with death becomes an ever greater concern. During the final hospitalizations, it is critical for the patient and family to make decisions regarding the level and intensity of care to be given as the patient deteriorates. In the adult patient, the decision making centers around the patient. Besides the decisions about mechanical ventilation and other extraordinary measures, it may be useful to discuss the desire of the patient to die at home or not. If these matters are discussed well in advance of the event, the decision whether to undertake mechanical ventilation is made well before respiratory failure supervenes and the judgment is clouded by the disordered biochemistry. In addition, decisions about organ (eye and skin) donation and necropsy are often made well before the fact and can have a calming effect on patients who value preparation and order. During hospitalizations, when the physician interacts with the patient daily, these considerations can be raised and discussed at leisure, and the patient has the opportunity to have second thoughts, late concerns, and discussions with family and friends and still return to the physician while the topic is open. These hospitalizations are thus important opportunities for decision making by patients and families, in conjunction with the physician, and for allowing the patient to assume control, when possible, of the events to occur at a time when the patient will be unable to participate fully. Hospitalizations are also opportunities for the physician and patient to establish mutual trust and respect, which gives rise to confidence in the patient that even the unforeseen will be dealt with as the patient would wish by the physician, who has acquired understanding of the patient's character, concerns, family priorities, and wishes. The current tendencies in health care coverage, however, force switching of physicians at the stroke of a clerk's pen and limit hospital care to times of acute illness with all subacute care delivered at home by rotating nurses unfamiliar with the issues of CF patients in general and the particular patient in particular, making this patient–physician familiarity and the confidence it engenders (in addition to the success of the treatment program itself) in jeopardy. Successfully bringing a life to closure, although not the prime goal of any physician, is still the last best service provided by the CF physician to the patient.

Acknowledgment

Support provided by P30 DK27651.

References

1. Copenhaver SC, Khan TZ, Wagener JS, et al. Airway inflammation in the absence of detectable *Pseudomonas aeruginosa* by culture and PCR in infants with cystic fibrosis. *Pediatr Pulmonol Suppl* 1994; 10:283.
2. Khan TZ, Copenhaver SC, Kirchner KK, et al. Serial assessment of airway inflammation in infants with cystic fibrosis identified through newborn screening. *Pediatr Pulmonol Suppl* 1994; 10:283.
3. FitzSimmons SC. The changing epidemiology of cystic fibrosis. *J Pediatr* 1993; 122:1–9.
4. Bedrossian CWM, Greenberg SD, Singer DB, et al. The lung in cystic fibrosis. A quantitative study including prevalence of pathologic findings among different age groups. *Hum Pathol* 1976; 7:195.
5. Kerem E, Reisman J, Corey M, Canny GJ, Levison H. Prediction of mortality in patients with cystic fibrosis. *N Engl J Med* 1992; 326:1187–1191.
6. Wilmott RW, Tyson SL, Matthew DJ. Cystic fibrosis survival rates. The influences of allergy and *Pseudomonas aeruginosa*. *Am J Dis Child* 1985; 139:699–671.
7. Demko CA, Byard PJ, Davis PB. Gender differences in cystic fibrosis: *Pseudomonas aeruginosa* infection. *J Clin Epidemiol* 1995; 48:1044–1050.
8. Lewin L, Byard P, Davis PB. Effect of *Pseudomonas cepacia* colonization on survival and pulmonary function of cystic fibrosis patients. *J Clin Epidemiol* 1990; 43:125–131.
9. Knoke J, Stern RC, Doershuk, Boat TF, Tucker AS, Matthews LW. Cystic fibrosis: the prognosis for five-year survival. *Pediatr Res* 1978; 12:676.
10. Olivier KN, Gilligan P, Yankaskas JR, Knowles MR. Pulmonary nontuberculous mycobacteria in cystic fibrosis. *Pediatr Pulmonol Suppl* 1994; 8:116–117.

11. Aitken ML, Burker W, McDonald G, et al. Nontuberculous mycobacterial disease in adult cystic fibrosis patients. *Chest* 1993; 103:1096–1099.

12. Schwartz RH, Johnstone DE, Holsclaw DS, Dooley RR. Serum precipitins to *Aspergillus fumigatus* in cystic fibrosis. *Am J Dis Child* 1970; 120:432–433.

13. Mearns M, Longbottom J, Batten J. Precipitating antibodies to *Aspergillus fumigatus* in cystic fibrosis. *Lancet* 1967; pp 538–539.

14. Simmonds EJ, Littlewood JM, Hopwood V, Evans EGV. *Aspergillus fumigatus* colonisation and population density of place of residence in cystic fibrosis. *Arch Dis Child* 1994; 70:139–140.

15. Physicians Desk Reference. 48th ed. Montvale, NJ. Medical Economic Data Production Company, 1994.

16. Cystic Fibrosis Foundation. Patient Registry 1993 Annual Data Report, Bethesda, MD: Cystic Fibrosis Foundation, 1994.

17. Schidlow DV, Taussig LM, Knowles MR. Cystic fibrosis foundation consensus conference report on pulmonary complications of cystic fibrosis. *Pediatr Pulmonol* 1993; 15:187–198.

18. Davis PB, di Sant' Agnese PA. Assisted ventilation for patients with cystic fibrosis. *JAMA* 1978; 239:1851–1854.

19. di Sant' Agnese PA, Davis PB. Adults with cystic fibrosis: 75 cases and a review of 232 cases in the literature. *Am J Med* 1979; 66:121–132.

20. Holsclaw DS, Grand RJ, Shwachman H. Massive hemoptysis in cystic fibrosis. *J Pediatr* 1970; 76:829–838.

21. Stern RC, Wood RE, Boat TF, Matthews LW, Tucker AS, Doershuk CF. Treatment and prognosis of massive hemoptysis in cystic fibrosis. *Am Rev Respir Dis* 1978; 117:825–828.

22. Fellows KE, Khaw K-T, Schuster S, Shwachman H. Bronchial artery embolization in cystic fibrosis; technique and long-term results. *J Pediatr* 1979; 95:959–963.

23. Trento A, Estner SM, Griffith BP, Hardesty RL. Massive hemoptysis in patients with cystic fibrosis: three case reports and a protocol for clinical management. Ann Thorac Surg 1985; 39:254–256.

24. Porter DK, Van Every MJ, Mack JW. Emergency lobectomy for massive hemoptysis in cystic fibrosis. *J Thorac Cardiovasc Surg* 1983; 86:409–411.

25. Spector ML, Stern RC. Pneumothorax in cystic fibrosis: a 26-year experience. *Ann Thorac Surg* 1989; 47:204–207.

26. Noyes BE, Orenstein DM. Treatment of pneumothorax in cystic fibrosis in the era of lung transplantation. *Chest* 1992; 101:1187–1188.

27. Stern RC, Borkat G, Hirshfeld SS, et al. Heart failure in cystic fibrosis: treatment and prognosis of cor pulmonale with failure of the right side of the heart. *Am J Dis Child* 1980; 134:267.

28. Moskowitz MB, Gewitz MH, Heyman S, Ruddy RM, Scanlin TF. Cardiac involvement in cystic fibrosis: early noninvasive detection and vasodilator therapy. *Pediatr Pulmonol* 1985; 5:139–148.

29. Moss AJ, Harper WH, Dooley RR, et al. Cor pulmonale in cystic fibrosis of the pancreas. *J Pediatr* 1965; 67:797.

30. Burghuber OC, Salzer-Muhar U, Bergmann H, Götz, M. Right ventricular performance and pulmonary haemodynamics in adolescent and adult patients with cystic fibrosis. *Eur J Pediatr* 1988; 148:187–192.

31. Wulffraat NM, De Graeff-Meeder ER, Rijkers GT, et al. Prevalence of circulating immune complexes in patients with cystic fibrosis and arthritis. *J Pediatr* 1994; 125:374–378.
32. Byard PJ. Relationship between clinical parameters and linear growth in children with cystic fibrosis. *Am J Hum Biol* 1989; 1:719–725.
33. Sung JH, Part SH, Mastri AR, Warwick WJ. Axonal dystrophy in the gracile nucleus in congenital biliary atresia and cystic fibrosis (mucoviscidosis): beneficial effect of vitamin E therapy. *J Neurophathol Exp Neurol* 1980; 39:584–597.
34. Hubbard VS, Dunn GF, Lester LA. Effectiveness of cimetidine as an adjunct to supplemental pancreatic enzymes in patients with cystic fibrosis. *Am J Clin Nutr* 1980; 33:2281–2286.
35. Heijerman HG, Lamers CBH, Dijkman JH, Bakker W. Ranitidine compared with dimethylprostaglandin E$_2$ analogue enprostil as adjunct to pancreatic enzyme replacement in adult cystic fibrosis. *Scand J Gastroenterol* 1990; 25(suppl 178):26–31.
36. McEvoy FA. Essential fatty acids and cystic fibrosis. *Lancet* 1975; 236.
37. L'Heureux PR, Isenberg JN, Sharp HL, Kopin I. Gallbladder disease in cystic fibrosis. *Am J Roentgenol* 1979; 128:953–956.
38. Shwachman H, Kowalski M, Khaw K-T. Cystic fibrosis: a new outlook. *Medicine* 1977; 56:129–149.
39. Roy CC, Weber AM, Morin CL, Combes JC, Nussle D, Megevant A, Lasalle R. Abnormal biliary lipid composition in cystic fibrosis: effect of pancreatic enzymes. *N Engl J Med* 1977; 298:1301–1305.
40. Weizman Z, Durie PR, Kopelman HR, Vesely SM, Forstner GG. Bile acid secretion in cystic fibrosis: evidence for a defect unrelated to fat malabsorption. *Gut* 1986; 27:1043–1048.
41. Strandvik B, Angelin B, Einarsson K. Bile acid kinetics and bile lipid composition in cystic fibrosis (abstract). *Scand J Gastroenterol* 1988; 23 (suppl 43):166.
42. Snouwaert JN, Brigman KK, Latour AM, Malouf NN, Boucher RC, Smithies O, Koller BH. An animal model for cystic fibrosis made by gene targeting. *Science* 1992; 257:1083–1088.
43. Angelico M, Gandin C, Canuzzi P, Bertasi S, Cantafora A, De Santis A, Quatrucci S, Antonelli M. Gallstones in cystic fibrosis: a critical appraisal. *Hepatology* 1991; 14(5): 768–775.
44. Sahl B, Howat J, Webb K. Ursodeoxycholic acid dissolution of gallstones in cystic fibrosis. *Thorax* 1988; 43:490–491.
45. Rosenstein BJ, Eigen H. Risks of alternate-day prednisone in patients with cystic fibrosis. *J Pediatr* 1991; 87:245–246.
46. Lanng S, Thorsteinsson B, Nerup J, Koch C. Diabetes mellitus in cystic fibrosis: effect of insulin therapy on lung function and infections. *Acta Paediatr* 1994; 83:849–853.
47. Sullivan MM, Denning CR. Diabetic microangiophathy in patients with cystic fibrosis. *Pediatrics* 1989; 84:642–647.
48. DCCT Research Group (1993). Diabetes Control and Complications Trial (DCCT): the effect of intensive treatment of diabetes on the development and progression of long-term complications in insulin-dependent diabetes mellitus. *N Engl J Med* 1993; 329:977–986.
49. Rubenstein S, Moss R, Lewiston N (1994). Constipation and meconium ileus equivalent in patients with cystic fibrosis. *Pediatrics* 78:473–479.

50. Khoshoo V, Udall JN. Meconium ileus equivalent in children and adults. *Am J Gastroenterol* 1994; 89(2):153–157.
51. Nagel RA, Javaid A, Meire HB, Wise A, Westaby D, Kavani J, Lombard MG, Williams R, Hodson ME. Liver disease and bile duct abnormalities in adults with cystic fibrosis. *Lancet* 1989; pp. 1422–1425.
52. Psacharopoulos HT, Howard ER, Portman B, Mowat AP, Williams R. Hepatic complications of cystic fibrosis. *Lancet* 1981; pp. 78–80.
53. Ring EJ, Lake JR, Roberts JP, Gordeon RL, LaBerge JM, Read AE, Sterneck MR, Ascher NL. Using transjugular intrahepatic portosystemic shunts to control variceal bleeding before liver transplantation. Ann Intern Med 1992; pp. 304–309.
54. Noble-Jamieson G, Valenta J, Barners ND, Friend PJ, Jamieson NV, Rasmussen A, Calne RY. Liver transplantation for hepatic cirrhosis in cystic fibrosis. *Arch Dis Child* 1994; 71:349–352.
55. Colombo C, Setchell KDR, Podda M, Crosignani A, Roda A, CurcioL, Ronchi M, Giunta A. Effects of ursodeoxycholic acid therapy for liver disease associated with cystic fibrosis. *J Pediatr* 1990; 117:482–489.
56. Cotting J, Lentze JJ, Reichen J. Effects of ursodeoxycholic acid treatment on nutrition and liver function in patients with cystic fibrosis and longstanding cholestasis. *Gut* 1990; 31:918–921.
57. Taussig LM, Lobeck CC, di Sant'Agnese PA, et al. Fertility in males with cystic fibrosis. *N Engl J Med* 1972; 287:586–589.
58. Kopito LE, Kosasky HJ, Shwachman H. Water and electrolytes in cervical mucus from patients with cystic fibrosis. *Fertil Steril* 1973; 24(7):512–516.
59. Canny GJ, Corey M, Livingstone RA, Carpenter S, Green L, Levison H. Pregnancy and cystic fibrosis. Obstet Gynecol 1991; 77(6):850–853.
60. Cohen LF, di Sant'Agnese PA, Friedlander J. Cystic fibrosis and pregnancy. *Lancet* 1980; pp. 842–844.
61. Grand RJ, Talamo RC, di Sant' Agnese PA, Schwartz RH. Pregnancy in cystic fibrosis of the pancreas. *JAMA* 1966; 195:993–1000.
62. Kotloff, RM, FitzSimmons SC, Fiel SB. Fertility and pregnancy in patients with cystic fibrosis. *Clin Chest Med* 1992; 13(4):623–635.
63. Corkey CWB, Newton CJL, Corey M, et al. Pregnancy in cystic fibrosis: a better prognosis in patients with pancreatic function? *Am J Obstet Gynecol* 1981; 140:737–742.
64. Alpert SE, Cormier AD. Normal electrolyte and protein content in milk from mothers with cystic fibrosis: an explanation for the initial report of elevated milk sodium concentration. *J Pediatr* 1983; 102(1):77–80.
65. Slesinski MJ, Gloninger MS, Costantino JP, Orenstein DM. Lipid levels in adults with cystic fibrosis. *J Am Dietetic Assn* 1994; 94:402–408.
66. Lake CR, Davis PB, Ziegler M, Kopin I. Electrolytes and norepinephrine levels in blood of patients with cystic fibrosis. *Clin Chim Acta* 1979; 92:141–146.
67. Davis PB, Shelhamer J, Kaliner M. Abnormal adrenergic and cholinergic sensitivity in cystic fibrosis. *N Engl J Med* 1980; 302:1453–1456.
68. Lieberman J, Rodbard S. Low blood pressure in young adults with cystic fibrosis. *Ann Intern Med* 1975; 82:806–808.
69. FitzSimmons, SC, Neglia JP, Lowenfels AB. Increased gastrointestinal cancer risk among patients with cystic fibrosis. *Pediatr Pulmonol Suppl* 1994; 10:172.

70.   Blair C, Cull A, Freeman CP. Psychosocial functioning of young adults with cystic fibrosis and their families. *Thorax* 1994; 49:798–802.
71.   Cowen L, Corey M, Simmons R, Keenan N, Robertson J, Levison H. Growing older with cystic fibrosis: psychologic adjustment of patients more than 16 years old. *Psychosom Med* 1984; 46(4):363–376.
72.   Walters S, Britton J, Hodson ME. Demographic and social characteristics of adults with cystic fibrosis in the United Kingdom. *Br Med J* 1993; 306:549–552.

13

Lung Transplantation

BLAKESLEE E. NOYES

St. Louis University School
of Medicine and
Cardinal Glennon Children's Hospital
St. Louis, Missouri

GEOFFREY KURLAND

University of Pittsburgh School
of Medicine and
Children's Hospital of Pittsburgh
Pittsburgh, Pennsylvania

BARTLEY P. GRIFFITH

University of Pittsburgh School of Medicine
University of Pittsburgh Medical Center
Presbyterian University Hospital
Pittsburgh, Pennsylvania

I. Introduction

The dramatic advances that have taken place in the care of the patient with cystic fibrosis (CF) over the last decade have raised hopes for an eventual cure of the disease. However, the fact remains that CF is a life-shortening disease, killing many patients before their 30s. Heart-lung and lung transplantation (hereafter referred to simply as lung transplantation) is an accepted mode of treatment for end-stage cardiopulmonary disease from a variety of causes (1) and, at this time, offers the only hope for survival in CF patients with terminal respiratory failure (2). Since this procedure was described by Reitz and colleagues in 1982 (3), more than 4000 lung transplant procedures have been performed worldwide, nearly a thousand of them in patients with CF (4). The first such CF procedure was a heart-lung transplant at Presbyterian University Hospital in 1983 (5). Nationwide 1-year survival rates for CF patients after lung transplantation are approximately 65%, but there is a great deal of variability in posttransplantation morbidity and mortality depending on certain recipient risk factors. In Pittsburgh, 20 lower-risk recipients fared much better, with a 1-year survival rate of 84.6% compared with 36.5% for 14 higher-risk recipients. High-risk recipients had respiratory tract organisms resistant to all antibiotics, body

Table 1 Indications for Hospitalization in the Cystic Fibrosis Lung Transplant Candidate or Recipient

Transplant evaluation
Transplant procedure
Posttransplant period
    Onset of new or increased respiratory symptoms, including cough, dyspnea, fever, or chest pain
    New infiltrates on chest radiograph
    Decline in forced vital capacity or forced expiratory volume in 1 second by more than 10%–15%
    Decline in oxygenation (by pulse oximetry or blood gas measurement)
    Treatment of infection diagnosed by culture of sputum or bronchoscopy specimen
    Treatment of rejection diagnosed by transbronchial or open lung biopsy
    Treatment of posttransplant lymphoproliferative disease
    Treatment of other complications

weight less than 80% of ideal weight for height, or both of these factors. Despite these problems, lung transplantation still offers hope for long-term survival and for an improved quality of life for many patients with CF. Transplantation-related issues have become major indications for hospitalization of the patient with CF (Table 1).

II. Criteria for Selection of Patients and Evaluation Process

Many lung transplant centers believe that potential recipients with CF should be those who would otherwise be likely to die within 2 years. Identifying such patients among the CF population has never been easy. Recently, several reports have provided better tools to estimate the prognosis in CF patients with impending respiratory failure. Kerem and colleagues found that 50% of their patients with a forced expiratory volume in 1 second (FEV_1) of less than 30% of predicted values died within 2 years (see Table 1 in Chapter 14), and they recommended that patients with an FEV_1 of less than 30% be referred to a transplant center for evaluation (6). Nixon et al. found that reduced levels of aerobic fitness as measured by peak oxygen consumption or work rate was associated with a worse prognosis (7). Colonization with *Burkholderia cepacia* (8) carries a negative prognosis, yet may be a contraindication to transplantation. Other negative prognostic factors that may warrant referral for lung transplantation include cor pulmonale with heart failure (1,9), the need for frequent and prolonged hospitalizations (6), and an intolerable quality of life (10). Better criteria are needed for the timing of transplant evaluation, because referral too late in a patient's course will more likely result in a poor outcome if the patient receives a transplant (11) or the patient will die while waiting for a donor.

Table 2 Outcome in 71 Cystic Fibrosis Patients Accepted for Lung Transplantation

	Died (29) Mean ±SD	Transplanted (42) Mean ±SD
Days[a]	234	378
BMI	17 ± 3	18 ± 3
FVC%[a]	34 ± 10	43 ± 16
FEV$_1$%	20 ± 6	24 ± 9
DLco	58 ± 29	61 ± 24
Paco$_2$	51 ± 8	51 ± 12
Pao$_2$	53 ± 9	59 ± 12
6-min walk (ft)	984 ± 356	885 ± 319

[a]$P < 0.05$
BMI=body mass index; FVC%=forced vital capacity as percent predicted; FEV$_1$%=forced expired volume in 1 second as percent predicted; DLco = diffusing capacity for carbon monoxide; Paco$_2$=partial pressure of carbon dioxide in arterial blood; Paco$_2$=partial pressure of oxygen in arterial blood; 6=min walk (ft)=the distance in feet walked in 6 minutes.

Review of 71 candidates accepted for lung transplantation at our center failed to show striking differences between those 42 who survived an average of 378 days to transplant and those 29 who died waiting an average of 234 days after candidacy. Table 2 suggests that reduced 6-minute walk distance, as well as lower FEV$_1$ and Pao$_2$, was predictive of poor outcome, but the interplay of many variables prevents using any single factor to predict outcome.

The list of contraindications (Table 3) to lung transplantation has shrunk considerably as experience with this procedure has grown. Although there remains some debate, the unfavorable results reported in patients whose tracheobronchial secretions harbor *B. cepacia* (12,13) make this finding a relative or absolute contraindication to lung transplantation. Some centers are reluctant to transplant patients with other very resistant organisms. Following transplantation, host pulmonary defenses are compromised for a number of reasons, including airway anesthesia leading to an absent or ineffective cough, diminished mucociliary clearance, and interrupted trafficking of immune effec-

Table 3 Relative Contraindications to Lung Transplantation in Cystic Fibrosis

Colonization of airway secretions with *Burkholderia cepacia* or other multiply resistant
    organisms
Active extrapulmonary infection
Prior pleural ablation (surgical or chemical)
Serious disease of other organ systems, especially the liver
Serious psychiatric disability, history of medical noncompliance
Current cigarette smoking
Inadequate financial resources

tor cells. These factors make it even more difficult than usual to combat organisms resistant to conventional antimicrobial agents. Thus, pan-resistant organisms, especially *B. cepacia*, which are likely to speed lung destruction and make life without a transplant impossible also complicate posttransplant survival, and, in some centers, are considered a contraindication to transplantation.

The technique of bilateral sequential lung transplantation via a transverse submammary thoracic incision decreases the need for cardiopulmonary bypass and provides better access to the pleural surfaces. This technique has made previous pleurectomy or pleurodesis for pneumothorax in CF patients a relative, rather than absolute, contraindication to lung transplantation. A previous pleural procedure complicates the surgical approach to lung transplantation, because of bleeding from the extensive pleural adhesions. The avoidance of cardiopulmonary bypass (and the heparinization required for bypass), as well as improved visibility and treatment of pleural bleeding sites, reduces the risk of perioperative hemorrhage substantially.

Liver disease is generally considered a contraindication to lung transplantation, although the group from Papworth Hospital has reported success with combined heart-lung-liver transplantation in CF patients (11). Most transplant centers in the United States and Canada are reluctant to consider these patients for transplantation because of the high risk and use of multiple organs.

Previously, diabetes mellitus and use of even low-dose corticosteroids rendered patients ineligible for lung transplantation. Most transplant centers no longer consider these contraindications.

On the other hand, serious psychiatric disabilities, current cigarette smoking, a history of noncompliance with medical regimens, and, in some centers, inadequate financial resources are all considered absolute or relative contraindications to transplantation.

Noninvasive mechanical ventilation using nasal positive pressure (BiPAP) has been successfully used as a bridge to transplantation for patients with severe ventilatory failure (14). We have avoided candidates who have required tracheal intubation and prolonged mechanical ventilation because they often have bacterial infections and are seriously deconditioned.

After review of medical records and chest films, patients undergo an evaluation process that includes consultations with the CF team, as well as with specialists in infectious disease, cardiology, neurology, otolaryngology, dentistry, and psychiatry. Professionals in social and financial services are also involved. Numerous laboratory, immunological, and radiographical studies are carried out to assess the medical status of the patient and to assess the appropriateness of a transplant. Blood and serum studies include, but are not limited to, complete blood count (CBC), electrolytes, blood sugar and glycosylated hemoglobin, renal and liver function, and serology for cytomegalovirus (CMV), Epstein-Barr virus, human immunodeficiency virus, hepatitis, and toxoplasmosis. Other tests include pulmonary function and exercise studies, echocardiogram, electrocardiogram, and ventilation–perfusion scans. The transesophageal echocardiogram, although excellent for identifying atrial septal defects, including patent foramen ovale, and for evaluating left and right ventricular function (15), is not routinely used in most centers.

Once the patient has been accepted as a transplant candidate, 24-hour paging and emergency air travel are arranged so that the patient can arrive at the transplant center within 4 hours of notification that donor organs are available. Some transplant centers require the patient to move to the vicinity of the transplant program. Most centers advocate aggressive pulmonary and nutritional rehabilitation, and some institute a supervised exercise program.

III. Living-Related Lung Donation

Unlike dialysis (kidney) and mechanical circulatory support (heart), an alternative bridge to transplant does not exist for people with end-stage lung disease. Patients with CF and respiratory failure can seldom survive conventional mechanical ventilation for the long times usually required to await donor organs (16). In addition to suffering the physical and emotional discomfort of mechanical ventilation (17), those who do survive are likely to lose ground in terms of muscular and cardiovascular conditioning and in nutritional status, and many will have worsened infection. Until techniques in xenograft transplantation or artificial lungs develop beyond their current very early experimental stages, living donor lobar transplantation seems to be the only alternative to death for the desperately ill patient with CF (18). In most of the very few cases in which this technique has been carried out, such lobes have been donated by relatives of the patient, but, in unusual cases, a close friend might appropriately serve as a donor. Transplantation of a whole lung from a living donor is technically feasible, but, in our opinion, entails too great a risk for donor mortality (approximately 5%) and morbidity. Lobectomy, on the other hand, probably carries a less than 1% mortality rate and minimal long-term morbidity. Because of their chronic airway bacterial colonization, recipients with CF need to have both native lungs removed. Because survival with one lobe is unlikely, these patients require two donors. The technique as it is currently applied (18) involves using the left lower lobe from one adult donor and the right lower lobe from another. The procedure is not unlike that used for whole lung transplantation because each lobe—like a whole lung—has artery, vein, and bronchus. These transplanted lobes have shown hemodynamics (pulmonary vascular resistance) and physiology (gas exchange) similar to those seen following bilateral whole lung transplantation. Short-term survival statistics have been comparable to figures for cadaveric whole lung transplantation (18).

IV. Pretransplant Period

A very limited donor organ pool has made the waiting time for lung transplantation 2 years or more in most transplant centers in North America, so pretransplant care is particularly important (and prolonged). Generally, patients with CF who are awaiting lung transplantation continue to be followed at their referring CF center and have outpatient visits at the transplant center once or twice a year. The referring CF physician, with consultation from the transplant center physicians, is often forced to deal with important issues during this pretransplant period. Such issues may include the occurrence of a pneumothorax, the emergence of resistant organisms (e.g., *B. cepacia, Stenotrophomonas maltophilia*), and the medical or surgical treatment of CF sinus disease.

The treatment of a pneumothorax during the transplant waiting period is controversial, and a stepwise approach has been advocated that starts with less aggressive intervention than was usually used in the CF patient before the advent of transplantation (3,4). A pleural ablative procedure may reduce the patient's candidacy for lung transplantation, or at least make transplantation more difficult and dangerous (19,20).

A potentially more vexing and often tragic problem is the appearance of antibiotic-resistant organisms in the sputum. As discussed, many transplant centers consider the presence of resistant organisms such as *B. cepacia* a contraindication to transplant because of the poor outcome of patients harboring these organisms (12,13). Sputum samples are sent to the transplant center for culture and sensitivity testing at regular intervals during the pretransplant waiting period. These cultures monitor for the emergence of resistant organisms and help guide the choice of antimicrobial agents in the posttransplant period. For pulmonary exacerbations, patients continue to be hospitalized at the referring center, and antibiotic therapy is chosen based on the results of the patient's previous sputum or throat culture. Because half or fewer of patients awaiting transplantation actually receive donor organs (21), "saving" antibiotics in the hopes of maintaining sensitivity to one or more agents in the event of transplantation is not warranted. In patients with pan-resistant organisms, it may be possible to withhold intravenous antibiotics for several months, enabling more susceptible organisms to reemerge (22). Although terribly ill CF patients may not tolerate 2 months with no intravenous antibiotics, we have been successful with this approach in a few patients (22).

A subject of some controversy is whether a surgical drainage procedure of the sinuses is warranted either before or immediately after lung transplantation. Bacterial colonization of the sinuses in CF patients represents a potential source of contamination of the allograft. This has led some groups to advocate sinus surgery for all CF patients who are lung transplant candidates (23). However, there are no prospective, controlled studies indicating that surgical drainage of the sinuses prevents or lessens the risk of infectious complications following lung transplantation in CF patients (24). Recent evidence suggests that the rate of infectious complications in carefully selected CF lung transplant recipients (i.e., patients who do not harbor antibiotic-resistant organisms) is no greater than that of non-CF recipients (11,25), arguing against the routine need for sinus surgery. Part of the improvement in outcome with relation to infection in CF patients is almost certainly due to aggressive antibiotic therapy in the immediate posttransplant period, minimizing the patient's immunosuppressive regimen, and paying close attention to mucus-clearance techniques in this high-risk population. If substantial colony counts of aspergillus are noted in any sputum or sinus culture, we begin treatment with oral itraconazole (100–200 mg/day). Amphotericin B by inhalation may also be considered. (For the amphotericin aerosol, 10 mL of sterile water is added to a 50-mg vial; 1 mL of this preparation is put in 2 mL of normal saline and nebulized for inhalation).

V. Surgical Approach

Heart-lung transplantation for end-stage respiratory failure in CF patients has, for the most part, been supplanted in the United States by bilateral sequential lung transplantation. Almost no CF patients, even those with right ventricular hypertrophy, require concomitant heart transplantation. Single lung transplant procedures, without double pneumonectomy, are contraindicated because of the near certainty of infectious contamination from the remaining diseased lung to the allograft. Single lung transplantation following double pneumonectomy has been reported (26), but is unlikely to be widely used. With bilateral single lung transplantation, the transthoracic surgical approach through the fourth intercostal space, or "clamshell" approach (Fig. 1), allows superb visualization of the pleural cavities, an obvious advantage in CF patients who frequently have extensive pleural disease and adhesions. In this procedure, the mainstem bronchus of the recipient's less severely affected lung is intubated for single-lung ventilation while the sicker lung is replaced. The endotracheal tube is then repositioned into the mainstem bronchus of the newly transplanted lung while the second lung is removed and replaced. Because the transplant procedure is carried out sequentially, cardiopulmonary bypass is usually not required unless an atrial septal defect is present or the recipient is either hemodynamically unstable or too small for bibronchial anastomoses. Avoiding cardiopulmonary bypass has the major advantage of avoiding the need for anticoagulation, thereby decreasing the risk of perioperative hemorrhage. Vascular anastomoses are made between main pulmonary arteries of donor and recipient, and cuffs of donor left atrium, containing ipsilateral pulmonary veins, are sutured to their respective sides and the host's left atrium. Bronchial anastomoses are made to the recipient airways as they emerge from the mediastinum. The donor airways

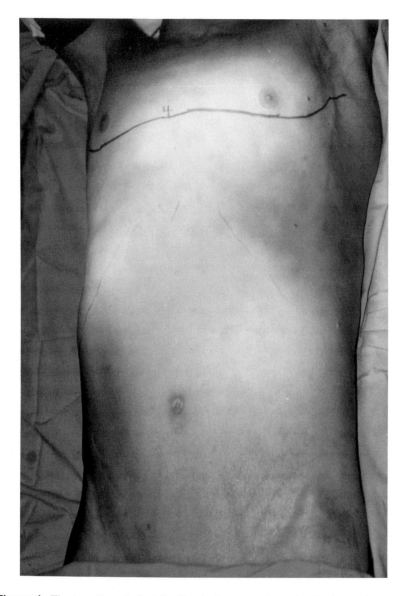

Figure 1 The transthoracic incision line is drawn on the patient's chest prior to lung transplantation.

are trimmed to one to two cartilage rings above the upper lobes. Bronchial arteries of the host are preserved and most use a telescoping anastomosis (27). This has reduced the incidence of airway dehiscence, a frequent complication when double-lung transplantation with a tracheal anastomosis was first introduced. In the CF patient, the anastomotic site is considered potentially contaminated from infected upper airway secretions, so careful handling of the airways is essential during the sequential procedure to avoid "seeding" the allograft or mediastinum with bacteria (13).

VI. Postoperative Considerations and Management

A. Immunosuppressive Protocol

The regimen of immunosuppression after lung transplantation is traditionally based on triple drug therapy centered around cyclosporine or tacrolimus (formerly FK506), methylprednisolone, and azathioprine. Cyclosporine or tacrolimus is administered as a continuous infusion at the time of transplant (2.5 mg/kg/day or 0.05 mg/kg/day, respectively) and for the first days after transplantation. Once the patient is tolerating oral medications, cyclosporine or tacrolimus is administered with pancreatic enzymes to help its absorption and decrease fluctuations in blood levels. It is assumed, but not yet demonstrated unequivocally, that administration of pancreatic enzymes helps absorption of these fatty compounds. Cyclosporine dosing is adjusted to achieve a random whole blood level of 500–700 ng/mL and tacrolimus to attain a trough whole blood value of 15–22 ng/mL. Methylprednisolone is given intraoperatively at a dose of 10 mg/kg and then at a dose of 7 mg/kg/day in three divided doses for the ensuing 3 days. Oral prednisone is then initiated at 2 mg/kg/day and tapered over the next several weeks to a dose of 0.1–0.3 mg/kg/day in those patients who show no ongoing or recurrent episodes of rejection. In some centers, the dose is tapered more quickly in CF patients than other lung recipients because of the perceived greater danger of infection in the CF recipient. In the absence of perioperative adult respiratory distress syndrome or pneumonia, azathioprine is administered at a dose of 1–2 mg/kg/day, either orally or parenterally. The dose of azathioprine is then adjusted to maintain peripheral white blood cell counts of more than 3000/mm^3 with absolute neutrophil counts of more than 1800/mm^3. In some circumstances, azathioprine has been omitted from the immunosuppressive regimen in CF patients in an attempt to lessen the frequency of infectious complications (28).

B. Antimicrobial Regimen

The antibiotic prophylaxis regimen in CF lung transplant recipients begins intraoperatively, and includes clindamycin, ceftazidime, and an aminoglycoside. The choice of posttransplant antibiotics is guided by the results of the recipient's pretransplant sputum culture and sensitivity testing. Antibiotics are continued for 10–14 days or longer, depending on posttransplant culture results and clinical status. Amphotericin B is administered for at least 48 hours in all recipients, with adjustments in the duration of therapy based on pretransplant cultures in the recipient as well as intraoperative cultures from both recipient and donor. In those from whom aspergillus has been recovered, amphotericin B administration is extended. In many CF patients, aerosolized high-dose tobramycin (600 mg three times a day) or colistin (75 mg three times a day) is also given after transplantation, particularly in patients whose pretransplant sputum cultures have revealed multiply resistant organisms.

Since cytomegalovirus disease in lung recipients has been associated with increased morbidity, including chronic rejection, prophylaxis for CMV infection is given to CMV-seropositive recipients and to CMV-negative recipients who receive lungs from a seropositive donor (29). Completely effective CMV prophylaxis has not yet been developed, but many transplant centers administer ganciclovir for 4 weeks or longer after transplant (10 mg/kg/day for 14 days, then 5 mg/kg/day) followed by high-dose acyclovir for an additional 3 months (650 mg/m^2 divided three times a day with dosage adjusted for the patient's creatinine clearance). Some centers are studying high-titer anti-CMV immunoglobulin as adjunctive prophylaxis. For candida prophylaxis, mycostatin (swish and swallow) is administered in the first days after transplant and continued indefinitely. To prevent *Pneumocystis carinii* pneumonia, oral trimethoprim/sulfamethoxazole 5 (TMP/SMZ) (mg/kg (three times a week) is started 2–4 weeks after transplant. In those patients who are allergic to or do not tolerate TMP/SMZ, weekly dapsone or monthly aerosolized pentamidine can be substituted.

Early in the postoperative period, oral feedings with pancreatic enzymes are initiated. Some transplant centers advocate the use of oral *N*-acetylcysteine to prevent the development of distal intestinal obstruction syndrome, a not uncommon occurrence in bedridden CF patients receiving narcotics for pain relief. Involvement of the CF center physicians is essential, because intensivists, surgeons, and intensive care unit nurses frequently (and understandably) focus their attention more on the transplant-related issues than on standard CF care, including digestive considerations. Aggressive pulmonary treatment, including the use of aerosolized bronchodilators, chest physical therapy, Flutter valve (see Chapter 4), incentive spirometry, and, occasionally, intermittent positive pressure breathing are initiated immediately after transplant. Bronchial drainage techniques are probably critical to decrease the incidence of infection in the allograft.

VII. Posttransplant Period

Flexible bronchoscopy, bronchoalveolar lavage (BAL), and transbronchial biopsy (TBBx) are invaluable tools in the diagnosis and monitoring of infection,

Table 4 Complications After Lung Transplantation in Patients with Cystic Fibrosis

---

Infection
    Bacterial, especially *Pseudomonas aeruginosa, B. cepacia*
    Viral, especially cytomegalovirus
    Fungal, especially aspergillus
    Parasitic, especially *P. carinii*
Rejection
    Acute
    Chronic
Posttransplant lymphoproliferative disease
Airway dehiscence
Bronchial stenosis
Diaphragmatic paresis
Vocal cord paresis
Hypertension
Distal intestinal obstruction syndrome, especially early after transplant

---

rejection, and other complications (Table 4) following lung transplantation (30). Bronchoscopy, BAL, and TBBx have generally been performed at 1–2 weeks (or before hospital discharge), at 1 month, 2 months, and every 3 months after transplantation in the first year, then every 4 months for subsequent years, and when clinically indicated. In recent years, the need for routine, scheduled BAL and TBBx has been questioned for the patient who is doing well clinically and whose pulmonary function has remained stable (31). Generally, a number of other studies are performed before TBBx, including pulmonary function and exercise tests, chest radiograph, and blood studies such as tacrolimus or cyclosporine levels, complete blood count with differential cell count, and determination of electrolytes, blood urea nitrogen and creatinine, liver function, prothrombin time and partial thromboplastin time, and serologic tests for CMV and Epstein-Barr virus. These studies and flexible bronchoscopy are generally performed in the outpatient setting. It is essential that the biopsy results be read by pathologists experienced in lung transplant pathology, because some grades of rejection might mistakenly be thought to suggest infection, with devastating results if treatment is based on this faulty interpretation.

After the transplant procedure, patients are sent home with digital electronic handheld microspirometers and are instructed to contact the transplant center if FVC or FEV_1 declines by 10% or more from their usual baseline for a 24-hour period (see Table 1). In addition, patients in whom cough, fever, dyspnea, radiographic infiltrates, or any other respiratory symptoms develop are generally examined and evaluated at the transplant center. Because infection and rejection are important causes of this constellation of symptoms, bronchoscopy with BAL and TBBx is usually performed. If an infectious complication is diagnosed by BAL or TBBx, antimicrobial agents are chosen on the basis of the culture and in vitro susceptibility results. In those patients with grade II or worse rejection as determined by transbronchial or open lung biopsy according to the criteria of Yousem et al. (32), methylprednisolone is administered as a single daily intravenous dose of 10 mg/kg for 3 days. After a treated episode of rejection, BAL, TBBx, and other studies are repeated 2 to 4 weeks later. Rejection that is refractory to courses of corticosteroid therapy receive lympholytic therapy, in the form of either rabbit or horse antithymocyte globulin or OKT3. Aerosolized cyclosporine for the treatment of rejection is being evaluated and may have a role in the treatment of refractory rejection.

Patients who survive more than a few months after transplant are at risk for development of chronic rejection, manifested clinically by severe airflow limitation and histologically by obliterative bronchiolitis (33). Several factors associated with an increased risk for chronic rejection include multiple or severe episodes of acute rejection and CMV pneumonitis. Chronic rejection tends to be recalcitrant to treatment with augmented immunosuppression unless it is detected early (33), and, with infection, it is the major cause of graft attrition and patient mortality after transplantation. Patients requiring treatment for episodes of infection or rejection are generally hospitalized at the transplant center. It is an irony that makes long-term care of the transplant recipient especially challenging that a complication of too much immunosuppression (i.e., CMV infection) seems to increase the risk of development of a complication of too little immunosuppression (i.e., chronic rejection).

Posttransplant lymphoproliferative disease (PTLD), an Epstein-Barr virus (EBV) driven lymphoma (usually B cell), is another common complication of the immunosuppressive transplant recipient that often requires inpatient care. Epstein-Barr virus disease is manifest clinically in a variety of fashions, from a self-limited, febrile, mononucleosis-type illness to PTLD itself, with widespread lymphadenopathy and multiple tumor masses. Although the allograft is the most common site of tumors, extrapulmonary lymphomas have been described. This disorder has been reported to occur in up to 22% of lung transplant recipients (28,30,34) and may be even more common in pediatric lung recipients. Intrapulmonary PTLD is diagnosed by transbronchial or open lung biopsy in conjunction with an acute increase in EBV titers. It is a cause of considerable morbidity and mortality in transplant recipients (34). Patients are usually hospitalized at the transplant center where a reduction in the immunosuppressive regimen (generally a discontinuation of azathioprine and prednisone and a reduction in tacrolimus or cyclosporine dose) is often successful in the treatment of PTLD. If lung nodules are the major manifestation, the course of the disease is often followed by chest computed tomography scans.

A myriad of other complications (30) (see Table 4) may affect lung recipients and may be severe enough to warrant hospitalization. Bronchial stenosis, occurring at the anastomotic site, may require placement of a surgical stent (35–37) or, in some cases, balloon catheter dilatation of the stenotic segment (38). Laser resection of intrabronchial granulation tissue is sometimes carried out. Vocal cord paresis and diaphragmatic paresis tend to complicate or prolong the initial posttransplant hospitalization but are not, in and of themselves, frequent indications for hospitalization afterwards. Complications of immunosuppressive agents may also occur. The most common such complication is hypertension and renal dysfunction with cyclosporine or tacrolimus administration.

VIII. Results

Early results of lung transplantation in CF patients in the United States compared with results in other patient groups were poor, with reported 1-year survival rates of 42% (39). The poor outcome in CF patients was attributed largely to complications from infection. As experience with these patients and this procedure has grown, the survival rates in CF patients is now comparable to those in other patient groups (11). As discussed, recent reports also suggest that the rate of infectious complications is similar to that of non-CF patients undergoing lung transplantation (25). Most transplant groups have reported dramatic improvements in pulmonary function (24,28) and exercise tolerance (24) in CF patients after lung transplantation. Several transplant centers have described a marked improvement in quality of life (40), and many lung transplant survivors are able to return to a full schedule of work and school.

IX. Future Considerations and Summary

Lung transplantation has been a lifesaving procedure for many patients with end-stage respiratory failure of cystic fibrosis who would otherwise have died. Nevertheless, there remains considerable morbidity and mortality associated with this procedure, particularly from infection and rejection. Donor organ shortages in the United States and elsewhere make this procedure available to only a limited number of CF patients, and many patients will die awaiting transplantation. The trend toward increased use of double-and single-lung transplant procedures for a variety of disorders will expand the number of possible recipients, but innovative approaches, such as xenotransplantation or living-related donation, will be needed if lung transplantation is to be offered to all potential recipients.

References

1. Griffith BP, Hardesty RL, Trento A, et al. Heart-lung transplantation: lessons learned and future hopes. Ann Thorac Surg 1987; 43:6–16.

2. Scott JP, Dennis C, Mullins P. Heart-lung transplantation for end-stage respiratory disease in cystic fibrosis patients. J Roy Soc Med 1993; 86:19–22.
3. Reitz BA, Wallwork JL, Hunt SA, et al. Heart-lung transplantation. N Engl J Med 1982; 306:557–64.
4. Hosenpud JD, Novick RJ, Breen TJ, Daily OP. The Registry of the International Society for Heart and Lung Transplantation: Eleventh Official Report—1994. J Heart Lung Transplant 1994; 13:451–70.
5. Cropp G, Griffith B, Hardesty R, et al. Heart-lung transplantation in cystic fibrosis. Cystic Fibrosis Club Abstracts 1984; 25:117.
6. Kerem E, Reisman J, Corey M, et al. Prediction of mortality in patients with cystic fibrosis. N Engl J Med 1992; 326:1187–91.
7. Nixon PA, Orenstein DM, Kelsey SF, Doershuk CF. The prognostic value of exercise testing in patients with cystic fibrosis. N Engl J Med 1992; 327:1785–1788.
8. Tablan OC, Chorba TL, Schidlow DV, et al. *Pseudomonas cepacia* colonization in patients with cystic fibrosis: risk factors and clinical outcome. J Pediatr 1985; 107:382–7.
9. Stern R, Borkat G, Hirschfeld S, et al. Heart failure in cystic fibrosis. Treatment and prognosis of cor pulmonale with failure of the right side of the heart. Am J Dis Child 1980; 134:267–272.
10. Orenstein DM, Kaplan RM. Measuring the quality of well-being in cystic fibrosis and lung transplantation. Chest 1991; 100:1016–1018.
11. Dennis C, Caine N, Sharples L, et al. Heart-lung transplantation for end-stage respiratory disease in patients with cystic fibrosis at Papworth Hospital. J Heart Lung Transplant 1993; 12:893–902.
12. Snell GI, de Hoyos A, Krajden M, et al. *Pseudomonas cepacia* in lung transplant recipients with cystic fibrosis. Chest 1993; 103:466–471.
13. Noyes BE, Michaels MG, Kurland G, et al. *Pseudomonas cepacia* empyema necessitatis after lung transplantation in two patients with cystic fibrosis. Chest 1994; 105:1888–91.
14. Kawai A, Paradis IL, Keenan RJ, et al. Lung transplantation at the University of Pittsburgh: 1982 to 1994. In: Terasaki, Cecka, eds. *Clinical Transplants 1994*. Los Angeles, CA. UCLA Tissue Typing Laboratory. In press.
15. Gorcsan J, Edwards TD, Ziady GM, Katz WE, and Griffith BP. Transesophageal echocardiography to evaluate patients with severe pulmonary hypertension for lung transplantation. Ann Thorac Surg 1995; 59:717–722.
16. Davis P, di Sant'Agnese P. Assisted ventilation for patients with cystic fibrosis. JAMA 1978; 239:1851–1854.
17. Jablonski R. If ventilator patients could talk. RN 1995; 58:32–34.
18. Starnes VA, Barr ML, Cohen RG. Lobar transplantation: indications, technique, and outcome. J Thorac Cardiovasc Surg 1994; 108:403–411.
19. Noyes B, Orenstein D. Treatment of pneumothorax in cystic fibrosis in the era of lung transplantation (editorial). Chest 1992; 101:1187–1188.
20. Schidlow D, Taussig L, Knowles M. Cystic Fibrosis Foundation Consensus Conference report on pulmonary complications of cystic fibrosis. Pediatr Pulmonol 1993; 15:187–198.
21. Sharples L, Hathaway T, Dennis C, et al. Prognosis of patients with cystic fibrosis awaiting heart and lung transplantation. J Heart Lung Transplant 1993; 12:669–674.

22. Bauldoff GS, Nunley D, Manzetti JD, Williams P, Iacono AT, Dauber JH, Keenan RJ, Griffith BP. Use of aerosolized colistin in patients with cystic fibrosis awaiting lung transplantation (abstr). Pediatr Pulmonol Suppl 1995; 12:257.

23. Lewiston N, King V, Umetsu D, et al. Cystic fibrosis patients who have undergone heart-lung transplantation benefit from maxillary sinus antrostomy and repeated sinus lavage. Transplant Proc 1991; 23:1207–1208.

24. Ramirez JC. Patterson GA, Winton TL, et al. Bilateral lung transplantation for cystic fibrosis. J Thorac Cardiovasc Surg 1992; 103:287–294.

25. Flume PA, Egan TM, Paradowski LJ, et al. Infectious complications of lung transplantation. Am J Respir Crit Care Med 1994; 149:1601–7.

26. Forty J, Hasan A, Gould FK, Corris PA, Dark JH. Single lung transplantation with simultaneous contralateral pneumonectomy for cystic fibrosis. Heart Lung Transplant 1994; 13:727–730.

27. Pasque M, Kaiser L, Dressler L, et al. Single lung transplantation for pulmonary hypertension: technical aspects and immediate hemodynamic results. J Thorac Cardiovasc Surg 1992; 103:475–482.

28. Noyes BE, Kurland G, Orenstein DM, et al. Experience with pediatric lung transplantation. J Pediatr 1994; 124:261–268.

29. Duncan S, Paradis I, Yousem S, et al. Sequelae of cytomegalovirus pulmonary infections in lung allograft recipients. Am Rev Respir Dis 1992; 146:1419–1425.

30. Kurland G, Orenstein DM. Complications of pediatric lung and heart lung transplantation. Curr Opin Pediatr. 1994; 6:262–271.

31. Fox J, Jessurun J, Kshettry V, Savik K, Hertz M. Clinically silent acute rejection following lung transplantation: the role of surveillance bronchoscopy (abstr). Am J Respir Crit Care Med 1994; 149:A1094.

32. Yousem S, Berry G, Brunt E, et al. A working formulation for the standardization of the nomenclature in the diagnosis of heart and lung rejection: Lung Rejection Study Group. J Heart Lung Transplant 1990; 9:593–601.

33. Glanville AR, Baldwin JC, Burke CM, et al. Obliterative bronchiolitis after heart-lung transplantation: apparent arrest by augmented immunosuppression. Ann Intern Med 1987; 107:300–304.

34. Armitage JM, Kormos RL, Stuart RS, et al. Post-transplant lymphoproliferative disease in thoracic organ transplant patients: ten years of cyclosporine-based immunosuppression. J Heart Lung Transplant 1991; 10:877–886.

35. Gaer JAR, Tsang V, Khaghani A, et al. Use of endotracheal silicone stents for relief of tracheobronchial obstruction. Ann Thorac Surg 1992; 54:512–516.

36. Sonett JR, Keenan RL, Ferson PF, Griffith BP, Landrenau R. Endobronchial management of benign, malignant, and lung transplant airway stenoses. Ann Thorac Surg 1995; 59;1417–1422.

37. Griffith BP, Magee MJ, Gonzalez IF, et al. Anastomotic pitfalls in lung transplantation. J Thorac Cardiovasc Surg 1994; 107:745–754.

38. Keller C, Frost A. Fiberoptic bronchoplasty. Chest 1992; 102:995–998.

39. Frist WH, Fox MG, Campbell PW, et al. Cystic fibrosis treated with heart-lung transplantation: North American results. Transplant Proc 1991; 23:1250–1256.

40. Busschbach JJV, Horikx PE, van den Bosch JMM, et al. Measuring the quality of life before and after bilateral lung transplantation in patients with cystic fibrosis. Chest 1994; 105:911–917.

14

Terminal Care

DAVID M. ORENSTEIN

University of Pittsburgh School of Medicine
and Children's Hospital of Pittsburgh
Pittsburgh, Pennsylvania

I. Introduction

The death of a patient with cystic fibrosis (CF) is often painful for the physicians and other members of the care team. They have usually known the patient and family for years, and have grown close to them. It is difficult to lose a friend, and difficult to watch a patient and family suffer. It may be hard for some to be witness to the defeat of Medicine by disease. As a family frequently does, the physician and medical team may force themselves through some thoughts: "Was this my fault?" "Should I have done more?" "Could I have done more?" "Am I missing something?" "Did I miss something a few months ago?" Even after those issues have been resolved, as they probably will be, with the conclusion that it was the ravages of a merciless disease that had been held at bay for as long as possible, it is still not easy. Because of these difficulties and despite best intentions, many staff members distance themselves from dying patients and their families (1,2).

But for the physician and care team, in addition to its very difficult aspects, terminal care can be rewarding as well. The team has the opportunity to make a tremendous contribution to the patient and family, to give care that may allow for the unlikely chance of recovery if that is possible, and for maximum

357

comfort, physical and emotional, for the patient and family if recovery is not possible. And these should be the goals of the terminal care of the patient with CF: to maintain the maximum possible comfort, physical and emotional, of the patient and family, while allowing for the chance of recovery, should that be possible. It can be a difficult tightrope to walk, because many of the treatments or interventions that might give the maximum chance for survival or that might extend life are also those that will interfere the most with comfort. Endotracheal intubation and mechanical ventilation stand out as obvious examples. Similarly, for the emotional well being of the patient and family, it makes sense never to take away all hope. Yet, it is cruel to hold out unreasonable hope of recovery, thereby denying a patient and family the opportunity to come to grips, together or separately, with the issues surrounding dying and to have the opportunity to put their affairs in order.

Because lung disease is the cause of death in more than 95% of patients with CF (3), this chapter deals with issues surrounding terminal care for a patient who is dying of respiratory disease. Care in the rare other forms of death in patients with CF is also discussed briefly.

II. Recognizing When a Patient Is Dying

Predicting the time of death in cystic fibrosis is extremely difficult. Patients thought unlikely to survive for hours have recovered and lived years more. Similarly, it is not rare for a reasonably healthy patient to decline and die within a few months. Among prognostic factors, low fitness on an exercise test is the strongest known correlate with poor survival (4). However, this report was an 8-year survival study and had highly significant results *for the population* of 100 patients; some individuals with poor fitness had good survival, and others with high fitness died early. In shorter-term studies, several pulmonary function and blood gas parameters have had fair predictive value, but, once again, *for a population*, with many individual exceptions (5). Table 1 lists several pulmonary function test values and their associated 1- and 2-year mortality rates. Young patients with a given low level of pulmonary function have a poorer prognosis than older patients, who have taken more years to arrive at the same level. Thus, for a forced expiratory volume in 1 second (FEV_1) of 20%–30% of predicted, the 2-year survival rate for patients 6–17 years old is 50%, whereas for patients 18–44 years old, it is 60%. If two patients of the same gender have the same FEV_1, and one is 15 years younger than the other, the younger one has 2.7 times the risk of the older patient of dying in the next 2 years (5).

However, despite this age difference in the prognosis for any given level of pulmonary function, it is not always true that the more rapidly lung function has declined to a given level, the worse the prognosis. In fact, a terrible pulmonary function test (PFT) result during an acute deterioration (associated

Table 1 One and Two-Year Mortality in Cystic Fibrosis

Pulmonary function test		1-yr Mortality (%)	2-yr Mortality (%)
FEV$_1$(% predicted)	<20	49	62
	20–30	25	45
	31–40	7	22
FVC (% predicted)	<30	50	75
	31–40	25	40
	41–50	10	28
PaO$_2$ (mm Hg)	<50	48	66
	50–55	24	38
	56–60	15	28
PaCO$_2$ (mm Hg)	>55	68	82
	51–55	30	49
	46–50	14	24

Source: Ref. 5.

with a viral infection or an automobile accident and forced immobility, for example) carries a much better prognosis than the same PFT arrived at through a gradual decline over months or years. This becomes an important point in deciding how aggressive to be in treating respiratory failure in a given patient.

Despite the difficulty in predicting the time of death, CF patients who are destined to die within days or weeks commonly share some clinical features. They have been oxygen dependent for some time, although they may or may not be dyspneic at rest. They have limited energy and little appetite. A trip to the bathroom may be a major effort. They may be difficult to arouse from sleep, particularly before noon. They have difficulty raising their very thick sputum and may become extremely dyspneic with paroxysmal cough. In the last days of life, they may even have diminished cough, despite copious lung mucus, which can be heard gurgling, even without the aid of a stethoscope. Most patients with CF who are dying assume a typical position for sleep: sitting in bed, usually cross-legged, leaning forward on pillows or a hospital bedside table. The assumption of this position is an ominous sign (Fig. 1). Carbon dioxide retention is another ominous finding, one that can be detected by measuring end-tidal carbon dioxide tension, obviating the need for arterial punctures. PaCO$_2$ of more than 55 mm Hg carries an 80% 2-year mortality rate (5). Carbon dioxide retention may be suggested by the patient's being difficult to arouse. It may be difficult to maintain oxyhemoglobin saturation levels of more than 90%, despite relatively high flows of oxygen by nasal cannula. Adjusting oxygen flow to maintain adequate oxygenation without dangerously depressing the hypoxic drive to breathe may be particularly difficult (however, see discussion on dyspnea).

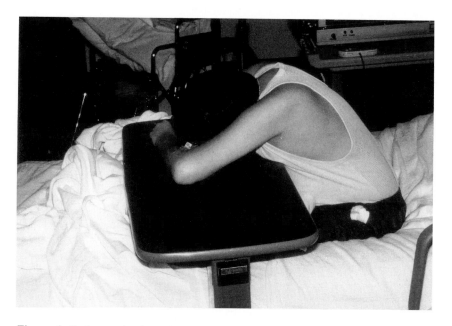

Figure 1   Patient posing in position often assumed by dying CF patients.

III.   Standard Care

Most aspects of standard CF care should continue, even—perhaps *especially*—
in what seem to be terminal stages. Fulfilling the principle of "First, do no
harm" requires the medical team to continue to carry out most standard CF care.
This approach maintains the maximum possible comfort, physical and emotional, of the patient and family, while allowing for the chance of recovery. If
there is any oral intake including fat, protein, or both, pancreatic enzymes
should be given. Because there is likely to be active pulmonary infection,
antibiotics (usually intravenous) should be continued, and monitoring for toxicity of these agents should also be continued. Chest physical therapy and aerosol
treatments for improving mucus clearance and decreasing bronchial obstruction
should also be continued. At some point, any or all of these parts of standard
care may interfere unreasonably with the dying patient's comfort. The point at
which the care becomes intolerable to the patient is the point at which that care
should be stopped. Patients differ in this regard. Some tolerate aerosols and
chest physical therapy, but not blood tests for aminoglycoside levels, for example, whereas others have no trouble with venepuncture, but chest physical therapy is intolerable, and still others cannot eat. None of these areas is an all-or-
none proposition, however. A patient may be able to accept modified chest

physical therapy, for example, with elimination of the head-down positions, or aerosol every 4 hours, but not every 2. The care team should continually attempt to define the most aggressive level of treatment that carries with it the minimum individual patient discomfort. Although it would be wrong to eliminate blood tests for drug toxicity in a relatively healthy 10-year-old patient, it would be equally wrong to insist on carrying out those tests in a dying patient who has requested being spared blood tests. And, although we insist on chest physical therapy for the large majority of patients with CF, despite its being considered boring and distasteful to many young patients, a dying patient should be allowed to refuse even this airway-clearing treatment.

IV. Transplantation

The advent of lung transplantation (see Chapter 13) has dramatically changed the approach to terminal care for CF patients. If the patient is on the transplant list, particularly if the patient is nearing the top of the list, there is usually much more emphasis on extending life (to await the donor organs) than easing suffering when those two goals are mutually exclusive. Thus, a number of centers have used various modes of mechanical ventilation as a "bridge" to transplantation (6,7), despite the realization that once mechanical ventilation is initiated, it is unlikely that the patient will ever be able to be weaned from it. The approach to nonterminal care (e.g., pneumothorax) has also been changed by the possibility of lung transplantation (8).

As the time approaches when life without mechanical ventilation will be impossible, the situation must be discussed with the patient and family. Some families insist on trying everything to allow the patient to survive to transplantation and a new life, whereas others decide that, with waiting times measured in many months, the chance of a successful transplant is not worth the discomfort of mechanical ventilation and the continued struggle to stay alive. The physician must be sensitive to the family's and patient's desires, even if the patient and family weigh the positives and negatives of each choice differently from the physician.

V. Hospital Versus Home Care

The idea of dying at home, surrounded by family and loved ones, including pets, seems appealing to many people, particularly as contrasted to dying in the big, impersonal, "high-tech" hospital, far from family and friends. In some centers, it is common for CF patients to die at home (9). Some appealing features of having the dying patient at home include the family's having more control, being closer to other family members (e.g., children), and there being less need for babysitting for siblings or other home-care arrangements because of frequent or prolonged hospital visits. There are more chances for parts of a more normal day-to-day life, such as eating home-cooked meals and having access to favorite toys, hobbies, pets, and friends. The family need not be split while one parent goes to the hospital. Home care is usually cheaper than hospital care.

Despite these considerable attractions and advantages of home care, for many—perhaps most—patients dying of CF, this is not the whole story. Home, familiar though it may be, may also be frightening to patient and parent. Both the patient and family may have grown comfortable over the years with hospital staff, and with knowing that, in the hospital, nurses and doctors are immediately available for whatever assessments need to be made and for whatever care needs to be given. Because of the availability of staff for monitoring the patient, family members may actually have a better opportunity to get rest and respite in the hospital than at home. In the home, the opportunity to make decisions can also be a burden: the family and patient *must* make many or most of the decisions, even what feel like medical decisions beyond their competence or comfort.

Hospice organizations are in place in many locations, and their services may make for an ideal compromise for some patients and families: skilled hospice nurses may be able to come into the home to continue to administer intravenous antibiotics, for example, and to remain in contact with both patient and physician for titrating treatments, including morphine (see discussion on dyspnea). Hospice nurses may be able to provide simple company for the patient, providing family members opportunities to shop, take a walk, or sleep.

VI. "Do Not Resuscitate" Orders

Once a patient is clearly dying, the patient's primary physician should speak with the patient and family about "do not resuscitate" (DNR) orders. As with most instances of information sharing and medical planning, particularly involving terminal care decisions and education, the patient's primary physician should conduct the conversations. And, as with most of these areas, the physician should ascertain what the patient and family understand about the patient's condition. Except in very unusual circumstances, it is inappropriate for a relative stranger, for example, a house officer who has known the patient and family for a matter of days, to be handling these issues instead of the physician who has known a patient and family for years.

Just as it may be very difficult for the physician to recognize with certainty when a patient is likely to be dying, it is extremely difficult for a patient and family to be able to make this judgment accurately. It is surprising how many families and patients underestimate or overestimate the severity of the situation. It is not rare for a relatively healthy child to be considered deathly ill by an overprotective family. More common is the opposite, that is, the very active application of denial, when a family or patient is extremely surprised when a physician brings up the possibility of a lung transplant, saying, for example, "I didn't think I was that bad." However, although they may not have discussed it among themselves or with the physician, in the last few weeks of a patient's life, most patients and families are aware that death is near.

In one study, only two of 16 "fatally ill" young children, including six with CF, had discussed death with their parents, but on projective testing, 63% produced stories related to death. Scores on this testing (10,11) correlated with the "degree to which the child had been given an opportunity to discuss fears and prognosis, ... suggest[ing] that open communication does not heighten death anxiety, but rather decreases feelings of isolation, alienation, and a perception that the disease is too terrible to talk about."

Once it is clear to the physician that long-term survival is unlikely, it is appropriate to review what should be done in the event of a respiratory or cardiac arrest. Under most hospitals' guidelines, personnel are required in such circumstances to initiate vigorous resuscitation efforts, including endotracheal intubation and mechanical ventilation, unless there are orders to the contrary. Because, for most patients with CF, mechanical ventilation is unlikely to provide any benefit (12) (see Section VIII), and because stopping mechanical ventilation is much more difficult than never starting, it is usually a mistake to initiate this treatment. Therefore, the entire medical team must be aware of the patient's and family's decision concerning advance directives. The only way to make this clear is through a written DNR order.

The DNR order must specify clearly which components of resuscitation are allowable. Allowable components that vary from patient to patient include bag and mask ventilation, cardiac drugs, chest compressions, tracheal intubation, and mechanical ventilation.

The need to include these orders is most often felt by house officers and nurses or others who are in the hospital when the primary attending physician might not be and are therefore the ones who might be forced to take aggressive and inappropriate actions. The residents and nurses may raise the issue before the attending physician has discussed resuscitation with the patient and family. In some instances, the attending physician may feel it is not an appropriate time for such a decision. Yet, opening this discussion may be a valuable opportunity to discuss something that has been prominently occupying a family's thoughts and sapping its energy. Families may often believe that this is not a subject to be discussed. Many families of children who have died have clear memories of the staff's withdrawing from the child and family as death approaches (2). Even families acutely worried about the impending death of a child might not have discussed this openly. In one study, only 19% of parents had discussed these issues with their children who were dying of cancer (13). Discussing a "do not resuscitate" order may open important communication between physician and patient, physician and family, and patient and family, and among various family members.

VII. Dyspnea, Hypoxemia, and Hypercapnia

If the lungs fail, hypoxemia and carbon dioxide retention occur. Each of these occurrences can bring symptoms and signs, summarized in the Table 2.

In different patients, different symptoms may predominate. In CF patients who are dying and have any of the symptoms listed in Table 2, the blood gas alterations should be the prime suspects as the underlying cause, but other pos-

Table 2 Signs and Symptoms of Altered Blood Gases[a]

Symptoms and signs of hypoxemia
    Cardiovascular
        Tachycardia
        Hypertension (if more severe, hypotension)
    Respiratory
        Tachypnea (if severe, depression of respiration)
        Dyspnea, particularly with exertion (if severe, may be present at rest)
    Neuromuscular
        Headache
        Weakness
        Behavioral changes
        Hyperreflexia
        If more severe, visual disturbance, somnolence, coma
    Miscellaneous
        Sweating
        Panic
        Anxiety
Symptoms and signs of hypercapnia
    Cardiovascular
        Flushed, hot hands and feet
        Bounding pulses
    Neurologic
        Confusion
        Drowsiness ("CO_2 narcosis")
        Muscular twitching (fine facial tremor, myoclonus, asterixis)
        If more severe, engorged retinal veins, papilledema, coma
    Miscellaneous
        Sweating
        Gastrointestinal upset
        Electrolyte depletion

[a]The signs and symptoms of hypercapnia (elevated carbon dioxide levels) largely reflect vascular dilation and sympathetic activity. The severity of the symptoms of hypercapnia depends more on the rapidity of the increase in Pa_{CO_2} than the absolute level thereof.
Source: Refs. 53 and 54.

sibilities should not be overlooked. For example, electrolyte disturbances are common in patients with respiratory failure (14), and hypomagnesemia, which is particularly common in CF (15), can cause twitching muscles. (See Chapter 6.)

In some dying patients, the cardinal symptom of hypercapnia— narcosis—predominates, whereas, in others, it is breathlessness, largely related to hypoxemia, that is most prominent. For patient comfort, CO_2 narcosis is not a problem; conversely, it is often helpful. Patients may not be awake or readily arousable, but they are not uncomfortable. On the other hand, when dyspnea is predominant, providing for patient comfort is a major challenge.

Dyspnea, the unpleasant sensation of difficult breathing and probably the most disturbing and most common of all the symptoms experienced by dying CF patients, is not completely understood. Studies suggest that it arises from (1) increased effort in response to increased work of breathing, (2) increased muscle force needed to maintain normal ventilation, or (3) increased ventilatory requirements (16). All of the following factors may be present in CF: (1) increased work of breathing because of airways narrowed by mucus or by varying degrees of mucosal edema or bronchospasm (17), (2) increased muscle force needed to overcome increased airway resistance and to compensate for the mechanical disadvantage at which the diaphragm is placed by pulmonary hyperinflation (18,19), and (3) increased ventilatory requirements because of the increased dead space and hypoxemia (20).

A. Oxygen

The primary treatment for dyspnea in terminally ill patients with CF is supplemental oxygen. Clearly, the hypoxemic patient may require oxygen to prevent tissue damage. [Haldane is said to have stated that "hypoxia not only stops the machine but wrecks the machinery" (21).] Supplemental oxygen also helps relieve dyspnea. In the patient with chronic respiratory failure, physicians often fear that oxygen will dangerously suppress the hypoxic respiratory drive. Fortunately, this is seldom the case. Adults with chronic obstructive pulmonary disease (COPD) and an acute elevation of their $PaCO_2$ increase their ventilatory response to hypoxemia. This suggests that such patients given oxygen with only partial correction of hypoxemia and with continued respiratory acidosis will have adequate ventilatory drive (22). In fact, when given oxygen, most such patients maintain their ventilation (23). They show an increase in oxygenation and a very small increase, no change, or (most commonly) a decrease in carbon dioxide tension. The ventilatory benefit may be accounted for in part by the bronchodilating effect of oxygen (23). Improvement in CO_2 tensions seen in terminally ill patients with CF who are given supplemental oxygen can also probably be explained by the greater effect of the extra oxygen on hypoxic ventilatory muscles than on ventilatory drive. That is, most CF patients with respiratory failure *improve* their $PaCO_2$ when they are given supplemental oxygen, probably indicating that the most important factor influencing their ventilation is not the drive to breathe but fatigued, hypoxic ventilatory muscles (24).

For terminally ill patients, oxygen should be administered with a goal of improving patient comfort rather than achieving a specific target PaO_2. Although an SaO_2 of 90% is reasonable, because this is at the upper bend of the oxyhemoglobin dissociation curve, where a small decrease in PaO_2 results in a large decrease in SaO_2 (25), it may not be achievable. The oxygen may be delivered via nasal cannulae or face mask. Some patients have distinct preferences, and these should be honored when possible. Some patients require very large flow rates for comfort. They may be anxious and continually ask for more oxygen. Particularly if they have an adequate SaO_2, it is worth a trial of increasing the volume of air, without increasing the oxygen concentration. A fan blowing on the face may also be helpful. This dependence on a high air flow to the face may have a psychological basis (equating air flow with oxygen supply), but may also have a physiological basis in that facial receptors in the distribution of the trigeminal nerve influence ventilation (26). In one study, cold air directed against the cheek decreased breathlessness in six healthy volunteers made dyspneic by increased inspiratory resistance and hypercapnia (27). Increased airflow to the face and body may also relieve the feeling of overheating often experienced by CF patients in respiratory failure.

No more oxygen should be used than is needed to provide for patient comfort, once the SaO_2 is more than 90%. Keeping inspired oxygen concentrations as low as possible minimizes the small chance of depressing hypoxic drive to breathe and the drying effects of oxygen, and prevents deconditioning of respiratory muscles.

B. Bronchodilators

The role of bronchodilators in CF in general is discussed more fully in Chapter 4. The role of these agents has not been studied in terminally ill CF patients, but it stands to reason that, for those patients with a substantial component of bronchospasm, they should help. In approximately 10% of patients with CF, particularly those with more severe lung disease, bronchodilators may actually cause a decrease in expiratory airflow, presumably a result of diminished bronchomotor tone in bronchiectatic airways, that is, airways whose cartilaginous support has been destroyed and whose patency relies on smooth muscle tone (28). However, most patients with CF either improve or show no change in expiratory airflow after bronchodilator inhalation.

C. Beta-2-Adrenergic Agonists

In addition to relaxing bronchial smooth muscle, beta-2 agents may have other effects relevant to control of dyspnea: mucociliary transport rates may be improved slightly (29) and ventilatory muscle contractility and endurance may be improved (30,31). Regardless of the mechanism, there is evidence in non-CF patients with COPD that these agents decrease dyspnea, even in patients with only a modest improvement in pulmonary function (26). On the other hand, by changing ventilation–perfusion relationships beta-agonists may worsen hypoxemia (32).

D. Theophylline

In contrast to beta-2 agonists, theophylline is a relatively poor bronchodilator, but—again, in non-CF patients with COPD—has been shown to decrease dyspnea significantly, even when there was no significant decrease in airflow obstruction (26,33). This effect might be caused by a direct effect of theophylline on ventilatory muscles (26,33). The notoriously narrow therapeutic window of theophylline, however, may be particularly small in CF (34) compared to other patient groups. Therefore, theophylline should be started at very low doses, with careful monitoring of gastrointestinal and nervous system symptoms.

E. Psychotropic Treatment

Dyspnea and anxiety are interrelated, with positive correlations between objective measures of each (35,36), and each making the other worse. This relationship has suggested the use of various psychotropic interventions to lessen dyspnea.

Relaxation, Hypnosis, and Other Psychophysical Techniques

Several kinds of interventions used in dyspneic patients may produce some relief. Relaxation techniques are based on the simple notion that people can focus attention on only one thing at a time (37). With these techniques, the patient focuses on decreasing muscle tension in various muscle groups, thus distracting primary attention from the effort of breathing. These techniques require the help of someone skilled in their application, but once taught, they may be sustained by the patient alone. An "in-between" approach that has been successful in decreasing panic attacks associated with dyspnea is the use of audio tapes with the instructor's voice giving guidance in relaxation (38). Hypnosis has been extremely helpful in decreasing dyspnea and anxiety in some dying CF patients. Skillful practitioners are essential, and not every institution has one. They may be pediatricians, family physicians, internists, psychologists, psychiatrists, social workers, or others. They use different strategies, but many provide the patient with the tools to induce self-hypnosis when the practitioner is not available. The strategies often include quiet surroundings, a word or image that is repeated or thought of repeatedly in a structured pattern, and perhaps the tensing and relaxing of individual muscle groups in succession (37). Other psychophysical techniques that have been used to lessen dyspnea include biofeedback, visual imagery, and meditation (37). The success of these techniques varies considerably among patients.

F. Opiates

Morphine ["God's own medicine," according to Sir William Osler (39)] is a cornerstone in the treatment of intractable dyspnea in the terminally ill patient with CF. Although there are no controlled studies on the use of morphine in terminally ill CF patients, its use has been shown clearly to decrease breathlessness and increase exercise tolerance in adults with COPD (40). Also in adults with COPD, Mahler (26) has stated, "The administration of opiates may provide a level of comfort and dignity otherwise not obtainable during the dying process." This is also true for patients with CF.

When using morphine to relieve dyspnea in the terminally ill patient with CF, the physician must keep in mind the potential for harm from this drug. Overdosing can cause fatal respiratory depression, and smaller doses can cause constipation, vomiting, and urinary retention. Patients with CF seem to be exceptionally sensitive to tiny doses of morphine, so that a very small dose may be effective, and a "normal" dose fatal. The heightened sensitivity may be explained by chronically elevated carbon dioxide levels and the insensitivity to CO_2 that may accompany that chronic retention: "the further imposition of the depressant effects of narcotics can be disastrous" (39). Another explanation may be indirectly related to carbon dioxide retention: acidosis increases the sensitivity to morphine (41).

Regardless of the mechanism of the apparent heightened sensitivity of terminally ill CF patients to morphine, it is prudent to start with a small dose and gradually increase the dose if the initial dose is ineffective. I begin with 0.1 mg of morphine intravenously. That is **not** 0.1 mg/kg, but rather a **total** dose of 0.1 mg. This dose will be effective in some patients. If it is not effective within 5–15 minutes, then doubling doses can be used every 5–15 minutes until an effective dose is reached.

Alternatively, a continuous morphine infusion can be used, starting with 0.20 mg/hr (again, this is a **total** dose, and **not** a per-kilogram dose). If the dose is ineffective, the infusion rate can be raised by 0.1 mg/hr. Reevaluation and dosage adjustments can be made every 30 minutes.

VIII. Mechanical Ventilation

Except in unusual patients with acute respiratory decompensation, such as in some infants (42,43), some patients with severe viral pneumonitis, and some

Table 3 Details to Be Attended to in Using BiPAP

Mask
    Size
    Fit (shape)
    Padding for nasal bridge; check for sores, leaks
Fio_2
Inspiratory pressure ("IPAP")
Expiratory pressure ("EPAP")
Timing

Changes in pressures can be made in increments of 2 cm H_2O, checking for patient comfort, chest wall movement, air movement (assessed by auscultation), and adequacy of gas exchange (Sao_2, end-tidal CO_2)

with trauma, mechanical ventilation is seldom beneficial in CF (12). Most patients with CF and respiratory failure have arrived at that state gradually and have very little reserve to call upon, and—unlike the adult with COPD (44)—cannot be "tided over" an acute respiratory infection time after time. In fact, it is seldom possible. In those few instances in which mechanical ventilation can be justified, great care must be taken to provide maximal patient comfort and safety (see Chapter 10). In some centers, endotracheal intubation and mechanical ventilation have been used as a short-term "bridge" to lung transplantation (7). Other centers have eschewed this approach, because the shortage of donor organs makes it impossible to predict the wait for a donor. These centers also recognize that the "stay alive at all costs to await transplantation" approach interferes with the patient's and family's ability to prepare for death with equanimity.

    Positive pressure ventilation delivered via face mask or nasal prongs can be a less invasive bridge to transplantation (6,45). This technique, with bilevel positive airway pressure (BiPAP), has not been met with universal success. It interferes with sleep in some patients and causes serious pressure sores in others. The tight face masks induce claustrophobia in some people, and always interferes with cough and airway clearance. However, with exquisite attention to detail (usually provided by respiratory therapists), it may be possible to provide ventilatory support for a few CF patients with chronic respiratory failure in a manner that is somewhat less invasive than traditional mechanical ventilation via an endotracheal tube. Table 3 lists some of the details that must be considered in using BiPAP.

IX. Dying from Nonrespiratory Causes

In a very few cases, patients with CF may die from nonrespiratory causes. As lung transplantation becomes more common, so too will death from transplant-related causes, including underimmunosuppression and overimmunosuppression. In 1995, "transplantation complication" had become the second leading cause of death among CF patients reported to the Cystic Fibrosis Foundation Data Registry (10.0% compared with 83.9% for "cardiorespiratory" and 1.6% for "liver disease/liver failure") (46). These problems are discussed in Chapter 13. Underimmunosuppression can lead to organ rejection and respiratory difficulties, perhaps failure and death. Overimmunosuppression has infection as its main complication. Infection can involve the transplanted lungs, but virtually any site can be affected. Sepsis can occur and can cause multiorgan failure. In the nontransplant patient with CF, most deaths that are not caused by the chronic pulmonary devastation of a lifetime of CF are related to liver disease. Details of liver disease in CF are discussed in Chapter 5. The aspects of the liver disease that can cause death are discussed here.

The hepatic disease of CF is primarily obstructive, with portal hypertension and its complications, including esophageal varices and hypersplenism. Bleeding from esophageal varices can be fatal, and life-threatening variceal hemorrhage can be the presenting symptom or sign of hepatic disease in patients with CF (47). In a tiny minority of patients, hepatocellular failure leads to death. In these patients, terminal care is merely supportive, and, for some patients, may be carried out at home.

X. Talking with the Family

As in all stages of CF, it is important for the physician to talk with the family throughout the terminal illness and after the patient dies. Several issues are of particular importance for discussion. These include the course of the patient's disease (life), autopsy, organ donation, funeral, and family (especially sibling) reactions.

A. Reviewing the Course

Even if death occurs in adulthood, parents often feel guilt for "not having done enough." It is worth reviewing the entire course of the patient's disease, because, in most cases, it is possible to point out that it was the devastation of the disease and not the parents' failings that led to the fatal outcome. Usually, parents do an amazing job of helping the patient stay alive and be functional and happy for as long as possible.

B. Autopsy

A postmortem examination can still yield information about an individual's life and death, even in a typical course in a disease as well understood as CF, and can, on occasion, provide information that might be relevant to others with the disorder. Many families find it difficult to grant permission for an autopsy. Some consider it mutilating and refuse because the patient "has been through too much already." Others may incorrectly believe that it will preclude an open casket funeral. It can be helpful to point out (gently) the fallacies in these beliefs. Some families may agree to a partial examination (e.g., thorax only). Most families are aware of the tremendous advances in the knowledge of the molecular and cellular bases of CF. They may not realize that many of the discoveries were made possible by the donation of tissue from CF patients who died. The need for CF tissue continues, and it is a moral obligation of all CF centers to be in contact with research centers that can use such tissue to continue basic CF research. Many (perhaps most) families will agree to removal of tissue samples (particularly trachea, bronchi, and liver) for research (see Organ Donation).

C. Organ Donation

Most dying patients and their families are aware of organ transplantation. They may have considered such a procedure for themselves. The CF patients are often acceptable donors for eyes and skin. Kidneys and heart valves may also be acceptable. The heart itself may be acceptable under certain circumstances. Many patients and families feel very good about organ donation. Patients who have been on a transplant waiting list may get special satisfaction from planning to give to someone else what they had been hoping to receive themselves.

There are special considerations for the harvesting of organs for donation that complicate the situation. For a heart to be viable, it must be removed while it is beating. In the most common non-CF setting, this occurs when a patient is brain-dead. The family has a chance to say goodbye while the patient is still on the ventilator; the patient is taken to the operating room, where the chest is opened, vessels clamped and resected, and preservation solution infused. For kidneys to be viable, the procedure is nearly as demanding: cannulae are placed in the femoral artery and vein, and preservation solution is infused. This procedure need not take place in the operating room while the heart is still beating, but it must be done within 15 minutes of cardiorespiratory arrest. Because the death of a patient with CF is typically not a brain death, but rather a cardiorespiratory arrest whose timing is not predictable with precision, these harvesting procedures may not be possible. Local organ procurement organizations are usually willing, however, to have teams on call if it is thought that a death and donation is imminent. These professionals are often helpful in talking with families and staff about the entire process. For skin, eye, and heart valves, harvesting can be accomplished anytime within 12 hours of cardiorespiratory arrest. For information about the organ procurement process in various geographic areas, the United Network for Organ Sharing (UNOS) can be contacted at 1-800-24-DONOR.

Some physicians choose to discuss obtaining tracheobronchial and hepatic tissue for basic CF research in terms of organ donation, because tissue is taken from the newly deceased and donated for someone else to use. In the case of research, this "organ donation" may help many people, and not just one recipient.

D. Funeral Arrangements

The physician is rarely involved in funeral arrangements but can sometimes facilitate some of the basics, such as telling the family how arrangements are made between hospital mortuary and funeral homes. In most hospitals, the mortuary personnel are able to call the family's chosen funeral home and make arrangements directly with them for transporting the body. Some families want a service with an open casket and need to know whether autopsy plans (if any) will interfere with that possibility (usually not).

The question often arises as to whether young siblings should attend funerals. Most experts agree that, although funerals can be upsetting to young children, they should be given the opportunity to go, because that is less upsetting than being boxed out of what is going on in the rest of the family (48). It may also be easier for the young sibling to understand and accept the older sibling's death if the child is allowed to attend the funeral.

E. Family Reactions

This chapter opened with some of the common reactions of family members to the death of a young person, such as "I didn't do enough," and "What did we do wrong?" There may also be relief at the end of a long ordeal, for the patient and for the family. Accompanying that may be guilt at that very feeling of relief. All of these feelings happen frequently, and normally, and it is worth talking with the family about their reactions, so that they can be reassured that what they are feeling is normal and healthy. In the rare cases in which there are other, unhealthy reactions (e.g., suicidal thoughts, tremendous anger), it is important for the physician to hear these as well to be able to direct the family to competent help. Family members may ask for anxiolytics or tranquilizers. In most cases, it is not wise to prescribe sedatives for someone whose medical history is not well known. In some cases, giving family members a small dose of diazepam may be justifiable.

The physician may be able to provide some small comfort in sharing with the family the high points of the patient's life and what made the patient special, and in lending a sympathetic ear. Obviously, it is not helpful to say, "Oh, you'll get over it," but it can be helpful to say, "I know it hurts terribly now and will hurt for a very long time. Gradually, with time, the sharp pain will ease, and it will be easier to think of all of the happy times and the warm memories. But you will never stop missing him (her), and that's right because there won't ever be another Johnny (Julie)."

It has been observed that the family often reacts as a unit to stress, for example, displaying "family pain" in response to terminal illness in the child (49,50). However, one of the often unrecognized stresses on families after the death of a loved one is that different family members may go through the same ups and downs at slightly different paces. In this scheme, one parent, for example, might be having a good day while the other is missing the child particularly painfully. It is easy for the parents to criticize each other for their different reactions, saying, for example, "You're so maudlin; snap out of it; get a life!" Or, "How can you be so cheerful? Didn't you love her? Don't you miss her?" It eases stress considerably for families to be told ahead of time to expect these times when one feels relatively good when the other feels bad, and to be patient with each other.

The reactions of siblings, especially those of young children, are worth addressing with the family. If the sibling has CF, it is worth stressing what is different about that child from the dying (or dead) sibling, and perhaps what is different about CF care that might make the outcomes different. It must also be addressed openly that it is perfectly understandable and normal for the surviving sibling to have "selfish" feelings and worries mixed in with feelings for the dead brother or sister. If the sibling does not have CF, a particularly common (nearly universal) feeling is a dual feeling of (1) gladness that the sibling who has stolen much of the parents' time (and apparent affection) during the prolonged illnesses and hospitalization is finally gone and (2) guilt at feeling that way. If the child is young enough, there may well have been enough "magical thinking" (51) to have convinced the child that he or she is partly to blame for the sibling's death, because there were certainly times when the child had *wished* the sibling dead. This possibility should be addressed explicitly with young children, even if they have not voiced the concerns themselves. If they have not felt that way, nothing is lost. If they have, it is useful to let them know that almost all children have, one time, wished for their siblings to be out of the way, and that it is not evil or naughty, and it did not cause the sickness or death. It may also be helpful to point out ways in which the surviving child was special to the patient.

In the emotional time immediately following a patient's death, it is easy and natural to focus on the patient's immediate family. There are almost always other people whose lives have been touched by the patient and who may need to be informed of the patient's death. This is likely to include a circle of friends with CF who have shared hospitalizations and other times, good and bad. It may be appropriate for a member of the staff to let such friends know of the patient's death. Center staff have been surprised by patients' expressed distress at not having been informed of another patient's death. On the other hand, it may be that those closest to the patient and family will have been in close touch throughout the ordeal, and will already know. It is impossible to notify everyone who might ever have known the patient or to guess which particular other patient will take one patient's death particularly hard.

In addition to other patients and families, staff members, including nurses and respiratory therapists, may have developed special attachments to patients, particularly those who have been in the hospital frequently. It may be worthwhile to have a ward meeting for staff who knew the patient to be able to talk about him or her and express their own grief (52).

Acknowledgment: I appreciate the help of Dr. Bill Cohen.

References

1. Maguire P. Barriers to psychological care of the dying. Br Med J 1985; 291:1711–1713.
2. Binger C, Ablin A, Feuerstein R, Kushner J, Zoger S, Mikkelsen C. Childhood leukemia: Emotional impact on patient and family. N Engl J Med 1969; 280:414–418.
3. Boat T, Welsh M, Beaudet A. Cystic fibrosis. In: Scriver C, Beaudet A, Sly W, Valle D, eds. The Metabolic Basis of Inherited Disease. Vol. 2. 6th ed. New York: McGraw-Hill, 1989:2649–2680).
4. Nixon P, Orenstein D, Kelsey S, Doershuk C. The prognostic value of exercise testing in patients with cystic fibrosis. N Engl J Med 1992; 327:1785–1788.
5. Kerem E, Reisman J, Corey M, Canny GJ, Levison H. Prediction of mortality in patients with cystic fibrosis. N Engl J Med 1992; 326(18):1187–1191.
6. Hodson M, Madden B, Steven M, Tsang V, Yacoub M. Noninvasive mechanical ventilation for cystic fibrosis patients—a potential bridge to transplantation. Eur Respir J 1991; 4:524–527.
7. Schidlow D, Taussig L, Knowles M. Cystic Fibrosis Foundation Consensus Conference report on pulmonary complications of cystic fibrosis. Pediatr Pulmonol 1993;15:187–198.
8. Noyes B, Orenstein D. Treatment of pneumothorax in cystic fibrosis in the era of lung transplantation (editorial). Chest 1992; 101:1187.
9. Fagan E, Harwood I. Home care for the dying patient. Proceedings of Eighth International Congress of Cystic Fibrosis. Toronto: Canadian Cystic Fibrosis Foundation, 1980:275–278.
10. Lloyd-Still D, Lloyd-Still J. The patient, the family, and the community. In: Lloyd-Still J, ed. Textbook of Cystic Fibrosis. Boston: John Wright PSG, 1983:433–445.
11. Waechter EH. Children's awareness of fatal illness. Am J Nursing 1971; 7:1168–1172.
12. Davis P, di Sant'Agnese P. Assisted ventilation for patients with cystic fibrosis. JAMA 1978; 239:1851–1854.
13. Goldman M, Christie D. Children with cancer talking about their own death, with their families. Pediatr Haematol Oncol 1993; 10:223–231.
14. Mellins R. Cardiorespiratory disorders in children. In: Winters R, ed. The Body Fluids in Pediatrics. Boston: Little, Brown, 1973:457–482.

15. Orenstein S, Orenstein D. Magnesium deficiency in cystic fibrosis. South Med J 1983; 76(12):1586.
16. Loughlin G. Dyspnea. In: Loughlin G, Eigen H, eds. Respiratory Disease in Children: Diagnosis and Management. Baltimore: Williams & Wilkins, 1994:195–200.
17. Davis P. Pathophysiology of the lung disease in cystic fibrosis. In: Davis P, ed. Cystic Fibrosis. New York: Marcel Dekker, 1993: 193–218.
18. Lands L, Desmond K, Demizio D, Pavilanis A, Coates A. The effects of nutritional status and hyperinflation on respiratory muscle strength in children and young adults. Am Rev Respir Dis 1990; 141:1506–1509.
19. Weiner P, Suo J, Fernandez E, Cherniack R. The effect of hyperinflation on respiratory muscle strength and efficiency in healthy subjects and patients with asthma. Am Rev Respir Dis 1990; 141:1501–1505.
20. Godfrey S, Mearns M. Pulmonary function and response to exercise in cystic fibrosis. Arch Dis Child 1971; 46(246):144–151.
21. Wollman H, Smith T. The therapeutic gases. Oxygen, carbon dioxide, and helium. In: Gilman L, Gilman A, Koelle G, eds. The Pharmacologic Basis of Therapeutics. 5th ed. New York: Macmillan, 1975:881–899.
22. Erbland M, Ebert R, Snow S. Interaction of hypoxia and hypercapnia on respiratory drive in patients with COPD. Chest 1990; 97:1289–1294.
23. Schmidt G, Hall J, Wood L. Ventilatory failure. In: Murray J, Nadel J, eds. Textbook of Respiratory Medicine. Vol. 2. 2nd ed. Philadelphia: WB Saunders, 1994: 2614–2635.
24. Jardim J, Farkas G, Prefaut G, Thomas D, Macklem P, Roussos C. The failing inspiratory muscles under normoxic and hypoxic conditions. Am Rev Respir Dis 1981; 124:274–279.
25. Block E. Oxygen therapy. In: Fishman A, ed. Pulmonary Diseases and Disorders. Vol. 3. 2nd ed. New York: McGraw-Hill, 1988:2317–2330.
26. Mahler D. Therapeutic strategies. In: Mahler D, ed. Dyspnea. Mount Kisco, NY: Futura Publishing, 1990:231–263.
27. Schwartzstein R, Lahive K, Pope A, et al. Cold facial stimulation reduces breathlessness in normal subjects. Am Rev Respir Dis 1987; 136:58–61.
28. Landau L, Phelan P. The variable effect of a bronchodilating agent on pulmonary function in cystic fibrosis. J Pediatr 1973; 82:863–868.
29. Wood R, Wanner A, Hirsch J, Farrell P. Tracheal mucociliary transport in patients with cystic fibrosis and its stimulation by terbutaline. Am Rev Respir Dis 1975; 111:733–738.
30. Nava S, Crotti P, Gurrieri G, Fracchia C, Rampulla C. Effect of a B_2-agonist (broxaterol) on respiratory muscle strength and endurance in patients with COPD with irreversible airway obstruction. Chest 1992; 101(1):133–140.
31. Suzuki S, Numata H, Sano F, Yoshiike Y, Miyashita A, Okubo T. Effects and mechanism of fenoterol on fatigued canine diaphragm. Am Rev Respir Dis 1988; 137:1048–1054.
32. Prendiville A, Rose A, Maxwell D, Silverman M. Hypoxaemia in wheezy infants after bronchodilator treatment. Arch Dis Child 1987; 62:997–1000.
33. Murciano D, Auclair M-H, Pariente R, Aubier M. A randomized, controlled trial of theophylline in patients with severe chronic obstructive pulmonary disease. N Engl J Med 1989; 320(23):1521–1525.
34. Shapiro G, Bauman J, Kanarek P, Beirman C. The paradoxical effect of adrenergic and methylxanthine drugs in cystic fibrosis. Pediatrics 1976; 58:740–743.

35. Gift A, Plaut S, Jacox A. Psychologic and physiologic factors related to dyspnea in subjects with chronic obstructive pulmonary disease. Heart Lung 1986; 15(6): 595–601.

36. Renfroe K. Effect of progressive relaxation on dyspnea and state anxiety in patients with chronic obstructive pulmonary disease. Heart Lung 1988; 17:408–413.

37. Kohlman-Carrieri V, Janson-Bjerklie S. Coping and self-care strategies. In: Mahler D, ed. Dyspnea. Mount Kisco, NY: Futura Publishing, 1990:201–230.

38. Horsman J. Using tape recordings to overcome panic during dyspnea. Respir Care 1978; 23:767–768.

39. Jaffe J, Martin W. Narcotic analgesics and antagonists. In: Goodman L, Gilman A, Gilman A, Koelle G, eds. The Pharmacological Basis of Therapeutics. 5th ed. New York: Macmillan Publishing, 1975:245–283.

40. Light R, Muro J, Sato R, et al. Effects of oral morphine on breathlessness and exercise tolerance in patients with chronic obstructive pulmonary disease. Am Rev Respir Dis 1980; 139:126–133.

41. Finck A, Berkowitz B, Hempstead J, Ngai S. Pharmacokinetics of morphine: effects of hypercarbia on serum and brain morphine concentrations in the dog. Anesthesiology 1977; 47(5):407–410.

42. Garland J, Chan Y, Kelly K, Rice T. Outcome of infants with cystic fibrosis requiring mechanical ventilation for respiratory failure. Chest 1989; 96:136–138.

43. Dinwiddie R. Good outcome after prolonged ventilation in an infant with cystic fibrosis. J R Soc Med 1989; 16(suppl 82):44–46.

44. Wagener J, Taussig L, Burrows B, Hernried L, Boat T. Comparison of lung function and survival patterns between cystic fibrosis and emphysema or chronic bronchitis patients. In: Sturgess J, ed. Perspectives in Cystic Fibrosis. Mississauga, Ontario: Imperial Press, 1980:236.

45. Padman R, Nadkarni V, Von Nessen S, Goodill J. Noninvasive positive pressure ventilation in end-stage cystic fibrosis: a report of seven cases. Respir Care 1994; 39(7):736–739.

46. Cystic Fibrosis Foundation. Cystic fibrosis foundation patient registry annual data report 1995. Bethesda, MD: Cystic Fibrosis Foundation, 1996.

47. Stern R, Stevens D, Boat T, Doershuk C, Izant R, Matthews L. Symptomatic hepatic disease in cystic fibrosis: incidence, course, and outcome of portal systemic shunting. Gastroenterology 1976; 70:645–649.

48. Simons J. Practical issues. In: Goldman A, ed. Care of the Dying Child. Oxford: Oxford University Press, 1993:115–131.

49. Chapman J, Goodall J. Helping a child to live whilst dying. Lancet 1980; 1:753–756.

50. Shapiro J. Family reactions and coping strategies in response to the physically ill or handicapped child: a review. Soc Sci Med 1983; 17(14):913–931.

51. Fraiberg S. The Magic Years. New York: Charles Scribner's Sons, 1959.

52. Black D. Bereavement. In: Goldman A, ed. Care of the Dying Child. Oxford: Oxford University Press, 1993:145–163.

53. Pasterkamp H. The history and physical examination. In: Chernick V, ed. Kendig's Disorders of the Respiratory Tract in Children. 5th ed. Philadelphia: WB Saunders, 1990:56–77.

54. Shneerson J. Ventilatory failure. Disorders of Ventilation. Oxford: Blackwell Scientific, 1988:47–49.

15

New Therapies for Cystic Fibrosis

THOMAS F. BOAT

University of Cincinnati College of Medicine
and Children's Hospital Medical Center
Cincinnati, Ohio

I. Introduction

For more than 50 years, the treatment of cystic fibrosis (CF) has been directed against its secondary effects, including abnormal or excessive mucus and infection in the lungs and malnutrition resulting from disordered digestion. This therapy must be judged effective, in that average life span has increased from several months to approximately 30 years.

Hospitalization is often used to intensify therapy or provide special types of care. Improvement of lung function and resolution of systemic symptoms have been well documented after the treatment of exacerbations of airways disease with intravenous antibiotics. Furthermore, the hospital has often been used as the setting to treat complications such as pneumothorax, severe hemoptysis, and the onset of hyperglycemia. Surgical care, when required for these or other complications, can be undertaken successfully, but often requires intensified chest therapy for and closed observation of the patient in a hospital setting.

A number of CF authorities have asked the question, "Have we come close to maximizing the benefits of standard therapy?" In a number of centers, longevity has not increased substantially over the last several years. Perhaps as a result of extended and intensive therapy, or perhaps as an outcome of prolonged survival, more and more patients are harboring multiply drug resistant organisms in their airways, such as *Pseudomonas aeruginosa* or *Burkholderia cepacia*, fungi, or mycobacteria. Current treatment of infection with these organisms is often not satisfactory. New therapies may be required if additional major advances are to be made in longevity or quality of life.

Fortunately, recent advances in the understanding of CF lung pathophysiology and the basic genetics of this disorder may lead to substantially more effective treatments. Some of these newly developed therapies are already being used experimentally. Those that have recently been approved or are likely to transcend the transition from experimental to standard therapy are, like those currently available, directed at the secondary effects of this disease. However, there will also be opportunities to improve organ function by circumventing the physiological defect at its cellular or molecular level. Both pharmacological and gene therapy approaches will be introduced.

Most efforts at identifying new effective therapies will target the lung disease, which accounts for most of the morbidity and nearly all the mortality. It may also be possible, however, to develop new therapies for gastrointestinal or genitourinary system disease, based on the emerging understanding of molecular pathogenesis.

The extent to which these new therapies will change the treatment of hospitalized patients is not yet clear. Ideally, they will decrease the need for hospitalization by stabilizing lung function and decreasing the rate of lung complications. However, some of the new therapies may be technology dependent and require prolonged hospitalization. One example is lung transplantation. In addition, it is likely that insertion of genetic material into airway epithelial cells will, at least initially, require hospitalization to monitor safety and efficacy.

The discussion of new therapies, whether currently available, under development, or in the planning stage, follows the pathophysiological scheme outlined in Figure 1. The figure presents a simplistic concept of the relationship between the abnormal CFTR gene and airways disease. Each new therapy discussed is identified based on its primary target within this pathophysiological scheme, starting with those that are most remote from the fundamental defect.

II. Replacing Irreversibly Damaged Lungs

Once structural damage in the form of diffuse, advanced bronchiectasis has occurred, options for control of pulmonary symptoms are limited. If the forced expiratory volume in 1 second (FEV_1) has consistently declined below 30% predicted and cor pulmonale is apparent, lung transplantation may offer an opportunity for extended survival (see Chapter 13) (1).

Initial efforts focused on combined heart-lung transplantation. With improved surgical techniques, double lung transplants have become increas-

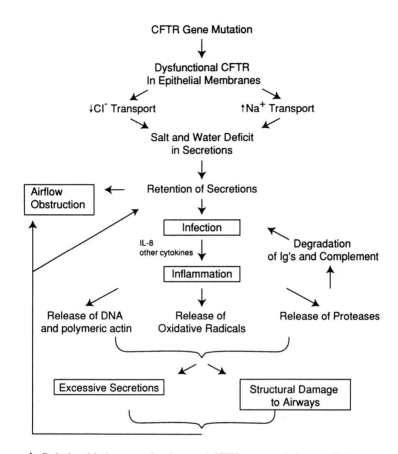

Figure 1 Relationship between the abnormal CFTR gene and airways disease.

ingly popular (2). Attempts to transplant single lungs for cystic fibrosis have been few and this approach is largely untested. Several children have successfully received lung lobes from living related donors.

Table 1 reviews the results of lung transplantation for patients with cystic fibrosis. Very few patients younger than 10 years of age have been lung transplant recipients. A substantial number of older children and adults do not survive the surgical procedure or the postoperative period; however, intermediate survival rate compares favorably with that of transplant for other major diagnoses that result in respiratory failure. A number of recipients have normal or near normal lung function at 1,2, and even 3 or more years after transplant.

Complications beyond the immediate postoperative period include infection of new airways with residual fungal organisms (aspergillus) or bacteria, especially those that have multiple drug resistance (3). The sinuses are thought

Table 1 Lung Transplant for CF: September 1994
International Registry

Number	466
Survival	
1 year	75%
2 years	65%
3 years	57%

Source: St. Louis Lung Transplant Registry.

to harbor organisms and serve as a reservoir to seed the donated lungs (4). However, recent results from one center demonstrate a low posttransplantation infection rate without special precautions (5). As has been the case with lung transplantation for other diagnoses, bronchiolitis obliterans is a manifestation of immunological rejection of the transplant (6), present to some degree in many recipients after several years, and is the major cause of death in those transplant recipients who survive the first year.

By far, the greatest obstacle to transplantation for lung failure in cystic fibrosis is availability of donor organs. Data in Table 2 document that, in 1993, three times as many CF patients were added to transplant wait lists as were lung transplant recipients. Xenografts could surmount this obstacle, but will not offer an alternative until methods are available to control the intense immunological reaction against animal organs. Patient characteristics that have been considered relative risks to lung transplantation for patients with cystic fibrosis include prior chest surgery, endocrine pancreatic insufficiency, poor nutrition, antimicrobial-resistant pulmonary pathogens, and documented noncompliance with therapy. High cost, including at some centers the requirement for the patient and often family members to move to a location near the center while they wait for a donor, has also been a deterrent.

Table 2 Bilateral Lung Transplantation CF—United States

1988	1
1989	0
1990	6
1991	23
1992	35
1993	83
1994	96
1994 (evaluated)	373
1994 (wait-listed)	300

Source: S. Fitzsimmons, Cystic Fibrosis Foundation, Bethesda, Maryland.

Liver transplant has been carried out in a small number of patients with end-stage liver disease (7). As with lung transplantation, the results are generally equivalent to experiences with other kinds of advanced liver disease. Pulmonary infection does not seem to worsen in the face of postoperative immunosuppression.

III. Treating Excessive Secretions

Airway gland secretion is under parasympathetic control, but there is no effective way of inhibiting reflex cholinergic stimulation systematically (such as with atropine) without incurring unacceptable side effects.

Aerosolization of a locally acting anticholinergic such as ipratropium bromide into CF airways has not been shown to be more effective than beta-agonist bronchodilators. A number of substances that are released by inflamed tissues, including neutrophil and bacterial proteases, as well as leukotrienes and cytokines, stimulate the release of mucus into airways (8–11). Potentially effective therapies might include inhibitors of these substances. So many factors can stimulate mucus production, however, that the use of a single agent is unlikely to be helpful. Control of infection or the inflammatory reaction to infection is presently the most effective approach.

An alternative approach is to provide for more effective clearance of secretions, especially from the smaller and more peripheral airways, where initial accumulation of mucus and the obstructive lesion is most severe. Equipment such as the Flutter device (12) has been shown to enhance mucus expectoration when compared with manual chest percussion, but this device has not been subjected to rigorous testing to ascertain whether sustained improvement of pulmonary function can be achieved. The suggestion that surfactant improves the surface properties of mucus and potentially its clearance offers yet another potential therapeutic avenue (13). Mucolytic agents are discussed in subsequent paragraphs.

IV. Reduction of Airflow Obstruction

Airflow obstruction is caused by mucus accumulation, airway wall inflammation and edema, a modest degree of bronchospasm, and, in patients with more advanced disease, airway collapse during expiration. Approaches to mucus clearance and the control of airway wall inflammation are discussed under Treating Excessive Secretions and under Antiinflammatory Drugs, respectively (see Chapter 4). Even though many patients with cystic fibrosis have some reversible airways obstruction and bronchodilators are widely used, no new or creative approaches to this aspect of CF care appear to be on the horizon. Beta-agonist bronchodilators increase resting energy expenditure and therefore may interfere with attempts to gain weight (14).

V. Enhancing Humoral Immune Responsiveness

Several studies show that the generation of uninhibited proteases in the airways results in degradation of immunoglobulins and complement (15–16), both of which play a role in airways surface immunity. Preliminary data suggest that intravenous infusion of large amounts of immunoglobulin in combination with intensive antibiotic therapy produces a salutary, albeit transient, effect on airways function (17). Some researchers have argued that the infusion of immunoglobulins containing high titers of antibodies to *P. aeruginosa* might be even more effective (18). Studies are underway to confirm the utility of this approach. Even if this therapy is shown to be effective, its benefits will need to be weighed against a substantial financial cost and possible immunological drawbacks (e.g., increased immune complex formation). Intravenous immunoglobulin therapy could become an adjunct to intensive antibiotic therapy, but its capacity to prevent exacerbations of lung infection and dysfunction should be investigated.

VI. Inhibition of Protease Activity

There is ample evidence that *P. aeruginosa* organisms and, perhaps more importantly, neutrophils release large amounts of proteases into the airways (8,9). Injurious effects of these proteases stem from their interference with immune function and stimulation of mucus secretion as well as disruption of ciliary activity and damage to structural components in the airways walls (19). It is likely that proteases contribute substantially to the development of bronchiolectasis and bronchiectasis. One strategy proposed by a number of investigators is to increase levels of protease inhibitors in the airway spaces. In preliminary studies, aerosolized alpha-1-antiprotease diminished the amount of free protease activity in CF airway secretions (20). Other investigators have suggested that the secretory leukocyte protease inhibitor (21) or other compounds that inhibit proteases might be more effective in CF lung disease. As yet, no definitive data from human studies confirm the efficacy of this approach. One problem is that aerosols are unlikely to deliver these drugs to the most damaged and obstructed airways where especially high levels of uninhibited protease activity might be expected. Aerosol delivery of these agents should work best if used early, before the onset of irreversible airways disease.

A more fundamental approach to the protease problem is to decrease the inflammatory response and the intensity of infection, thereby reducing the amount of proteases released. These approaches are discussed in Sections IX and X.

VII. Controlling Oxidative Injury

One mechanism by which inflammatory cells kill bacteria is the generation of oxidative radicals such as superoxide and peroxidase. In addition, macrophages can generate nitric oxide, which, in turn, can be converted to peroxynitrites, also strong oxidative compounds. Patients with cystic fibrosis may be deficient in antioxidants (22), including glutathione, a reducing agent that protects against oxidation. They might be well served by having an abundance of other antioxidative compounds such as vitamin E and beta-carotene (23) in their cells and body fluids. No serious harmful effects from supplemental administration of these compounds are known and they are relatively inexpensive. The administration of these substances on a daily basis to provide at least normal levels appears to be reasonable. However, no studies have been conducted to demonstrate that this approach improves or stabilizes lung function.

Compounds under development selectively inhibit the inducible nitric oxide synthase (24). These compounds may prove effective in reducing inflammatory injury to CF airways. Similar to the protease inhibitors, antioxidants will more likely be efficacious if used early, while CF lungs are relatively healthy, rather than after lung disease has reached advanced stages.

VIII. Enhancement of CF Mucus Clearance by Degrading DNA and Polymerized Actin

The high DNA content of sputum from patients with cystic fibrosis contributes substantially to the sticky and difficult-to-clear properties of their secretions (25). It has been demonstrated that inhalation of human recombinant DNase by patients with mild to moderate lung disease improves pulmonary function and maintains at least a modest degree of improvement over several months (26). The response to this drug varies among patients, but, on average, significant improvement has been documented in all studies. Use of compounds such as DNase might be useful as an adjunct for the treatment regimen of the hospitalized patient who has increased mucus secretion and accumulation. However, the only study that has combined DNase treatment with more intensive antibiotic and mucus clearance therapy at the time of pulmonary exacerbation (27) has failed to show clear efficacy over the standard antibiotic and lung clearance therapy. A few patients may benefit from this therapy, and continuing DNase therapy for patients already taking this drug during hospitalization has no obvious drawbacks. Furthermore, a 2-week study of patients with advanced lung

Table 3 Treatment of Severe Lung Disease with rhDNase for 3 Months

	DNase	Placebo
Number of subject	162	158
FVC: % improvement	12.4	7.3
FEV$_1$ % improvement	9.4	2.1
Voice alternation	18.4	6.2
Deaths	9	6

Source: C. Johnson: Report to the North American Cystic Fibrosis Conference, October, 1994, Orlando, Florida.

disease, as defined by a forced vital capacity (FVC) of less than 40% predicted, failed to demonstrated a beneficial effect of DNase on pulmonary function (28). A follow-up placebo-controlled, double-blind study using a 3-month treatment period for individuals with an FVC of less than 40% predicted showed, on average, a modest improvement in pulmonary function (Table 3). Most of this effect could be explained by substantial improvement of a relatively small number of subjects. Survival did not improve with DNase treatment. Based on studies to date, it is likely that aerosolized DNase in the amounts currently used (2.5 mg once or twice daily) will work best when administered in a sustained fashion to patients who have less extensive structural damage to their airways and mild to moderate airflow obstruction.

Recent evidence suggests that polymerized actin, released by polymorphonuclear leukocytes in the airways, inhibits mucus clearance in CF patients (29). Gelsolin is a naturally occurring protein that depolymerizes actin and has been shown to reduce the viscosity of CF secretions (30). Studies are underway to determine whether this compound might be efficacious for patients with CF, in a manner similar to that demonstrated for DNase. In vitro studies suggest beneficial effects that are additive to those of DNase. Thymosin beta-4, a small peptide, appears to have similar effects on actin and may also have therapeutic potential. It is possible that a combination of DNase and an agent that interferes with actin polymerization would be particularly beneficial in the treatment of CF lung disease characterized by excessive, difficult-to-clear, purulent secretions.

IX. Antiinflammatory Drugs

For a number of years, caretakers of patients with CF have speculated that the predominant cause of progressive airways disease is not infection per se, but rather the accompanying inflammatory response. Based on this premise, several studies of sustained corticosteroid therapy were undertaken. The first, a small study of alternate-day prednisone therapy given to young and relatively healthy patients, appeared to demonstrated an improved outcome (31). A follow-up multicenter trial revealed modest benefits over 4 years but also demonstrated an unacceptable rate of corticosteroid side effects, especially hyperglycemia and suppression of growth (32). Based on this result, a similar study was conducted to determine whether nonsteroidal antiinflammatory drugs would provide benefit with less risk (33). This study also targeted patients with mild lung disease and treated them with ibuprofen at a dose determined to provide serum concentrations of 50–100 μg/mL. During the 4-year study, a substantial decrease in the rate of progression of lung disease as assessed by pulmonary function testing could be demonstrated. Insufficient numbers of patients were enrolled in the study to demonstrate efficacy for older patients. Patients with advanced lung disease were not studied. The authors stressed the importance of achieving serum levels within a carefully defined range to minimize adverse effects. As with DNase and other drugs, application of this therapy is more likely to be useful if started early and given continuously. Use of this therapy solely as an adjunct to therapy for hospitalized patients seems problematic.

A recent report suggests that pentoxifylline, a compound that has several antiinflammatory effects including antagonism of tumor necrosis factor-alpha and interleukin-1-beta, as well as antagonism of neutrophil migration into infected lungs, prevented progression of lung disease as assessed by pulmonary function over a 6 month period (34). Sputum neutrophil elastase concentrations also decreased modestly for treated cases. This study included small numbers of subjects and observations were made over a relatively short period. Follow-up studies should indicate whether pentoxifylline will be a useful adjunct to current CF therapy.

Future studies should be directed at the antagonism of the cytokines that mediate the inflammatory response. The ability to inhibit the generation of interleukin-8, a potent chemoattractant for neutrophils (21), might be particularly useful. Antagonism of interleukin-1 receptor has also been suggested as a useful pharmacological intervention (35). However, suppression of the polymorphonuclear chemoattractant leukotriene B4 by supplementing omega-3 fatty acids in the diet for 6 weeks did not improve pulmonary function (36). Theoretically, any of these approaches could help suppress the exuberant inflammatory response that appears to underlie pulmonary exacerbations of CF, especially if used early in the course of the lung disease.

X. Improved Control of Infection

Infection is an important, perhaps the most important, pathogenetic mechanism for progression of lung disease in CF. Frequent and intensive use of antimicrobial agents has been a cornerstone of CF therapy over many years. This approach has undoubtedly contributed to the extended life span of people with

CF. The emergence of organisms in the airways that are highly resistant to the usual antimicrobial agents, whether given orally or intravenously, has become a major challenge for CF therapy. Undoubtedly, new antimicrobial agents will be formulated, although activity along these lines seems to be less productive than it was 10–20 years ago. Use of synergistic combinations of antimicrobials may prove beneficial. Immunization to boost antimicrobial defenses has been considered for many years. Recent work with the herpes virus suggests that immunization may be effective in controlling chronic infection as well as preventing primary infection (37). If so, this approach to therapy is worthy of further consideration. Of interest in this regard is an observation that immunological capacity to clear mucoid *P. aeruginosa* may be an important determinant of progression of lung disease in CF patients (38). There is not yet any reliable way to enhance the elimination of mucoid organisms.

A fundamental mechanism of bacterial colonization is adherence of organisms to airway epithelial cells. Adherence of *P. aeruginosa* to epithelial cells is significantly greater in patients homozygous for ΔF508 than those with other mutations of the CFTR gene (39). Increasing efforts have been directed toward identifying the adhesive molecules and devising methods for interfering with the bacterial adherence. If successful, such therapy could be beneficial, both for treatment of pulmonary exacerbations and for inhibiting early bacterial colonization.

While there are differences of opinion about the pathogenetic contributions of viruses, it is likely that both respiratory syncytial virus (40) and adenovirus (41) contribute substantially to pulmonary exacerbations and may set off a cascade of events leading to a loss of pulmonary function. Therefore, use of rapid detection methods and antiviral compounds may become a more important part of CF therapy. However, immunization approaches seem more likely to be efficacious in the long run. Better treatments also are needed for control of fungi and nontuberculous mycobacteria. Along these lines, the use of itraconazole may be particularly useful in controlling the inflammatory effects of aspergillosis colonization in patients who experience episodes of allergic bronchopulmonary aspergillosis (42).

XI. Correction of Salt and Water Deficits in Secretions

Transient addition of salt and water to the airway surface liquids may be possible using aerosol inhalation of saline. However, it is difficult to aerosolize large amounts of liquids into the airways. Distribution is also a problem, in that deposition will likely occur in greatest amounts where it is least needed. It is more likely that hydration objectives in the airways can be achieved by altering chloride and sodium transport.

XII. Inhibiting Sodium Transport Across Epithelial Membranes

One physiological abnormality of cystic fibrosis airway epithelial cells is the excessive absorption of sodium from airway surface liquids into epithelial cells. The extra sodium is pumped across the basolateral membrane into the interstitial fluid by a Na^+ / K^+ ATPase. Sodium transport across the apical membrane can be inhibited by the diuretic amiloride (43). This has been demonstrated both in vitro and in vivo, in animal and human studies. A pilot study in adults with cystic fibrosis demonstrated that this drug is safe when given by aerosol (44). Furthermore, a small number of patients taking amiloride by aerosol three or four times a day for 6 months experienced a slower decline in pulmonary function (FVC, FEV_1) than did control subjects given vehicle. Chronic administration to six patients increased sodium and chloride content of CF sputum and favorably altered sputum viscoelasticity and clearance (45). If it is efficacious and if safety can be confirmed, amiloride may be an important therapeutic adjunct to current treatment programs. Its benefits will be most easily documented with chronic use. One study suggested that cough clearance improves after a single 3-mL inhalation of 10^{-3} M amiloride to stable CF subjects with a wide range of lung dysfunction (46), raising the possibility of efficacy as an acute, adjunctive therapy. However, even though short-term safety has been established in children younger than 12 years of age, no evidence has been found for rapid (up to 4 weeks) improvement. In one study, amiloride did not result in a greater overall improvement in hospitalized patients with acute exacerbations of chest disease (47).

XIII. Drugs that Enhance Chloride Secretion

A fundamental physiological defect in cystic fibrosis airway epithelial cells is failure of the CFTR protein to function as a chloride channel (48). Consequently, chloride cannot be secreted onto the apical surface, impairing the ability of CF epithelia to hydrate surface secretions. However, there are alternative epithelial cell channels for translocating chloride ions from the intracellular to the luminal compartment. One such channel can be upregulated by triphosphate nucleotides such as adenosine triphosphate (ATP) and uridine 5-triphosphate (UTP) (49). It is likely that these substances act through selective apical receptors that increase calcium concentrations within the cell (49). Calcium may be the intracellular signal that opens these alternative chloride channels. Studies by Knowles and colleagues (50) have demonstrated that UTP, when applied to the apical surface of CF respiratory epithelium, can stimulate a chloride current. Furthermore, studies of UTP aerosolization into the airways of patients with cystic fibrosis have demonstrated enhanced clearance of mucus from the peripheral airways (51). Additional clinical trials will further assess the efficacy as well as the safety of UTP as a therapeutic agent in cystic fibrosis. Combined UTP and amiloride therapy may be especially effective in stimulating secretion of salt and water and achieving adequate hydration of secretions at the epithelial surface. Once again, this inhalation approach to therapy is most likely to be helpful when the airways are relatively clear of accumulated mucus and infection, but it is not impossible that these drugs would also be a useful adjunct to intensive antibiotic therapy.

XIV. Correction of Dysfunctional CFTR

Mutations of the CFTR protein can have several adverse effects, including failure to synthesize a mature CFTR molecule, failure to transport CFTR from the endoplasmic reticulum through the Golgi where it is modified to the apical membrane, failure of CFTR activation by ATP or phosphorylation mechanisms, and failure of the CFTR to form functional channels in the apical membrane (52). It is possible that pharmacological manipulation could result in enhancement of CFTR delivery to the apical membrane and improvement of CFTR function. For example, there is in vitro evidence that selected phosphodiesterase inhibitors (e.g., milrinone) in combination with beta-agonists greatly increase intracellular activities of protein kinase A and partially activate chloride channel function of mutated CFTR (53). If this effect can be achieved in vivo, at least some CFTR mutations might be treatable.

Alternatively, normal CFTR could be delivered exogenously to CF airway epithelial cells with a carrier that would allow it to be integrated into apical membranes. Preliminary studies have demonstrated that, although insertion of protein is not highly efficient, anion transport properties can be imparted to CF airway epithelial cells by in vitro protein transfer (54). Whether this approach can ever be clinically effective at an affordable cost remains to be determined. As with many other therapies, protein replacement would ideally be started early in life, before the onset of structural damage to airways.

XV. Gene Therapy

The ultimate goal for cystic fibrosis therapy is to transfer normal CFTR genes into relevant cells in such a way that they are stably integrated into the genome and express CFTR protein normally. Now that the CFTR gene can be cloned readily, the material for gene transfer studies and, ultimately, therapy is available. However, a safe and effective vehicle that can be used to deliver CFTR into airway epithelial cells is not yet available. Table 4 lists the kinds of vectors have been used experimentally.

Table 4 Vectors for Transfer of the
CFTR Gene to Airway Epithelial Cells

Viral
Adenovirus
Adeno-associated virus
Retrovirus
Nonviral
Naked DNA
Cationic liposomes
Polymeric IgA
Surfactant proteins (A,B,C)
Lectins (e.g., concanavalin A)

The adenovirus has been studied most extensively (55,56). Parts of the virus genome are removed to create a replication-deficient virus and to make room for the insertion of the CFTR gene as well as appropriate promoter elements. Several different adenovirus–CFTR constructs have been devised and tested. It is clear that the adenovirus will target receptors on cultured human respiratory epithelial cells, that the adenovirus construct is internalized, and that CFTR expression occurs promptly. There is a suggestion that cell injury is required for this process in vivo. Most data are consistent with expression that is episomal and transient. An immunological response is generated to cells that have been genetically manipulated; cytotoxic lymphocytes subsequently destroy these airway epithelial cells. The epithelium rapidly regenerates and expression of the transferred gene is lost. The therapeutic use of this construct would require repeat administration. Several additional concerns have surfaced. The first is that repeated treatment may be precluded by the immunological surveillance system (57). Another is that when using virus construct in the amounts needed for expression, airway inflammation occurs and ranges from mild at lower doses to exuberant at higher doses (58). Human studies suggest that there is substantial lung inflammation and injury at the application site (59). As a result, new adenovirus constructs are being developed with the hope that they can deliver the CFTR gene with less toxicity (60). Whether this is achievable is open to question.

Another promising vector is the adeno-associated virus. This virus has a genome that is just big enough to accommodate the CFTR gene. The adeno-associated virus has the theoretical advantage of not being able to replicate, unless an adenovirus infects the cell simultaneously. A considerable technical challenge has been the generation of enough adeno-associated virus to perform an adequate number of experiments. Nevertheless, work to date suggests that the adeno-associated virus can efficiently transfer CFTR to airway epithelial cells and that expression is detectable in rabbit airways for up to 6 months after administration of the construct (61). Initial animal experiments suggest, however, that replication of this virus may occur and that it appears in other organs, an unforeseen outcome that could be troublesome. Retrovirus vectors, although potentially capable of stable integration of CFTR (62), require dividing cells that are present in exceedingly small numbers in uninjured mature airway epithelium cells.

Other vehicles for CFTR transfer include cationic liposomes and receptor-mediated delivery of a protein-DNA construct. Both of these approaches are relatively inefficient, but are less likely to have adverse side effects. Early human studies with liposome-mediated CFTR gene transfer suggest that some expression and functional correction can be achieved (63). Approaches to receptor-mediated gene transfer include the use of CFTR gene conjugated to polymeric IgA (64), which is recognized by receptors on the basolateral membrane of the epithelial cell. Therefore, this construct is delivered by the vascular route. Another carrier that deserves further study is surfactant-associated proteins (65), which are normally recycled by airways epithelial cells using a receptor-mediated process. When placed in the airways, DNA conjugated with polylysine to these naturally occurring airway products should spread evenly throughout the conducting airways before uptake.

References

1. Kerem E, Reisman J, Corey M, Canny GJ, Levison H. Prediction of mortality in patients with cystic fibrosis. N Engl J Med 1992;326:1187–1197.
2. Shennib H, Noirclerc M, Ernst P, Metras D, Mulder S, Giudicelli R, Lebel F, Dumon JF. Double-lung transplantation for cystic fibrosis. Ann Thorac Surg 1992; 54:27–32.
3. Snell GI, de Hoyos A, Krajde M, Winton T, Maurer JR. *Pseudomonas cepacia* in lung transplant recipients with cystic fibrosis. Chest 1993; 103:466–471.
4. Lewiston N, King V, Umetsu D, Starnes V, Marshall S, Kramer M, Theodore J. Cystic fibrosis patients who have undergone heart-lung transplantation benefit from maxillary sinus antrostomy and repeated sinus lavage. Transplant Proc 1991; 23:1207–1208.
5. Flume PA, Egan TM, Paradowski LJ, Detterbeck FC, Thompson JT, Yankaskas JR. Infectious complications of lung transplantation: impact of cystic fibrosis. Am J Respir Crit Care Med 1994; 149:1601–1607.
6. Scott JP, Higenbotam TW, Sharples L, Clelland CA, Smyth RL, Stewart S, Wallwark J. Risk factors for obliterative bronchiolitis in heart-lung transplant recipients. Transplantation 1991, 51:813–817.
7. Mieles LA, Orenstein D, Teperman L, Pedesta L, Koneru B, Starzl T. Liver transplantation in cystic fibrosis. Lancet 1989; 1:1073.
8. Klinger JD, Tandler D, Liedtke CM, Boat TF. Proteinases of *Pseudomonas aeruginosa* evoke mucin release by tracheal epithelium. J Clin Invest 1984; 74: 1669–1678.

9. Nadel JA. Protease actions on airway secretions: relevance to cystic fibrosis. Ann NY Acad Sci 1991; 624:286–296.
10. Cohan VL, Scott AL, Dinarello CA, Prendergast RA. Interleukin-1 is a mucus secretagogue. Cellular Immunology 1991; 136:425–434.
11. Hoffstein ST, Malo PE, Bugelski P, Wheeldon EB. Leukotriene D4 induces mucus secretion from goblet cells in the guinea pig respiratory epithelium. Exp Lung Res 1990; 16:711–725.
12. Konstan MW, Stern RC, Doershuk CF. Efficacy of the Flutter device for airway mucus clearance in patients with cystic fibrosis. J Pediatr 1994; 124:689–693.
13. Rubin BK, Ramirez OE, Dian T, Albers GM, Rejent AJ, Noyes BE, Kleinhenz ME, Jeng I. Surfactant improves the mucociliary and cough clearability of CF sputum in vitro. Am J Respir in Crit Care Med 1994; 149:A670.
14. Vaisman N, Levy LD, Pencharz PB, Tan YK, Soldin SJ, Canny GJ, Hahn E. Effect of salbutamol on resting energy expenditure in patients with cystic fibrosis. J Pediatr 1987; 111:137–139.
15. Fick RB, Nagel GP, Squier SU, Wood RE, Gee JBL, Reynolds HY. Proteins of the cystic fibrosis respiratory tract: fragmented immunoglobulin G opsonic antibody causing defective opsonophagocytosis. J Clin Invest 1984; 74:236–248.
16. Tosi MF, Zakem H, Berger M. Neutrophil elastase cleaves C3bi on opsonized *Psuedomonas* as well as CR1 on neutrophils to create a functionally important opsonin receptor mismatch. J Clin Invest 1990; 86:300–308.
17. Winnie GB, Cowan RG, Wade NA. Intravenous immune globulin treatment of pulmonary exacerbations in cystic fibrosis. J Pediatr 1989; 114:309–314.
18. Van Wye JE, Collins MS, Baylor M, Pennington JE, Hsu Y-P, Sampanvejsopa V, Moss RB. *Pseudomonas* hyperimmune globulin passive immunotherapy for pulmonary exacerbations in cystic fibrosis. Pediatr Pulmonol 1990; 9:7–18.
19. Bruce MC, Poncz L, Klinger JD, Stern RC, Tomashefski JF Jr, Dearnborn DG. Biochemical and pathologic evidence for proteolytic destruction of lung connective tissue in cystic fibrosis. Am Rev Respir Dis 1985; 132:529–535.
20. McElvaney NG, Hubbard RC, Birrer P, Chernick MS, Caplan DB, Frank MM, Crystal RG. Aerosol alpha 1-antitrypsin treatment for cystic fibrosis. Lancet 1991; 337:392–394.
21. McElvaney NG, Nakamura H, Birrer P, Herbert CA, Wong WL, Alphonso M, Baker JB, Catalano MA, Crystal RG. Modulation of airway inflammation in cystic fibrosis: in vivo suppression of interleukin-8 levels on the respiratory epithelial surface by aerosolization of recombinant secretory leukoprotease inhibitor. J Clin Invest 1992; 90:1296–1301.
22. Langley SC, Brown RK, Kelly FJ. Reduced free radical-trapping capacity and altered plasma antioxidant status in cystic fibrosis. Pediatr Res 1993; 33:247–250.
23. Homnick DN, Cox JH, De Loof MJ, Ringer TV. Carotenoid levels in normal children and in children with cystic fibrosis. J Pediatr 1993; 122:703–707.
24. Szabo C, Southan GJ, Thiemermann C. Beneficial effects and improved survival in rodent models of septic shock with S-methylisothiourea sulfate, a potent and selective inhibitor of inducible nitric oxide synthase. Proc Nat Acad Sci USA 1994; 91: 12472–12476.
25. Shak S, Capon DJ, Hellmiss R, Marsters SA, Baker CL. Recombinant human DNase I reduces the viscosity of cystic fibrosis sputum. Proc Natl Acad Sci USA 1990; 87:9188–9192.

26. Fuchs HJ, Borowitz DS, Christiansen DH, Morris EM, Nash ML, Ramsey BW, Rosenstein BJ, Smith AL, Wohl ME. Effect of aerosolized recombinant human DNase on exacerbation of respiratory symptoms and on pulmonary function in patients with cystic fibrosis. N Engl J Med 1994; 331:637–642.

27. Wilmott R. A phase II double-blind, multicenter study of the safety and efficacy of aerosolized recombinant human DNase I in hospitalized patients with CF experiencing acute pulmonary exacerbations. Pediatr Pulmonol 1993; S9:154.

28. Shah PL, Scott SF, Hodson ME. Report on a multicenter study using aerosolized recombinant human DNase I in the treatment of cystic fibrosis patient with severe pulmonary disease. Pediatr Pulmonol 1993; (suppl 9):157–158.

29. Stossel TP, Allen PG, Janmey PA, Kas J, Sheils CA. Actin, DNA and mucolysis of CF sputum in vitro. Pediatr Pulmonol 1994; S10:102.

30. Vasconcellos CA, Allen PG, Wohl ME, Drazen JM, Janmey PA, Stossel TP. Reduction in viscosity of cystic fibrosis sputum in vitro by gelsolin. Science 1994; 263:969–971.

31. Auerbach HS, Williams M, Kirkpatrick JA, Colten HR. Alternate day prednisone reduces morbidity and improves pulmonary function in cystic fibrosis. Lancet 1985; 2:686–688.

32. Rosenstein BJ, Eigen H, Schidlow DV. Alternate day prednisone in patients with cystic fibrosis. Pediatr Res 1993; 31:A2289.

33. Konstan MW, Byard PJ, Hoppel CL, Davis PB. Effect of high-dose ibuprofen in patients with cystic fibrosis. N Engl J Med 1995; 332:848–854.

34. Aronoff SC, Quinn FJ, Carpenter LS, Novick WJ Jr. Effects of pentoxifylline on sputum neutrophil elastase and pulmonary function in patients with cystic fibrosis: preliminary observations. J Pediatr 1994; 125:992–997.

35. Wilmott RW, Kassab JT, Kilian PL, Benjamin WR, Douglas SD, Wood RE. Increased levels of interleukin-1 in bronchoalveolar washings from children with bacterial pulmonary infections. Am Rev Respir Dis 1990; 142:365–368.

36. Kurlandsky LE, Bennink MR, Webb PM, Ulrich PJ, Baer LJ. The absorption and effect of dietary supplementation with omega-3 fatty acids on serum leukotriene B4 in patients with cystic fibrosis. Pediatr Pulmonol 1994; 18:211–217.

37. Stanberry LR. The concept of immune-based therapies in chronic viral infections. J Acquir Immune Defic Syndr 1994; 7(suppl l)1: S1–S5.

38. Parad RB, et al. A model for predicting pulmonary outcome in cystic fibrosis from genotype, mucoid *Pseudomonas aeruginosa* (MPA) colonization status, and the presence of antibody to MPA. 8th North American Cystic Fibrosis Conference, Late Breaking Science Session 1994; S 5.4.

39. Zar H, Saimon L, Quittell L, Prince A. Binding of *Pseudomonas aeruginosa* to respiratory epithelial cells from patients with various mutations in the cystic fibrosis transmembrane regulator. J Pediatr 1995; 126:230–233.

40. Abman SH, Ogle JW, Butler-Simon N, Rumack CM, Accurso FJ. Role of respiratory syncytial virus in early hospitalizations for respiratory distress of young infants with cystic fibrosis. J Pediatr 1988; 113:826–830.

41. Nicolai T, Rosenecker J, Richman-Eisenstat JBY, Harms K-H, Bertele RM, Mutius Ev, Adam D. Adenovirus infection and decreased lung function in cystic fibrosis patients. Am J Respir Crit Care Med 1994; 149:A665.

42. Denning DW, Van Wye JE, Lewiston NJ, Stevens DA. Adjunctive therapy of allergic bronchopulmonary aspergillosis with itraconazole. Chest 1991; 100:813–819.

43. Knowles M, Gatzy J, Boucher R. Increased bioelectric potential difference across respiratory epithelia in cystic fibrosis. N Engl J Med 1981; 305:1489–1495.

44. Knowles MR, Church NL, Waltner WE, Yankaskas JR, Gilligan P, King M, Edwards LJ, Helms RW, Boucher RC. A pilot study of aerosolized amiloride for the treatment of lung disease in cystic fibrosis. N Engl J Med 1990; 322:1189–1194.

45. Tomkiewicz RP, App EM, Zayas JG, Ramirez O, Church N, Boucher RC, Knowles MR, King M. Amiloride inhalation therapy in cystic fibrosis: influence on ion content, hydration and rheology of sputum. Am Rev Respir Dis 1993; 148:1002–1007.

46. App EM, King M, Helfesrieder R, Kohler D, Matthys H. Acute and long term amiloride inhalation in cystic fibrosis lung disease. Am Rev Respir Dis 1990; 141:605–612.

47. Bowler IM, Kelman B, Worthington D, Littlewood JM, Watson A, Conway SP, Smye SW, James SL, Sheldon TA. Nebulised amiloride in respiratory exacerbations of cystic fibrosis: a randomised controlled trial. Arch Dis Child 1995; 73:427–430.

48. Anderson MP, et al. Generation of cAMP-activated chloride currents by expression of CFTR. Science 1991; 251:679–682.

49. Mason SJ, Paradiso AM, Boucher RC. Regulation of transepithelial ion transport and intracellular calcium by extracellular ATP in human normal and cystic fibrosis airway epithelium. Br J Pharmacol 1991; 103:1649–1656.

50. Knowles MR, Clark LL, Boucher RC. Activation by extracellular nucleotides of chloride secretion in the airway epithelia of patients with cystic fibrosis. N Engl J Med 1991; 325:533–538.

51. Bennett WD, Olivier KN, Zeman KL, Hohneker KH, Boucher RC, Knowles MR. Acute effect of aerosolized uridine 5-triphosphate (UTP) plus amiloride on mucociliary clearance in cystic fibrosis. Am J Respir Crit Care Med 1994; 149:A670.

52. Welsh MJ, Smith AK. Molecular mechanisms of CFTR chloride channel dysfunction in cystic fibrosis. Cell 1993; 73:1251–1254.

53. Kelly TJ, et al. cAMP-dependent chloride transport in epithelial cells homozygous for the ΔF508 mutation. Pediatr Res 1994; (suppl 10):239.

54. Bagley RG, et al. Delivery of purified, functional CFTR to epithelial cells in vitro using influenza hemagglutinin. 8th North American Cystic Fibrosis Conference, Late Breaking Science Session 1994; S 5.3.

55. Rosenfeld MA, Yoshimura K, Trapnell BC, Yoneyama K, Rosenthal ER, Dalemans W, Fukayama M, Bargon J, Stier LE, Stratford-Perricaudet L, Perricaudet M, Guggino WB, Pavirani A, Lecocq J-P, Crystal RG. In vivo transfer of the human cystic fibrosis transmembrane conductance regulator gene to the airway epithelium. Cell 1992; 68:143–155.

56. Zabner J, Couture LA, Gregory RJ, Graham SM, Smith AE, Welch MJ. Adenovirus-mediated gene transfer transiently corrects the chloride transport defect in nasal epithelia of patients with cystic fibrosis. Cell 1993; 75:207–216.

57. Morsy MA. Progress toward human gene therapy. JAMA 1993; 270:2338–2345.

58. Yei S, Mittereder N, Wert S, Whitsett JA, Wilmott RW, Trapnell BC. In vivo evaluation of the safety of adenovirus-mediated transfer of the human cystic fibrosis transmembrane conductance regulator cDNA to the lung. Hum Gene Ther 1994; 5:731–744.

59. Crystal RG, McElvaney NG, Rosenfeld MA, Chu CS, Mastrangeli A, Hay JG, Brody SL, Jaffe HA, Eissa NT, Danel C. Administration of an adenovirus containing the human CFTR cDNA to the respiratory tract of individuals with cystic fibrosis. Nature Genetics 1994; 8:4251.

60. Yang Y, Nunes FA, Berencsi K, Gonczol E, Engelhardt JF, Wilson JM. Inactivation of E2a in recombinant adenoviruses improves the prospect for gene therapy in cystic fibrosis. Nature Genetics 1994; 7:362–369.

61. Flotte TR, Afione SA, Conrad C, McGrath SA, Solow R, Oka H, Zeitlin PC, Guggino WB, Carter BJ. Stable in vivo expression of the cystic fibrosis transmembrane conductance regulator with an adeno-associated virus vector. Proc Natl Acad Sci U S A 1993; 90:10613–10617.

62. Englehardt JF. In vivo retroviral gene transfer into human bronchial epithelia xenografts. J Clin Invest 1992; 90:2598–2607.

63. Caplen NJ, Alton EW, Middleton PG, Dorin JR, Stevenson BJ, Gao X, Durham SB, Jeffrey PK, Hodson ME, Coutelle C. Liposome-mediated CFTR gene transfer to the nasal epithelium of patients with cystic fibrosis. Nature Medicine 1995; 1: 39–46.

64. Ferkol T, Kaetzel CS, Davis PB. Gene transfer into respiratory epithelial cells by targeting the polymeric immunoglobulin receptor. J Clin Invest 1993; 92:2394–2400.

65. Morris RE, Ciraolo G, Korfhagen T, Baatz JE, Whitsett JA, Ross GF. Receptor-mediated transfection of lung adenocarcinoma cells in culture using surfactant protein A:poly-L-lysine conjugates. Pediatr Pulmonol 1994; (suppl 10):231.

AUTHOR INDEX

Italic numbers give the page on which the complete reference is listed.

A

Abdul-Karim, F. J. W., 217, *230*
Abernathy, R. S., 13, *38*
Ablin, A., 357, 363, *374*
Ablin, A. R., 276, *281*
Abman, S. H., 31, 32, *41,*142, *170,* 176,
    186, *206, 208,* 386, *392*
Abramowski, C. R., 34, *42*
Abramowsky, C., 167, *173*
Accurso, F., 142, *170*
Accurso, F. J., 31, 32, 33, 34, *41, 42,*
    177, 186, *206, 208,* 386, *392*
Ackerman, V., 285, *296*
Adam, E. J., 266, *278*
Adams, E., 189, 190, *208*
Adams, K. S., 216, 217, *229*
Adelstein, E. H., 12, *37*
Adrian, T. E., 216, *229*
Afione, S. A., 390, *394*
Ahmad, T., 217, *230*
Aitken, M. L., 28, *40,* 321, *337*

Akwari, O. E., 218, *230*
Al Essa, S., 17, *39*
Al-Hafidh, A. S., 275, *281*
al-Saleh, Q., 141, *169*
Alagappan, V., 216, *229*
Albers, G. M., 381, *391*
Albert, D., 255, 259, *277*
Albo, V. C., 276, *281*
Alexander, M. F., 285, *297*
Allan, J. L., 251, *277*
Allen, J. R., 176, 177, *206*
Allen, P. G., 96, 112, *130, 132,* 384, *392*
Alpert, S. E., 291, *297,* 333, *339*
Alphan, G., 6, *36*
Alphonso, M., 382, 385, *391*
Altman, D. H., 254, 255 *277*
Alton, E. W., 390, *394*
Alton, E. W. F. W., 28, 30, *41*
Altshuler, R., 20, *39*
Amendola, M., 140, *169*
Ament, M. F., 117, *133*
Amini, S. B., 199, *210*

395

SUBJECT INDEX